Temporomandibular Joint Disorders: A Guide to Diagnosis and Treatment

Temporomandibular Joint Disorders: A Guide to Diagnosis and Treatment

Editor: Darwin Miller

MURPHY & MOORE
www.murphy-moorepublishing.com

www.murphy-moorepublishing.com

MURPHY & MOORE

Cataloging-in-Publication Data

Temporomandibular joint disorders : a guide to diagnosis and treatment / edited by Darwin Miller.
p. cm.
Includes bibliographical references and index.
ISBN 978-1-63987-519-1
1. Temporomandibular joint--Diseases. 2. Temporomandibular joint--Diseases--Diagnosis.
3. Temporomandibular joint--Diseases--Treatment. 4. Jaws--Diseases. 5. Joints--Diseases.
6. Temporal bone--Diseases. I. Miller, Darwin.
RK470 .T46 2022
617.522--dc23

Murphy & Moore Publishing,
1 Rockefeller Plaza,
New York City, NY 10020, USA

ISBN 978-1-63987-519-1 (Hardback)

Contents

Preface ... VII

Chapter 1 **Importance of Bone Markers and Radiological Status on Clinical Signs of Temporomandibular Joint Disorders** ... 1
Oksana Ivask, Ülle Voog-Oras and Edvitar Leibur

Chapter 2 **Surgical Approaches to the Temporomandibular Joint** ... 22
Mohammad Esmaeelinejad and Maryam Sohrabi

Chapter 3 **Reconstruction of TMJ with Prosthesis Joint** ... 36
José Thiers Carneiro Junior, Dênis Pimenta e Souza, Diogo Souza Ferreira Rubim de Assis, Paulo Hemerson de Moraes and Francisco de Sousa Neves Filho

Chapter 4 **Benign Tumors of Temporomandibular Joint** ... 54
Mehmet Emre Yurttutan, Ayşegül Tüzüner Öncül and Hakan Alpay Karasu

Chapter 5 **Myofascial Pain Dysfunction Syndrome: Etiology, Diagnosis, and Treatment** ... 79
Serdar Gözler

Chapter 6 **Internal Derangements of the Temporomandibular Joint: Diagnosis and Management** ... 108
Ufuk Tatli and Vladimir Machon

Chapter 7 **Optimizing the Management Outcomes in Patients with Temporomandibular Disorder** ... 129
Buket Aybar, Yusuf Emes and Guhan Dergin

Chapter 8 **Temporomandibular Joint Pathology and its Indication in Clinical Orthodontics** ... 141
Bakr M.Rabie, Jeremy Ho and Qianfeng Li

Chapter 9 **Osteoarthritis of the Temporomandibular Joint: Clinical and Imagenological Diagnosis, Pathogenic Role of the Immuno-Inflammatory Response, and Immunotherapeutic Strategies Based on T Regulatory Lymphocytes** ... 165
Gustavo Monasterio, Francisca Castillo, Daniel Betancur, Arnoldo Hernández, Guillermo Flores, Walter Díaz, Marcela Hernández and Rolando Vernal

Chapter 10 **JVA, Mastication and Digital Occlusal Analysis in Diagnosis and Treatment of Temporomandibular Disorders** ... 194
Serdar Gözler

Permissions

List of Contributors

Index

Preface

The joint which connects the jawbone to the skull is termed as the temporomandibular joint. The disorders of this joint can lead to pain in the muscles which control movement of the jaw as well as the jaw joint itself. This pain could be due to several reasons, such as arthritis, injury to the jaw or genetics. It could also be a combination of these reasons. A few symptoms of temporomandibular joint disorders are locking of the joint, tenderness in the jaw, ache in and around the ear, and difficulty in chewing food. It can be treated through physical therapy or medications. Severe cases might even require surgery for the management of temporomandibular joint disorders. This book contains some path-breaking studies related to the clinical management of temporomandibular joint disorders. It consists of contributions made by international experts. This book aims to equip students and experts with the advanced topics and upcoming concepts in this area.

This book is the end result of constructive efforts and intensive research done by experts in this field. The aim of this book is to enlighten the readers with recent information in this area of research. The information provided in this profound book would serve as a valuable reference to students and researchers in this field.

At the end, I would like to thank all the authors for devoting their precious time and providing their valuable contribution to this book. I would also like to express my gratitude to my fellow colleagues who encouraged me throughout the process.

Editor

1

Importance of Bone Markers and Radiological Status on Clinical Signs of Temporomandibular Joint Disorders

Oksana Ivask, Ülle Voog-Oras and Edvitar Leibur

Abstract

This chapter describes the diagnostics of temporomandibular joint disorders (TMDs) with the main focus on the radiographic changes and the role of different bone markers as procollagen type I N-terminal propeptide (P1NP), C-telopeptide crosslaps of type I collagen (CTX-1) as well as vitamin D (25(OH)D) in the pathogenesis of TMDs. From our population-based study, 47% subjects had TMJ problems where pain is commonly accompanied by stiffness, sounds and functional limitations, resulting in a decreased quali-ty of life, and thus exert a significant negative impact on activities of daily living (ADL). Assessment of individual pain level is important in the evaluation of TMD. Radiographic examination is commonly used for assessment of TMJ problems. Orthopantomograph (OPTG) is the most routine method for assessment of bone structural changes as erosions, flattening and osteophytes of the condyle and temporal part of TMJ. It is found that sub-jects with increased levels of P1NP, CTX-1 have less TMJ pain/discomfort. Increased levels of CTX-1 would probably cause an immediate increase of P1NP which is known as a sensitive marker of bone formation. TMJ radiographic changes seem to be related to the low level of 25(OH)D level.

Hence, the aim of this chapter is to critically review the evidence of possible association between TMJ pain and bone radiographic changes with main focus on the role of different bone markers and vitamin D.

Keywords: Activities of daily living, biochemical markers, OPTG, osteoporosis, pain measurement, temporomandibular joint disease, vitamin D

1. Introduction

Temporomandibular joint disorders (TMDs) present an important health problem. It has been estimated that approximately 20% to 30% of the adult population will experience temporomandibular joint (TMJ) dysfunction [1,2].

The most signs and symptoms include facial and jaw pain which can be initiated by jaw movements, TMJ sounds and functional disability. Radiological investigation often shows the displacement of the disc from its normal location, or osteoarthritic changes in the TMJ. Many researches focus on the role of biochemical mediators in development and progression of TMJ pain and dysfunction. There has been found association between bone markers (procollagen type I N-terminalpropeptide (P1NP), C-telopeptide crosslaps of type I collagen (CTX-1) as well as vitamin D (25(OH)D) and TMD [3,4,5]. Several biochemical markers of bone turnover can be used to predict individual bone loss on risk for TMJ pathologies [6].

The globally increasing prevalence of TMD calls for a more detailed knowledge on the relationship between bone markers and vitamin D in the pathogenesis of TMJ disorders. The Northern Europe population has a high risk for D-hypovitaminosis [7]. There is still a lack of the knowledge of the specific impact of TMJ pain on daily activities in patients with clinical involvement of the TMJ. Hopefully, the new knowledge of the TMJ etiopathogenesis will help predict TMJ bone destruction. Additional vitamin D consumption might be suggested to avoid TMJ dysfunctions and thereby reduce pain level. A multidimensional understanding of the etiopathogenesis of TMJ pathologies detected at an earlier stage would help improve diagnostics and apply evidence-based treatment.

2. Temporomandibular joint disorders and pain

2.1. TMJ pain

Pain in the jaw musculature is the most commonly reported pain of nondental origin in the orofacial region [8]. The TMJ pain is common among all age groups [9]. Chronic craniofacial pain conditions with a prevalence of approximately 10–15% are increasing in the adult population [10,11,12]. The prevalence of TMJ pain across lifetime is still debated, but there seems to be a peak of the pain at approximately 45 years of age for women, although also elderly people may suffer from TMD pain [13]. Pain is always a subjective experience, and the impact of chronic pain is not just a sensory experience but also an emotional experience [14,15,16].

Chronic pain may be nociceptive, neuropathic, ischemic, visceral or exhibit a combination of different etiologies. Nociceptive pain may result from the stimulation of nociceptors at the nerve endings and is characteristically present in TMDs. Stress, somatic distress and depression may be potential etiological risk factors for TMDs-related pain. In chronic pain, psychological factors may become more obvious and prominent [17]. In a population-based study, 47% subjects had TMJ problems where pain is commonly accompanied by stiffness, sounds and functional limitations, which result in a decreased quality of life, and thus exert a significant negative impact on activities of daily living (ADL) [5]. The following everyday activities such as eating, talking, yawning and laughing were more disturbed [18,19,20]. It was found that the impact of TMJ pain/discomfort was the greatest on eating (ADL 9) in 68% of the men and 77% of the women and smallest on performing daily household chores (ADL 3) in 37% of the men and in 61% of the women (Table 1) [5].

	Median	IQR	% pos.	Median	IQR	% pos.
ADL questions		Male			Female	
ADL1	0	4	45	3	5	74
ADL2	0	3	37	2	4	68
ADL3	0	3	37	2	4	61
ADL4	1	5	50	4	6	68
ADL5	0	3	37	2	5	74
ADL6	0	3	45	3	5	67
ADL7	1	5	50	3	6	67
ADL8	2	5	53	3	5	74
ADL9	3	7	68	3	4	77
ADL11	0	3	50	3	6	68
ADL12	1	4	58	3	4	75

IQR = interquartile range, % pos: percentage of observations exceeding zero, ADL scale: 0–12, socialize with family and close friends? (ADL 1), perform daily work? (ADL 2), perform daily household chores (preparing meals, cleaning, taking care of small children)? (ADL 3), sit in a company or participate in other social activities (e.g. parties)? (ADL 4), exercise (walk, bicycle, jogging, etc.)? (ADL 5), perform hobbies (read, fish, knit, play an instrument)? (ADL 6), sleep at night? (ADL 7), concentrate (ADL 8), eat (chew, swallow)? (ADL 9), talking (laughing, singing)? (ADL 10), yawn, open mouth wide? (ADL 11), how much does the pain/discomfort affect your daily activities? (ADL 12) where 0 = activity without any pain/discomfort at all and 12 = activity impossible due to pain/ discomfort.

Table 1. The influence of temporomandibular joint pain/discomfort on activities of daily living

2.2. Temporomandibular joint Disorders (TMD)

Temporomandibular joint disorders refer to several clinical conditions that involve muscles of mastication and TMJ or both [21]. Also, TMD are associated with disc displacement [22]. The etiology of TMD is multifactorial, being related to factors such as stress, muscle hyperactivity, arthrogenous factors, parafunctions or the anatomy of the TMJ [23]. The knowledge of the pathogenesis on a molecular level of disorders of the TMJ has been improved by allowing a possibility to use these data for the evidence-based treatment [24-26].

Signs and symptoms of TMD may include pain, impaired jaw function, malocclusion, deviation or deflection, limited range of motion, joint noise and locking. Headache, tinnitus, visual changes and other neurologic complaints may also accompany TMD. It has been found that 28% of the adult population have signs of temporomandibular joint disorder, with higher prevalence in women at reproductive ages [11,27–29]. Women report more pain, TMJ pain of longer duration, higher clinical and experimental pain intensity and lower pain thresholds [30]. Together with arthralgia of the temporomandibular joints, it is collectively referred to as 'temporomandibular disorder' [8].

The TMJ involvement may occur in systemic rheumatic diseases (rheumatoid arthritis, psoriatic arthritis, etc.), secondary from the neighbouring regions (otitis, maxillary sinusitis, tonsillitis), trauma (chronic), prevalence of dental arch defects, e.g. missing of molar teeth, malocclusion, endocrinological disturbances, odontogenic infections [31]. Many specific bacteria and several inflammatory mediators play an important role in the pathogenesis of TMJ diseases [32-34]. These inflammatory mediators drive catabolic pathways, inhibit matrix synthesis and promote cellular apoptosis. The bone loss at the TMJ condyle involves a common resorptive pathway: cytokine-activated osteoblasts promote activity of osteoclasts, which in turn result in the secretion of enzymes that are responsible for the breakdown of hydroxyapatite and collagen [35].

The most common form of TMJ arthritis is osteoarthritis (OA). It is one of the chronic diseases that involves TMJ [2]. The OA is classified as follows: (a) primary, which is idiopathic, i.e. factors are unknown; (b) secondary, where local and systemic factors are identified. It is mentioned that in secondary OA systemic causes are related to ethnicity, nutritional factors, genetics, hormonal status and bone metabolism, where as local causes include obesity, mechanical environment, overloading of articular cartilage and acute joint injury [36,37]. Most scientists regard osteoarthritis as an inflammatory process, being the most frequent TMJ disorder, characterized by proliferative changes in the synovia and primary degeneration of the cartilage and surrounding tissues with destruction of the bone structures and causing TMJ pain [24,38]. Nowadays, it is increasingly recognized that OA is a disease of the whole joint that affects all articular structures, including articular cartilage, subchondral bone, synovium, tendons, ligaments and menisci. The role of bone and articular soft tissues in the pathophysiology of OA has been widely overlooked [39].

3. Diagnostics of temporomandibular joint disorders

3.1. Activities of Daily Living (ADL) and the Visual Analogue Scale (VAS)

The impact of pain on the health status and quality of life in patients with chronic inflammatory joint diseases has been recognized, but there is a lack of knowledge about the specific impact of TMJ pain on daily activities in patients with clinical involvement of the TMJ [18]. Assessment of the individual level of daily activities is important in the evaluation of TMD. There are several scales for assessing patients' TMJ functions and for describing the particulars of their disability and the fact how their current status reflects in their day-to-day activities.

The term 'activities of daily living'(ADL) has been used to denote activities undertaken as part of a person's daily functions [40]. The ADL scale by Katz et al. [41] was primarily designed to measure the ability to carry out every day activities necessary for daily living. It has been validated and modified for specific use in patients with TMJ disorders [18,42–44]. Use of an ADL questionnaire is a very convenient method for pain assessment. This questionnaire is very simple and easy to handle and it can be recommended for future clinical trials in patients with TMJ disorders [45,46]. Only a few systematic reviews have addressed to daily activities or quality of life in relation to management of TMJ disorders. It is concluded that the use of specific questionnaires is justified for assessment of the character of TMJ pain [5].

The visual analogue scale (VAS) is a single-item scale to measure pain intensity [47]. The VAS is a continuous scale comprised of a horizontal or vertical line, usually 10 cm (100 mm) in length, anchored by two verbal descriptors, one for each symptom extreme. For pain intensity, the scale is most commonly anchored by 'no pain' (score of 0) and 'pain as bad as it could be' or 'worst imaginable pain' (score of 100 [100-mm scale; 48,49]. The VAS was initially used in psychology by Freud in the early 1900s and was elaborated in rheumatology through a series of investigations by Huskisson et al. in the late 1970s [50]. The scale has a high degree of sensitivity and validity because slight changes in pain intensity can be detected; however, it can also be confusing in a way for both very young and elderly patients [51,52]. The VAS scale has been used in several TMJ studies [53–56].

3.2. Radiographic imaging

Radiographic examination is commonly used for assessment of TMJ problems. Radiographic changes of the TMJ can be evaluated by orthopantomography, computed tomography and magnet resonance imaging [57,58] among other techniques, as well as by ultrasonography [59].

3.2.1. Orthopantomography (OPTG)

Orthopantomography (OPTG) is most commonly used for assessment of bone changes in the TMJ. By evaluating OPTGs, the following radiographic signs of bone structural changes can be detected, such as presence of erosions, flattening and osteophytes of the TMJ condyle as well as of temporal bone [60,61]. OPTGs give the possibility to describe structural changes in bone in different regions as alveolar cortical thickness of the mandible, lamina dura width, alveolar bone hight, mandibular bone mineral density (BMD) and status of teeth [62–66]. The studies have shown that mandibular cortical shape on OPTGs may be an indicator of bone turnover and spine BMD [67–70].

The most visible radiographic sign in the TMJ by OPTG is erosion (Figure 1).

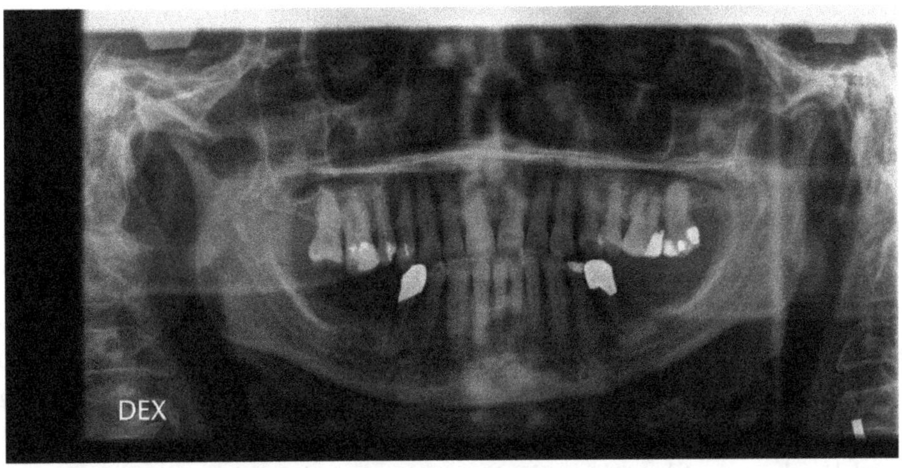

Figure 1. Ortopantomograph. Subchondral bony erosions of the right mandibular condyles are visible. Narrowing of both temporomandibular joint spaces and an irregularity of joint surfaces is observed.

The mandibular cortical erosion has been significantly associated with increased N-telopeptide cross-links of type I collagen and alkaline phosphatase levels [71]. Recent investigations have shown that radiographic examination including OPTG may be an effective tool as primary changes appear in alveolar bone for the early diagnosis of osteoporosis [4,72–75]. OPTGs could be useful as a simple screening method to estimate bone structure changes in the TMJ as well as to provide valuable information about the quality of the jaw bone such as joint space narrowing, osteophytes, subchondral sclerosis and subchondral cysts [76].

The total sum of radiographic changes in the TMJ is observed in 57% of the participants. Erosions occurred in 80%, flattening occurred in 37% and osteophytes occurred in 5% of the participants (Figure 2) [77].

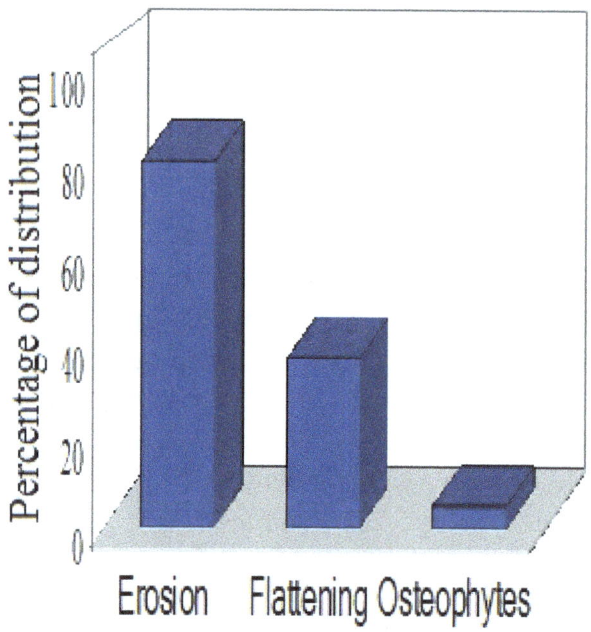

Figure 2. Distribution of radiographic changes.

3.2.2. *Computed Tomography (CT)*

The first report of TMJ computed tomography (CT) was published by Suarez et al. in 1980 [78] and this method is superior to plain transcranial or transmaxillary imaging for detecting bone changes. CT allows detailed three-dimensional examination of the TMJ and it is capable to detect even small bone changes not demonstrable by conventional tomographic procedures [2,79]. According to Rohlin and Petersson [80], the changes can be investigated by CT as follows: erosion – a local area with decreased density of the cortical joint surface including or not including adjacent subcortical bone, sclerosis – a local area with increased density of the cortical bony joint surface that may extend into the subcortical bone, subchondral pseudocyst (a well-defined local area of bone rarefication underneath an intact cortical outlining of the joint surface; Figure 3) and flattening (a flat bony contour deviating from the convex form osteophyte – a marginal bony outgrowth; Figure 4).

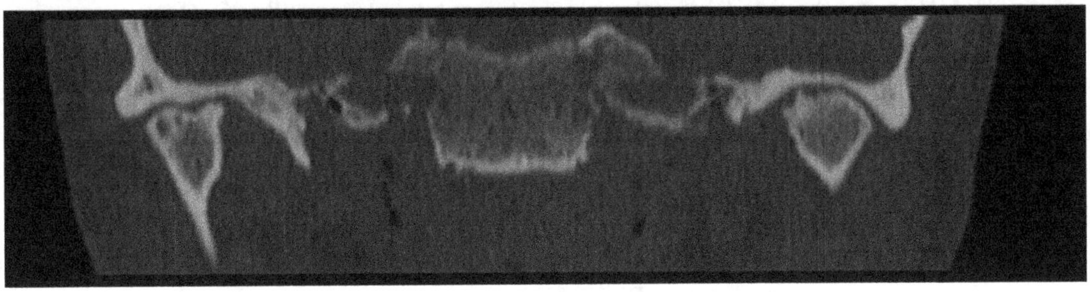

Figure 3. Osteoarthritis of TMJ. Bilateral signs of erosions on the surfaces of the condyles in a coronal view of the CT. Subchondral cyst in the right condyle. The joint spaces are asymmetric.

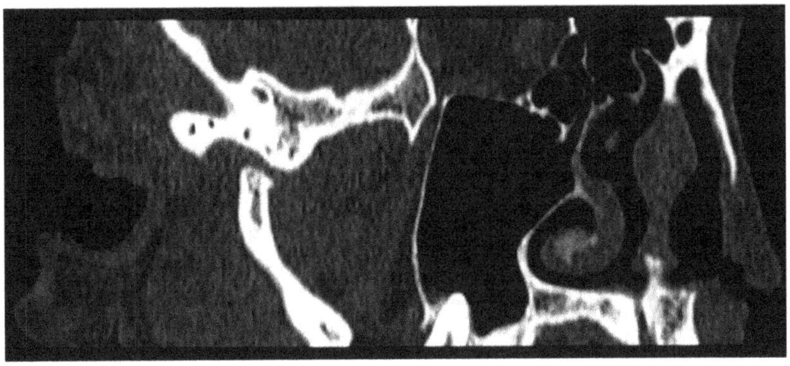

Figure 4. Sagittal view of the CT, right TMJ in an open mouth position. Sign of flattening of the mandibular condyle.

The CT allows to diagnose TMJ fractures, ankylosis, dislocation, neoplasms and growth abnormalities such as condylar hyperplasia [81]. The first choice for TMJ pathology diagnostics is OPTG; the CT imaging must improve treatment planning and prognosis.

4. The role of bone markers, vitamin D and osteoporosis in the pathogenesis of TMD

4.1. C-Telopeptidecrosslaps of type I collagen (CTX-1) and procollagen type I N-terminal Propeptide (P1NP)

Although several markers have been described to measure bone metabolism, it has been difficult to differ between the different mechanisms of bone resorption. These assays measure, in serum or in urine, enzymes or matrix proteins synthesized or degraded by bone cells [6]. It is stated that the most sensitive markers of bone resorption are C-telopeptidecrosslaps of type I collagen (CTX-1) and C-terminal telopeptide of type I collagen (1CTP), which are released from bone by different enzymatic pathways. The key osteoclastic enzyme for systemic bone resorption is generated by cathepsin K. The 1CTP is generated by matrix-metalloproteinases which plays an important role in collagen degradation associated with systemic inflammatory disease [82]. Procollagen type I N-terminal propeptide (P1NP) is a sensitive marker of bone formation. P1NP is synthesized by osteoblasts from type I procollagen precursor proteins. These precursors have large extension domains at both ends. While type I collagen is being synthesized, type I aminoterminal and carboxyterminal propeptides, PINP and PICP, respectively, are enzymatically removed and released into the circulation [83]. As bone is the major structure synthesizing type I collagen, PINP and PICP reflect bone formation [84]. Bone markers provide information beyond that of a single bone density measurement and on the cellular process leading to bone loss [85]. However, some of the few studies have not reported relationship between biomarkers and BMD [86]. Serum bone biomarkers are associated not only with systemic BMD loss but also with alveolar bone loss [87]. Biomarkers have the potential to provide an early warning of the initiation of breakdown of the articular matrix, which in future could lead to earlier treatment to prevent joint destruction that leads to disability [88].

The markers of joint tissue metabolism have opened new possibilities for earlier diagnosis of radiographic changes in joints and of OA [89,90]. It is found [77] that subjects with increased levels of P1NP, CTX-1 have less TMJ pain/discomfort. Increased levels of CTX-1 would probably cause an immediate increase of P1NP, which is known as a sensitive marker of bone formation. Subjects with a lower BMD had significantly less occluding pairs of teeth (Figure 5).

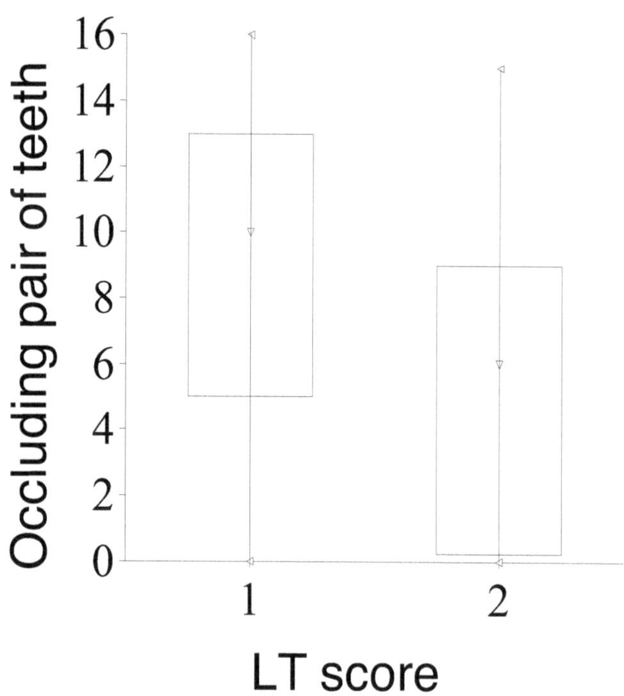

Figure 5. Relationship between occluding pair of teeth and LT score. Box plot showing the relationship between occluding pair of teeth and LT score. Box number 1 – subjects with normal mineral density. Box number 2 – subjects with lower LT score.

There are not enough data about the bone characteristics of patients with TMJ disorders. There still remains the question whether osteopenia in the TMJ area of the mandible is a local manifestation of osteoporosis having similar aetiology and risk factors, or it is an independent process depending primarily on factors that cause bone structural changes in the TMJ [75]. All these points to the need for additional studies which would evaluate the influence of potential contributing factors to further define the relationship between bone markers and TMJ disorders in population.

4.2. Vitamin D (25(OH)D)

Vitamin D (25(OH)D) plays an important role in calcium and bone metabolism inhibiting cytokine production and cell proliferation in various tissues [91]. Low levels of vitamin D lead to compensatory elevation of parathyroid hormone, which can cause lowering of BMD and eventually osteoporosis [92,93]. Vitamin D is related to musculoskeletal functioning and has been associated with a lower incidence of several cancers and autoimmune diseases. Studies have also shown that vitamin D has a role in neuromuscular function [94-96].

A majority of studies examined the association between serum 25(OH)D concentration and physical performance in community-dwelling older adults [93,95,97–99]. In particular, elderly people have a higher risk of vitamin D insufficiency, but it affects all age groups [100,101]. Low levels of 25(OH)D in young people can be partly explained by inadequate dietary sources and low activity in the daytime. It is estimated that vitamin D inadequacy is present in 36% of healthy young adults and in 57% of general medicine inpatients in the United States [102,103]. Vitamin D insufficiency seems a common health problem for people who live in countries at high latitudes where sunshine hours are short in the winter. Also Vitamin D levels are affected by modifiable and non-modifiable factors such as diet, time outdoors, skin pigmentation, sunbathing habits and medications [104,105,106]. Limited clinical research has focused on the specific effects of vitamin D deficiency on jaw pain. It is reported that vitamin D deficiency can cause predisposition to TMJ disorders [5,77,107,108].

A number of studies have addressed the relationship between sex hormones and TMDs and between low levels of vitamin D and pain all over the body but have not described the relationship between vitamin D and TMDs.

It was found [5] that lowering of 25(OH)D correlated negatively with activities of daily living such as social life with family (ADL 1), other social activities (ADL 4), exercising (ADL 5), performing hobbies (ADL 6), concentrating (ADL 8), eating (ADL 9), how much the pain/ discomfort affects daily activities (ADL 12; Fig. 6). The women had lower 25(OH)D level compared to the men.

4.3. Osteoporosis

Osteoporosis is one of the most common human bone diseases affecting millions of people, including over one-third of females above the age of 65 years and generally characterized by low bone mass, with increase in bone fragility and susceptibility to fracture. According to the World Health Organization, osteoporosis is considered to be present when BMD is 2.5 standard deviations (SD) below the young normal. Osteopenia is defined as bone density levels between 1 SD and 2.5 SD below normal BMD. Osteopenia is a reduction in bone mass due to imbalance

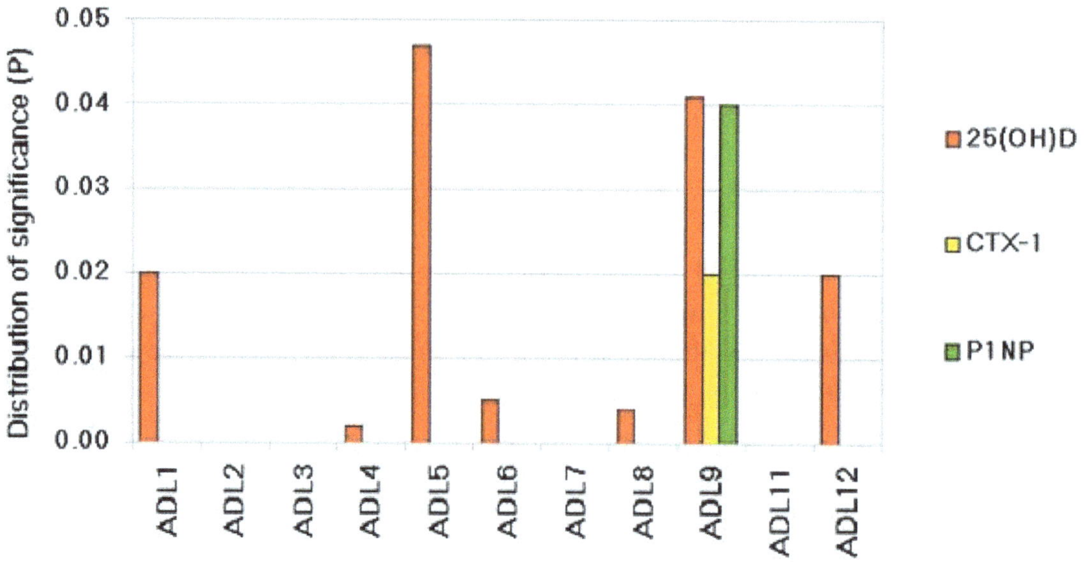

Figure 6. Distribution of significance between ADL data and bone characteristics. Relationship between bone characteristics and activities of daily living.

between bone resorption and formation, favouring resorption, resulting in demineralization and leading to osteoporosis [109]. The risk factors for osteoporosis are: sex, age, low body mass, early menopause, race, heredity, physical inactivity, lack of calcium intake, smoking and alcohol consumption [66].

The association between osteoporosis and oral bone disease was found already in 1960 [110]. Osteoporosis can affect all craniofacial and oral structures [76]. Osteoporosis is reported to cause bone loss in the alveolar processes of the maxilla and the mandible, which provides bony framework for tooth anchorage [111]. Some researchers have investigated whether dental radiographs could play a role in the detection of individuals with osteoporosis [112]. Bone mass in the jaw might be related to that of other skeletal sites in which osteoporosis was a significant problem [113,114]. The association between systemic osteoporosis and oral health remains controversial [115] while studies in this area are limited. Therefore, the relationship between systemic osteoporosis and oral health is still a complex problem of great interest for a large number of researchers and clinicians. Some epidemiological studies found that non-osteoporotic women's mandibular bone mass was not affected by age but was significantly associated with skeletal bone mass at the spine and wrist. The trabecular pattern was a highly significant predictor of future skeletal fracture risk [63,116]. Biochemical markers of bone turnover can be used to predict individual bone loss and therefore, they may help to alert patients to the risk of pathologies in the TMJ [4]. Thus, studies which evaluate the above mentioned contributing factors to define relationship between TMJ pain and several bone characteristics and ADL in population are justified.

The radiographic changes in the TMJ seem to be related to BMD. The patients with severe erosion of the cortex had significantly lower BMD values. In a population-based study was found out of 95 participants, 42% had abnormally low values of LT score. Among them osteoporosis was observed in 10.4% and osteopenia in 31.6% [77].

5. Conclusion

It is demonstrated that pain/discomfort originating from the TMJ is influenced by the biochemical markers of bone turnover. TMJ radiographic changes and teeth loss seem to be related to the low levels of BMD and 25(OH)D. The finding leads to the possible role of 25(OH)D in lowering of BMD in the TMJ and eventually osteoporosis. These findings indicate that presence of lowering BMD seems to be as one of the predictors for TMJ bone destruction.

Associations between TMJ pain/discomfort with vitamin D with the activities of daily living is evident. Subjects with lower 25(OH)D values experienced difficulties in performing physical exercises, engaging hobbies, they have problems with eating, participating in static social gatherings or other social activities. The social life of these persons is disrupted to a considerable degree. The median value of TMJ pain in the male as well as in the female group was relatively high considering that the study sample consisted of voluntary participants. Comparing the different sexes, we found highly significant correlations between female gender in following activities of daily living: social life, performing daily work, performing daily household chores, exercising, performing hobbies and yawning and opening the mouth wide. The same correlations in male were less significant.

Low 25(OH)D level can predict TMJ bone destruction and additional vitamin D consumption might be suggested to avoid TMJ dysfunction.

It is found that subjects with increased levels of P1NP, CTX-1 have less TMJ pain/discomfort. Increased levels of CTX-1 would probably cause an immediate increase of P1NP, which is known as a sensitive marker of bone formation.

Correlation between these two markers is probably due to equal shift / balance in a normal bone metabolism, where osteoblasts are acting simultaneously with osteoclasts.

The tight interaction and coordination between different aspects of TMD can be as a puzzle for health professionals. Based on obtained knowledge, the accuracy of diagnosis, quality of treatment as well as care for TMD can improve in the nearest future.

Acknowledgements

The study was financially supported by targeted funding project IUT2-8, by grant 6591 of the Estonian Science Foundation, by the European Union through the European Social Fund and by Ermst Jaakson Memorial Scholarship.

Author details

Oksana Ivask[1*], Ülle Voog-Oras[1] and Edvitar Leibur[2]

*Address all correspondence to: oksana.ivask@kliinikum.ee

1 Department of Stomatology, University of Tartu, Estonia

2 Departments of Stomatology and InternalMedicine, University of Tartu, Estonia

References

[1] Guo C, Shi Z, Revington P. Arthrocentesis and lavage for treating temporomandibular joint disorders. Cochrane Database Systemat Rev 2009;7(4):CD004973.

[2] Lee JY, Kim DJ, Lee SG, Chung JW. A longitudinal study on the osteoarthritic change of the temporomandibular joint based on 1-year follow-up computed tomography. J Cranio-Maxillo-Facial Surg 2012;40(8):e223–8.

[3] Israel HA, Langevin CJ, Singer MD, Behrman DA. The relationship between temporomandibular joint synovitis and adhesions: pathogenic mechanisms and clinical implications for surgical management. J Oral Maxillofacial Surg 2006;64(7):1066–74.

[4] Vlasiadis KZ, Damilakis J, Velegrakis GA, Skouteris CA, Fragouli I, Goumenou A, Matalliotakis J, Koumantakis EE. Relationship between BMD, dental panoramic radiographic findings and biochemical markers of bone turnover in diagnosis of osteoporosis. Maturitas 2008;59(3):226–33.

[5] Jagur O, Kull M, Leibur E, Kallikorm R, Lember M, Voog-Oras U. The associations of TMJ pain and bone characteristics on the activities of daily living. Open J Stomatol 2012;2(12):237–43.

[6] Garnero P, Ferreras M, Karsdal MA, Nicamhlaoibh R, Risteli J, Borel O, Qvist P, Delmas PD, Foged NT, Delaisse JM. The type I collagen fragments ICTP and CTX reveal distinct enzymatic pathways of bone collagen degradation. J Bone Miner Res 2003;18(5):859–67.

[7] Kull M Jr, Kallikorm R, Tamm A, Lember M. Seasonal variance of 25-(OH) vitamin D in the general population of Estonia, a Nothern European country. BMC Public Health 2009;9:22–33.

[8] Okeson JP. Management of Temporomandibular Disorders and Occlusion. In: St. Louis. Mosby; 2003; pp. 413–435.

[9] Helkimo M. Studies on function and dysfunction of the masticatory system. I. An epidemiological investigation of symptoms of dysfunction in Lapps in the north of Finland. Acta Odontol Scandinav 1974;32(4):225–65.

[10] Dworkin SF, Huggins KH, LeResche L, Von Korff M, Howard J, Truelove E, et al. Epidemiology of signs and symptoms in temporomandibular disorders: clinical signs in cases and controls. J Am Dental Assoc 1990;120(3):273–81.

[11] LeResche L. Epidemiology of temporomandibular disorders: implications for the investigation of etiologic factors. Crit Rev Oral Biol Med 1997;8(3):291–305.

[12] John MT, Dworkin SF, Mancl LA. Reliability of clinical temporomandibular disorder diagnoses. Pain 2005;118(1–2):61–9.

[13] Svensson P, Jadidi F, Arima T, Baad H, Sessle BJ. Relationships between craniofacial pain and bruxism. J Oral Rehab 2008;35(7):524–47.

[14] Kelley P, Clifford P. Coping with chronic pain: assessing narrative approaches. Social Work 1997;42(3):266–77.

[15] Thomas SP. A phenomenologic study of chronic pain. West J Nurs Res 2000;22(6): 6836–99.

[16] Tjakkes GH, Reinders JJ, Tenvergert EM, Stegenga B. TMD pain: the effect on health related quality of life and the influence of pain duration. Health Quality Life Outcomes 2010;28:46.

[17] Zakrzewska JM. Trigeminal neuralgia. In: Zakrzewska JM, Harrison SD. (Eds.) Assessment and Management of Orofacial Pain, 1st edn. Amsterdam: Elsevier Sciences; 2002; pp. 267–370.

[18] Voog U, Alstergren P, Leibur E, Kallikorm R, Kopp S. Impact of temporomandibular joint pain on activities of daily living in patients with rheumatoid arthritis. Acta Odontol Scandinav 2003a;61(5):278–82.

[19] Bessa-Nogueira RV, Vasconcelos B, Niederman R. The methodological quality of systematic reviews comparing temporomandibular joint disorder surgical and non-surgical treatment. BMC Oral Health 2008;26:8–27.

[20] De Boever JA, Carlsson GE, Klineberg IJ. Need for occlusal therapy and prosthodontic treatment in the management of temporomandibular disorders. Part I. Occlusal interferences and occlusal adjustment. J Oral Rehab 2000;27(5):367–79.

[21] Peck CC, Goulet JP, Lobbezoo F, Schiffman EL,Alstergren P, Anderson GC, de Leeuw R, Jensen R, Michelotti A, Ohrbach R, Petersson A, List T. Expanding the taxonomy of the diagnostic criteria for temporomandibular disorders. J Oral Rehab 2014;41(1):2–23.

[22] Barkin S, Weinberg S. Internal derangements of the temporomandibular joint: the role of arthroscopic surgery and arthrocentesis. J (Canad Dental Assoc) 2000;66(4): 199–203.

[23] Yáñez-Vico RM, Iglesias-Linares A, Torres-Lagares D, Gutiérrez-Pérez JL, Solano-Reina E. Association between condylar asymmetry and temporomandibular disorders using 3D-CT. Med Oral, Patol Oral y Cirugia Bucal 2012;17(5):e852–8.

[24] Holmlund AB, Axelsson S. Temporomandibular arthropathy: correlation between clinical signs and symptoms and arthroscopic findings. Int J Oral Maxillofacial Surg 1996;25(3):266–71.

[25] Kumagai K, Hamada Y, DDS, Holmlund AB, Gotoh A, Nakaoka K, et al. The levels of vascular endothelial growth factor in the synovial fluid correlated with the severity of arthroscopically observed synovitis and clinical outcome after temporomandibular joint irrigation in patients with chronic closed lock. Oral Surg Oral Med Oral Pathol Oral Rad Endodontics 2010;109(2):185–90.

[26] Guarda-Nardini L, PavanCk, Arveda N, Ferronato G, Manfredini D. Psychometric features of temporomandibular disorders patients in relation to pain diffusion, location, intensity and duration. J Oral Rehab 2012a;(39):737–73.

[27] Bagis Bhttp://www.medsci.org/v09p0539.htm – coraddress, Aydogan E, Turgut S, Durkan R, Özcan M. Gender difference in prevalence of signs and symptoms of temporomandibular joint disorders: a retrospective study on 243 consecutive patients. Int J Med Sci 2012;9(7):539–44.

[28] Rezaii T, Hirschberg AL, Carlström K, Ernberg M. The influence of menstrual phases on pain modulation in healthy women. J Pain 2012;13(7):646–55.

[29] Sipila K, Näpänkangas R, Könönen M, Alanen P, Siominen AL. The role of dental loss and denture status on clinical signs of temporomandibular disorders. J Oral Rehab 2013;40(1):15–23.

[30] Rezaii T, Ernberg M. Infuence of oral contraceptives on endogenous pain control in healthy women. Experiment Brain Res 2010;203(2):329–38.

[31] Tallents RH, Macher DJ, Kyrkanides S, Katzberg RW, Moss ME. Prevalence of missing posterior teeth and intraarticular temporomandibular disorders. J Prosthet Dentist 2002;87(1):45–50.

[32] Kim SJ, Park YH, Hong SP, Cho BO, Park JW, Kim SG. The presence of Bacteria in the synovial fluid of the temporomandibular joint and clinical significance: preliminary study. J Oral Maxillofacial Surg 2003;61(10):1156–61.

[33] Voog Ü, Alstergren P, Eliasson S, Leibur E, Kallikorm R, Kopp S. Inflammatory mediators and radiographic changes in temporomandibular joints with rheumatoid arthritis. Acta Odontol Scandinav 2003b;60:57–65.

[34] Hamada Y, Holmlund AB, Kondoh T, Nakaoka K, Sekiya H, Shiobara N, et al. Severity of arthroscopically observed pathology and levels of inflammatory cytokines in the synovial fluid before and after visually guided temporomandibular joint irrigation correlated with the clinical outcome in patients with chronic closed lock. Oral Surg Oral Med Oral Pathol Oral Radiol Endodontics 2008;106(3):343–9.

[35] Gunson MJ, Arnett GW, Milam SB. Pathophysiology and pharmacologic control of osseous mandibular condylar resorption. J Oral Maxillofacial Surg 2012;70(8):1918–34.

[36] Jordan JM, Kingtom RS, LaneNe, Nevitt MC, Zhang Y, Sowers MF, et al. Systemic risk factors for osteoarthritis. In: Felson DT, conference chair. Osteoarthritis: new insights. Part I: The disease and its risk factors. Annal Internal Med 2000;133(8):637–9.

[37] Kang SC, Lee DG, Choi JH, Kim ST, Kim YK, Ahn HJ. Association between estrogen receptor polymorphism and pain susceptibility in female temporomandibular joint osteoarthritis patients. Int J Oral Maxillofacial Surg 2007;36:391–4.

[38] Emshoff R. Clinical factors affecting the outcome of arthrocentesis and hydraulic distension of the temporomandibular joint. Oral Surg Oral Med Oral Pathol Oral Radiol Endodontics 2005;100(4):409–14.

[39] Brandt KD, Doherty M, Lohmander LS. Definition and classification of osteoarthritis.In: Brandt KD, Doherty M, Lohmander LS. (Eds.) Osteoarthritis. New York: Oxford University Press; 2003.

[40] Bucks SR, Haworth J. Bristol activities of daily living scale: a critical evaluation. Expert Rev Neurotherapeutics 2002;2(5):669–76.

[41] Katz S, Ford AB, Moskowitz RW, Jackson BA, Jaffe MW. Studies of illness in the aged. The index of ADL: a standardized measure of biological and psychological function. JAMA 1963;185:914–9.

[42] List T, Helkimo M. A scale for measuring the activities of daily living (ADL) of patients with craniomandibular disorders. Swed Dental J 1995;19(1–2):33–40.

[43] Kaselo E, Jagomägi T, Voog Ü. Malocclusion and the need for orthodontic treatment in patients with temporomandibular dysfunction. Stomatologija, Baltic Dental Maxillofacial J 2007;9(3):79–85.

[44] Karibe H, Goddard G, Aoyagi K, Kawakami T, Warita S, Shimazu K, Rudd PA, McNeill C. Comparison of subjective symptoms of temporomandibular disorders in young patients by age and gender.Cranio 2012;30(2):114–20.

[45] Murakami K, Segami N, Okamoto I, Takahashi K, Tsuboi Y. Outcome of arthroscopic surgery for internal derangement of the temporomandibular joint: long-term results covering 10 years. J Cranio-Maxillo-Facial Surg 2000;28(5):264–71.

[46] Undt G, Murakami K, Clark GT, Ploder O, Dem A, Lang T, et al. Cross–cultural adaptation of the JPF-Questionnarie for German speaking patients with functional temporomandibular joint disorders. J Cranio-Maxillo-Facial Surg 2006;34(4):226–33.

[47] McCormack HM, Horne DJ, Sheather S. Clinical applications of visual analogue scales: a critical review. Psychol Med 1988;18(4):1007–19.

[48] Burckhardt CS, Jones KD. Adult measures of pain: The McGill Pain Questionnaire (MPQ), Rheumatoid Arthritis Pain Scale (RAPS), Short-Form McGill Pain Questionnaire (SF-MPQ), Verbal Descriptive Scale (VDS), Visual Analog Scale (VAS), and West Haven-Yale Multidisciplinary Pain Inventory (WHYMPI). Arthritis Care Res 2003;49:S96–104.

[49] Hawker GA, Mian S, Kendzerska T, French M. Measures of adult pain: Visual Analog Scale for Pain (VAS Pain), Numeric Rating Scale for Pain (NRS Pain), McGill Pain Questionnaire (MPQ), Short-Form McGill Pain Questionnaire (SF-MPQ), Chronic Pain Grade Scale (CPGS), Short Form-36 Bodily Pain Scale (SF-36BPS), and Measure of Intermittent and Constant Osteoarthritis Pain (ICOAP). Arthritis Care Res 2011;63(11):S240–52.

[50] Sokka T. Assessment of pain in patients with rheumatic diseases. Best Practise Res Clin Rheumatol 2003;17(3):427–49.

[51] Gagliese L, Weizblit N, Ellis W, et al. The measurement of postoperative pain: a comparison of intensity scales in younger and older surgical patients. Pain 2005;117(3): 412–20.

[52] Williamson A, Hoggart B. Pain: a review of three commonly used pain rating scales. J Clin Nurs 2005;14(7):798–804.

[53] Ahn HJ, Lee YS, Jeong SH, Kang SM, Byun YS, KIM BI. Objective and subjective assessment of masticatory function for patients with temporomandibular disorder in Korea. J Oral Rehab 2011;38(7):475–81.

[54] Rusanen J, Silvola AS, Tolvanen M, Pirttiniemi P, Lahti S, Sipilä K. Pathways between temporomandibular disorders, occlusal characteristics, facial pain, and oral health-related quality of life among patients with severe malocclusion. Eur J Orthodontics 2012;34(4):512–7.

[55] Edefonti V, Bravi F, Cioffi I, Capuozzo R, Ammendola L, Abate G, Decarli A, Ferraroni M, Farella M, Michelotti A. Chronic pain and weather conditions in patients suffering from temporomandibular disorders: a pilot study. Commun Dentist Oral Epidemiol 2012;40(1):56–64.

[56] Guarda-Nardini L, Cadorin C, Frizziero A, Ferronato A, Manfredini D. Comparison of 2 hyaluronic acid drugs for the treatment of temporomandibular joint osteoarthritis. J Oral Maxillofacial Surg 2012b;70(11):2522–30.

[57] Ohnuki T, Fukuda M, Iino M, Takahashi T. Magnetic resonance evaluation of the disk before and after arthroscopic surgery for temporomandibular disorders. Oral Surg Oral Med Oral Pathol Oral Radiol Endodontics 2003;96(2):141–8.

[58] Whyte AM, McNamara D, Rosenberg I, Whyte AW. Magnetic resonance imaging in the evaluation of temporomandibular joint disc displacement. Int J Oral Maxillofacial Surg 2006;35(8):696–703.

[59] Landes CA, Sader R. Sonographic evaluation of the ranges of condylar translation and of temporomandibular joint space as well as first comparison with symptomatic joints. J Cranio-Maxillo-Facial Surg 2007;35(8):374–81.

[60] Rohlin M. Åkerman S, Kopp S. Tomography as an aid to detect macroscopic changes of the temporomandibular joint. Acta Odontol Scandinav 1986;44(3):131–40.

[61] Helenius L, Hallikainen D, Meurman J, Koskimies S, Tervahartiala P, Kivisaari L, Hietanen J, Suuronen R, Lindqvist C, Lerisalo-Repo M. HLA-DRB1 alleles and temporomandibular joint erosion in patientes with rheumatic disease. Scand J Rheumatol 2004;33:24–9.

[62] Leibur E, Jian JL, Söder PÖ. Alveolar bone level on intraoral and panoramic radiographs analysed by a computerized image system. Oral Surg Oral Diag 1995;6(2):13–7.

[63] Jeffcoat MK, Lewis CE, Reddy MS, Wank CY, Redford M. Post-menopausal bone loss and its relationship to oral bone loss. Periodontology 2000;23:94–102.

[64] Jonasson G, Bankvall G, Kiliaridis S. Estimation of skeletal bone mineral density by means of the trabecular pattern of the alveolar bone, its interdental thickness and the bone mass of the mandible. Oral Surg Oral Med Oral Pathol Oral Radiol Endodontics 2001;92(3):346–52.

[65] Krejc CB, Bissada NF. Womens health issues and their relationship to periodontitis. J Am Dental Assoc 2002;133(3):323–8.

[66] Hardanti S, Azhari, Oscandar F. Description of mandibular bone quality based on measurements of cortical thickness using Mental Index of male and female patients between 40-60 years old. Imaging Sci Dentist 2011;41(4):151–3.

[67] Balcikonyte E, Balciuniene I, Alekna V. Panoramic radiographs in assessment of the bone mineral density. Stomatologija, Baltic Dental and Mafillofacial J 2004;6:17–9.

[68] Vlasiadis KZ, Skouteris CA, Velegrakis GA, Fragouli I, Neratzoulakis JM, Damilakis J, et al. Mandibular radiomorphometric measurements as indicators of possible osteoporosis in postmenopausal women. Maturitas 2007;58(3):226–35.

[69] Taguchi A. Panoramic radiographs for identifying individuals with undetected osteoporosis. Jap Dental Sci Rev 2009;45(2):109–20.

[70] Hastar E, Yilmaz HH, Orhan H. Evaluation of mental index, mandibular cortical index and panoramic mandibular index on dental panoramic radiographs in the elderly. Eur J Dentist 2011;5(1):60–7.

[71] Taguchi A, Tsuda M, Ohtsuka M, Kodama I, Sanada M, Nakamoto T, et al. Use of dental panoramic radiographs in identifying younger postmenopausal women with osteoporosis. Osteoporosis Int 2006;17(3):387–94.

[72] Bonnick SL, Shulman L. Monitoring osteoporosis therapy: bone mineral density, bone turnover markers, or both? Am J Med 2006;119(4 Suppl 1):25–31.

[73] Jagelaviciene E, Kubilius R. The relationship between general osteoporosis of the organism and periodontal diseases. Medicina 2006;42(8):613–8.

[74] Miliuniene E, Alekna V, Peciuliene V, Tamulaitiene M, Maneliene R. Relationship between mandibular cortical bone height and bone mineral density of lumbar spine. Stomatologija. Baltic Dental Maxillofacial J 2008;10(2):72–5.

[75] Khatoonabad MJ, Aghamohammadzade N, Taghilu H, Esmaeili HF, Khamnei J. Relationship among panoramic radiography findings, biochemical markers of bone turnover and hip BMD in the diagnosis of postmenopausal osteoporosis. Iran J Radiol 2011;8(1):23–8.

[76] Aggarwal A, Panat SR. Identification of postmenopausal women at risk of osteoporosis using panoramic and intraoral radiographs – a review. Minerva Stomatol 2012;61(7–8):323–8.

[77] Jagur O, Kull M, Leibur E, Kallikorm R, Loorits D, Lember M, Voog-Oras U. Relationship between radiographic changes in the temporomandibular joint and bone mineral density: a population based study. Stomatologija 2011;13(2):42–8.

[78] Suarez FR, Bhussry BR, Neff PA, Huang HK, Vaughn D (1980). A preliminary study of computerized tomographs of the temporomandibular joint. Compend Continuing Edu Gen Dentist 1980;1(3):217–22.

[79] Larheim TA, Westesson P, Sano T. Temporomandibular joint disk displacement: comparison in asymptomatic volunteers and patients. Radiology 2001;218(2):428–32.

[80] Rohlin M, Petersson A. Rheumatoid arthritis of the temporomandibular joint:radiologic evaluation based on standard reference films. Oral Surg Oral Med Oral Pathol 1989;67(5):594–9.

[81] Barghan S, Tetradis S, Mallya SM. Application of cone beam computed tomography for assessment of the temporomandibular joints. Austral Dental J 2012;57(Suppl 1): 109–18.

[82] Chopin F, Garnero P, le Henanff A, Debiais F, Daragon A, Roux C, Sany J, Wendling D, Zarnitsky C, Ravaud P, Thomas T. Long term effects of infliximab on bone and

cartilage turnover markers in patients with rheumatoid arthritis. Annal Rheumatic Dis 2008;67(3):353–7.

[83] Calvo MS, Eyre DR, Gundberg CM. Molecular basis and clinical application of biological markers of bone turnover. Endocrine Rev 1996;17(4):333–68.

[84] Delmas PD. Clinical use of biochemical markers of bone remodeling in osteoporosis. Bone 1992;13(suppl 1):S17–21.

[85] Åkesson K, Vergnaud P, Gineyts E, Delmas Obrant KJ. Impairment of bone turnover in elderly women with hip fracture. Calcif Tissue Int 1993;53(3):162–9.

[86] Cosman F, Nieves J, Wilkinson C, Schnering D, ShenV, Lindsay R. Bone density change and biochemical indices of skeletal turnover. Calcif Tissue Int 1996;58(4):236–43.

[87] Payne JB,Stoner JA, Lee HM, Nummikoski PV, Reinhardt RA, Golub LM. Serum bone biomarkers and oral/systemic bone loss in humans. J Dental Res 2011;90(6):747–51.

[88] Kraus VB, Burnett B, Coindreau J, Cottrell S, Eyre D, Gendreau M, Gardiner J, et al. Application of biomarkers in the development of drugs intended for the treatment of osteoarthritis. Osteoarthritis Cartilage 2011;19(5):515–42.

[89] Garnero P, Ayral X, Rousseau JC, Christgau S, Sandell LJ, Dougados M, et al.Uncoupling of type II collagen synthesis and degradation predicts progression ofjoint damage in patients with knee osteoarthritis. Arthritis Rheumatism 2002;46(10):2613–24.

[90] Kumm J, Tamm A, Lintrop M, Tamm A. The value of cartilage biomarkers in progressive knee osteoarthritis: cross-sectional and 6-year follow-up study in middle-aged subjects. Rheumatol Int 2012;33(4) 903–11.

[91] Dietrich T, Joshipura K. Association between serum concentrations of 25-hydroxyvitamin D 3 and periodontal disease in the US population. Am J Clin Nutrit 2004;80(1): 108–13.

[92] Kwon J, Suzuki T, Yoshida H, Kim H, Yoshida Y, Iwasa H. Concomitant lower serum albumin and vitamin D levels are associated with decreased objective physical performance among Japanese community-dwelling elderly. Gerontology 2007;53(5):322–8.

[93] Annweiler C, Beauchet O, Berrut G, Couris C, Fantino B, Bonnefoy M, Herrmann FR, Schott AM. Is there a relationship between serum vitamin D insufficiency and reduced muscle strength among older women? Results from baseline assessment of EPIDOS study. J Nutrit Health Aging 2009;13:90–5.

[94] Bischoff HA, Borchers M, Gudat F, Duermueller U, Theiler R, Stahelin HB, et al. In situ detection of 1,25-dihydroxyvitamin D3 receptor in human skeletal muscle tissue. Histochem J 2001;33(1):19–24.

[95] Bischoff-Ferrari HA, Dietrich T, Orav EJ, Dawson-Hughes B. Positive association between 25-hydroxy vitamin D levels and bone mineral density: a population-based study of younger and older adults. Am J Med 2004;116(9):634–9.

[96] Bischoff-Ferrari HA. The 25-hydroxyvitamin D threshold for better health. J Steroid Biochem Molecul Biol 2007;103(3–5):614–9.

[97] Dukas L, Staehelin HB, Schacht E, Bischoff HA. Better functional mobility in community-dwelling elderly is related to D-hormone serum levels and to daily calcium intake. J Nutrition Health Aging 2005;9(5):347–51.

[98] Gerdhem P, Ringsberg KA, Obrant KJ, Akesson K. Association between 25-hydroxy vitamin D levels, physical activity, muscle strength and fractures in the prospective population-based OPRA Study of Elderly Women. Osteoporos Int 2005;16:1425–31.

[99] Houston DK, Cesari M, Ferrucci L, Cherubini A, Maggio D, Bartali B, Johnson MA, Schwartz GG, Kritchevsky SB. Association between vitamin D status and physical performance: the InCHIANTI study. J Gerontol Ser A Biol Sci Med Sci 2007;62(4): 440–6.

[100] Chapuy MC, Preziosi P, Maamer M, Arnaud S, Galan P, Hercberg S, et al. Prevalence of vitamin D insufficiency in an adult normal population. Osteoporos Int 1997;7(5): 439–43.

[101] Lappe JM, Davies KM, Travers-Gustafson D, Heaney RP. Vitamin D status in a rural postmenopausal female population. J Am College Nutrit 2006;25(5):395–402.

[102] Holick MF. High prevalence of vitamin D inadequacy and implications for health. Mayo Clin Proc 2006;81(3):353–73.

[103] Holick MF. Vitamin D deficiency. New Engl J Med 2007;357(3):266–81.

[104] Sherman SS, Hollis BW, Tobin JD. Vitamin D status and related parameters in a healthy population: the effects of age, sex, and season. J Clin Endocrinol Metabolism 1990;71(2):405–13.

[105] Budak N, Ciçek B, Sahin H, Tutus A. Bone mineral density and serum 25-hydroxyvitamin D level: is there any difference according to the dressing style of the female university students. Int J Food Sci Nutrit 2004;55(7):569–75.

[106] Bolek-BerquistJ, Elliott ME, Ronald E,Gemar D, Engelke J, Lawrence SJ, Hansen KE. Use of a questionnaire to assess vitamin D status in young adults. Public Health Nutrit 2009;12(2):236–43.

[107] Abdel-Fattah RA. Evaluating TMJ Injuries, Volume 1. New York: Wiley Law Publications; 1992; pp. 105–112.

[108] Shen M, Luo Y, Niu Y, Chen L, Yuan X, Goltzman D, Chen N, Miao D. 1,25 (OH) 2D deficiency induces temporomandibular joint osteoarthritis *via* secretion of senescence – associated inflammatory cytokines. Bone 2013;55(2):400–9.

[109] Wactawski-Wende J, Grossi SG, Trevisan M, Genco RJ, et al. The role of osteopenia in oral bone loss and periodontal disease. J Periodontol 1996;67(10):1076–84.

[110] Groen JJ, Duyvensz F, Halsted JA. Diffuse alveolar atrophy of the jaw (non-inflammatory form of paradental disease) and presenile osteoporosis. Gerontol Clin 1960;2:68–86.

[111] Wactawski-Wende J, Hausmann E, Hovey K, Trevisan M, Grossi S, Genco RJ. The association between osteoporosis and alveolar crestal height in postmenopausal women. J Periodontol 2005;76(11):116–1124.

[112] Nackaerts O, Jacobs R, Devlin H, Pavitt S, Bleyen E, Yan B, et al. Osteoporosis detection using intraoral densitometry. DentoMaxillo Facial Radiol 2008;37(5):282–7.

[113] Kim JY, Nah KS, Jung YH.Comparison of panorama radiomorphometric indices of the mandible in normal and osteoporotic women. Kor J Oral Maxillofacial Radiol 2004;34:69–74.

[114] Hua Y, Nackaerts O, Duyck J, Maes F, Jacobs R. Bone quality assessment based on cone beam computed tomography imaging. Clin Oral Implants Res 2009;20(8):767–71.

[115] Makker A, Singh MM, Mishra G, Singh BP, Jain GK, Jadhav S. Relationship between bone turnover biomarkers, mandibular bone mineral density, and systemic skeletal bone mineral density in premenopausal and postmenopausal Indian women. Menopause 2012;19(6):642–9.

[116] Jonasson G, Sundh V, Ahlqwist M, Hakeberg M, Björkelund C, Lissner L. A prospective study of mandibular trabecular bone to predict fracture incidence in women: a low-cost screening tool in the dental clinic. Bone 2011;49(4):873–9.

2

Surgical Approaches to the Temporomandibular Joint

Mohammad Esmaeelinejad and Maryam Sohrabi

Abstract

The temporomandibular joint (TMJ) acts as a sliding hinge between mandible and temporal bone. Disorders of temporomandibular joint are intolerable for the patients in severe cases. Furthermore, surgical treatment of temporomandibular joint problems is a challenge for surgeons in some cases. In that order, it is critical for the surgeon to choose the best surgical approach in treating the temporomandibular joint diseases. There are several surgical approaches in the management of temporomandibular joint problems including some pros and cons. So, in this chapter, we aim to present a comprehensive review of surgical approaches to the temporomandibular joint.

Keywords: facial nerve, mandible, mandibular condyle, superficial musculoaponeurotic system, temporomandibular joint

1. Introduction

Exact diagnosis and appropriate treatment plan are two important fundamentals of successful surgical results. Planning the treatment of temporomandibular joint (TMJ) problems is not an exception. TMJ is a hinge that connects the mandible to the temporal and serves the movement of lower jaw. TMJ problems such as disc derangement, pathologic lesions, and traumatic injuries would have a significant influence on quality of life of the patients.

Treatment of TMJ diseases is still one of the controversial issues in maxillofacial surgery field. It is important to choose the best surgical technique to solve the problem and rehabilitate the TMJ function. There are several surgical approaches to the TMJ mentioned in the literature and a maxillofacial surgeon should know the technical aspects of these surgical procedures.

This chapter is based on recent investigations reported in the literature and briefly presents the different aspects of available surgical approaches to TMJ including their indications, techniques, and benefits.

2. Applied anatomy

TMJ is a synovial joint between the head of mandibular condyle and the temporal glenoid fossa. The space between the head of mandibular condyle and the glenoid fossa of temporal bone is divided into two separate cavities by the articular disc (**Figure 1**). The inferior compartment is involved in the hinge movement of the joint, while the superior joint space participates in the translation movement.

The postglenoid process and articular eminence are the posterior and anterior limitations of the articular space, respectively. TMJ is surrounded by a fibrous capsule called articular capsule, and its extension is the articular disc (**Figure 2**).

The movements of TMJ are restricted by three main ligaments. The temporomandibular ligament is the lateral portion of articular capsule. This fan-shaped ligament is responsible for synchronizing the condyle and articular disc. The other two ligaments are sphenomandibular and stylomandibular ligaments which are involved in controlling the mandibular movements (**Figure 2**).

2.1. Regional nerves

The most common anatomical structure facing during the approaches to the TMJ is the facial nerve. The main trunk of facial nerve exits the stylomastoid foramen and after passing about 2 cm distance divides into two main branches of temporofacial and cervicofacial divisions (**Figure 3**) [1]. The distance from the bony part of external auditory canal to the bifurcation is 1.5–2.8 cm (mean is 2.3 cm) [2]. The assumed line connected from the tragus to the

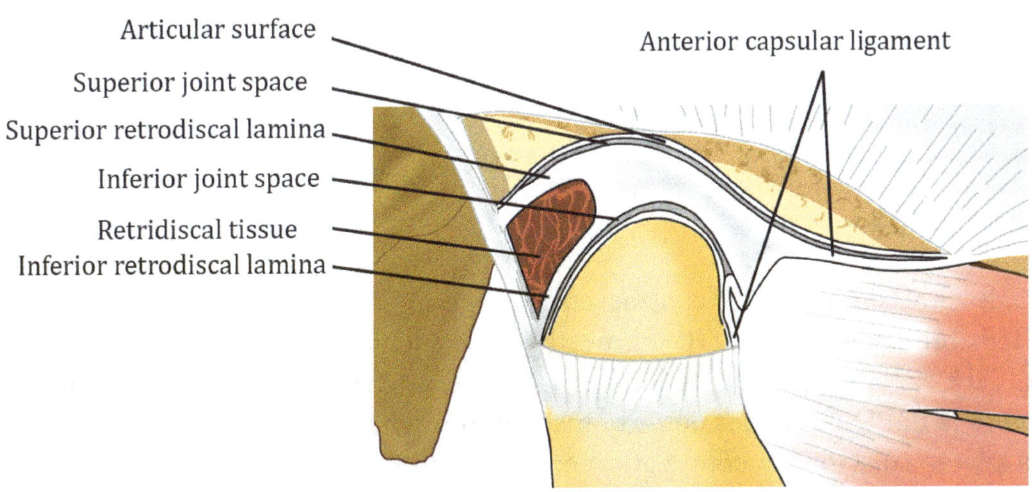

Figure 1. Anatomy of the TMJ.

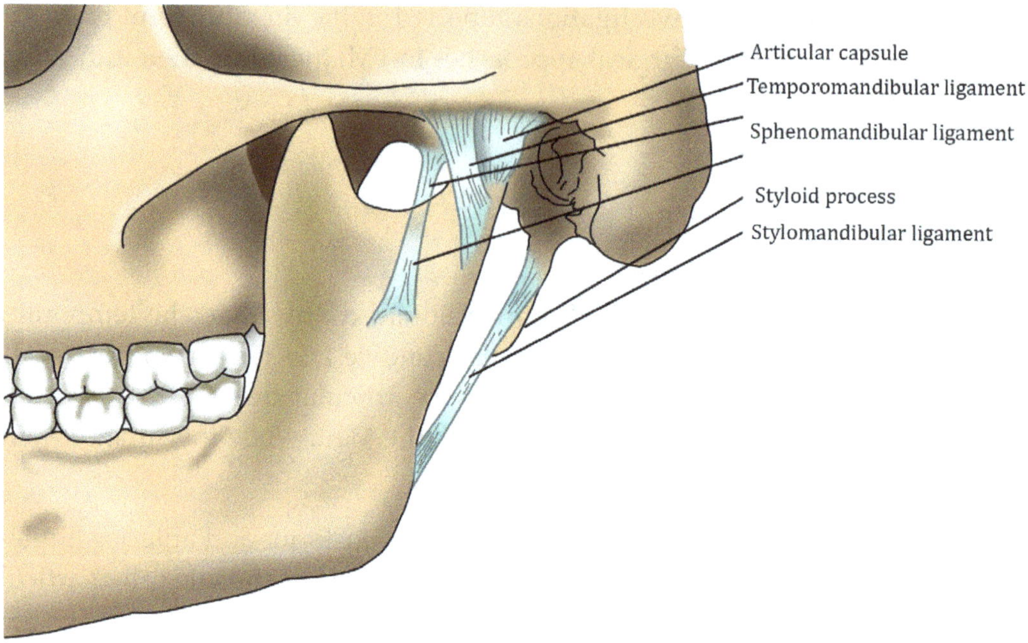

Figure 2. Anatomy of the articular ligaments.

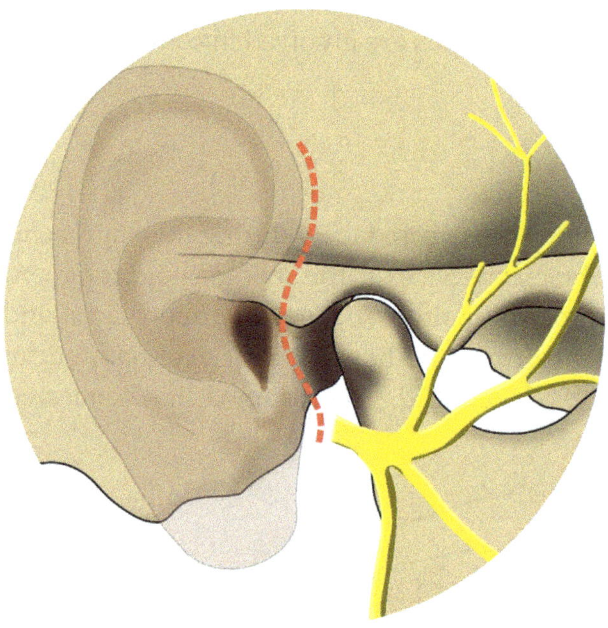

Figure 3. Anatomy of the facial nerve.

lateral palpebral commissure is considered the superior limit of temporal branch of the facial nerve. This branch of facial nerve is mostly located under this oblique line [3]. Temporal branch is the most susceptible branch of facial nerve that would be damaged during the approaches to the TMJ [4]. This nerve branch lies under the surface of temporoparietal fascia [5]. The average distance of bony part of external auditory canal to the location where temporal branch of facial nerve crosses the zygomatic arch is almost 2 cm (8–35 mm). In some surgical approaches to the subcondylar area, the most important anatomical structure that should be preserved is the marginal mandibular branch of the facial nerve. This branch is superior to the mandibular inferior border in 74% of the cases [6]. The maximum distance to the mandibular inferior border is 1.2 cm; in other patients that marginal mandibular branch of facial nerve is located beneath the inferior border of the mandible. This branch is located superior to the facial artery and vein immediately deep to the superficial layer of the deep cervical fascia.

The branches of trigeminal nerve are other critical structures adjacent to the TMJ. The auriculotemporal branch supplies sensation to the anterior external meatus and the temporal and preauricular region skin. This branch of trigeminal nerve passes behind the neck of mandibular condyle (**Figure 4**).

2.2. Anatomy of regional vessels

Maxillary artery and superficial temporal artery are two last branches of external carotid artery and important structures adjacent to the TMJ. The surgeons usually face the superficial temporal artery during the preauricular approaches. This terminal branch of external carotid artery runs posterolateral to the mandibular condyle within the temporoparietal fascia (**Figure 5**).

Maxillary artery is important in condylectomy procedure. Middle meningeal artery is a branch of internal maxillary artery that passes medial to the mandibular condyle and could be damaged during the surgical procedures on TMJ.

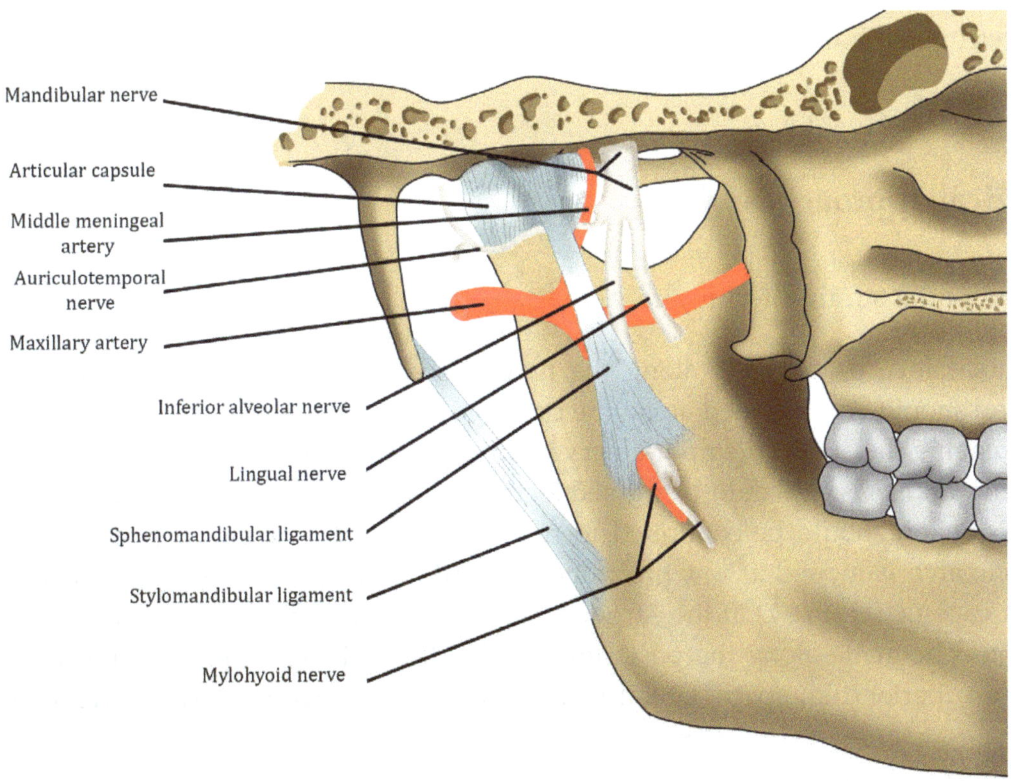

Figure 4. Relation of trigeminal nerve to the TMJ.

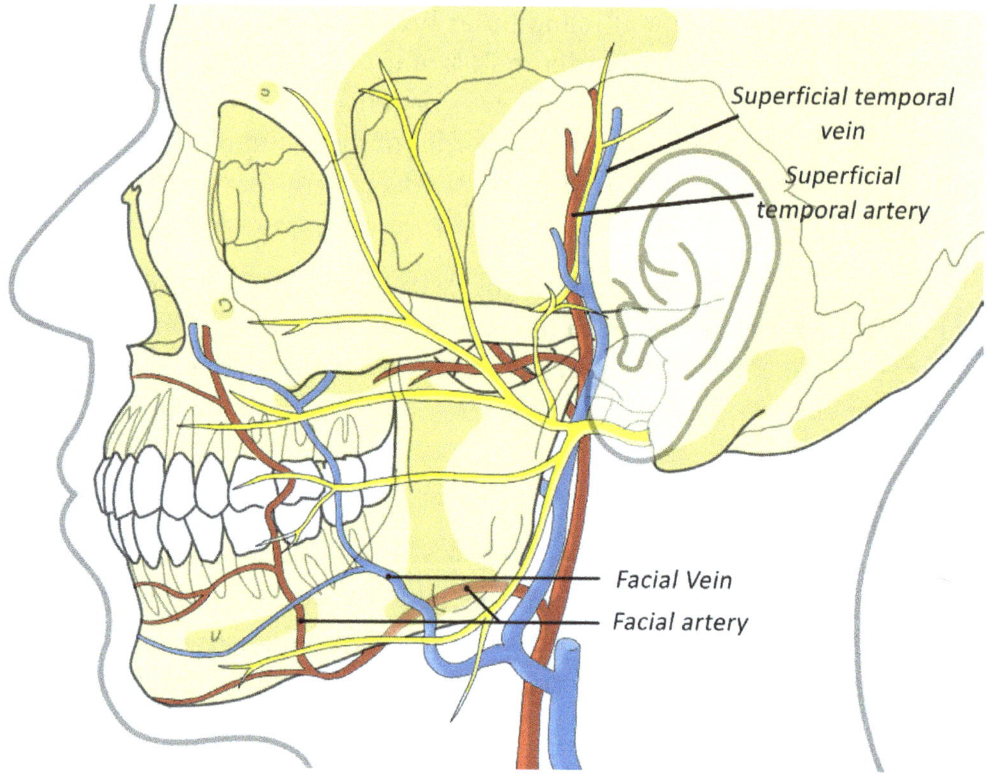

Figure 5. Vascular anatomy of the face encountered during surgical procedures of the TMJ.

The important vein that the surgeon usually encounters in surgical treatment of the TMJ problems is retromandibular vein which is formed from the superficial temporal and the maxillary veins.

3. Surgical approaches

3.1. Preauricular surgical technique

Preauricular incision is made along the natural crease anterior to the tragus (**Figure 6**). Dissection should be continued along the cartilage of external auditory canal in order to prevent damaging the auriculotemporal nerve and superficial temporal artery. Superficial layer of the temporalis fascia would be incised 2 cm above the zygomatic arch in an oblique line. Blunt dissection should be continued to reach the zygomatic arch. The periosteum of the zygomatic arch is incised at this time, and it should be reflected laterally to achieve to the articular capsule (**Figure 7**). If the surgeon needs to expose the superior joint space, the incision should be made along the posterior slope of the articular eminence. Incising the disc along the superior joint space, lateral recess allows the surgeon to expose the inferior joint space.

In some cases, to maximize the exposure to the TMJ, preauricular incision is modified to a question mark pattern presented by Al-Kayat and Bramley (**Figure 8**).

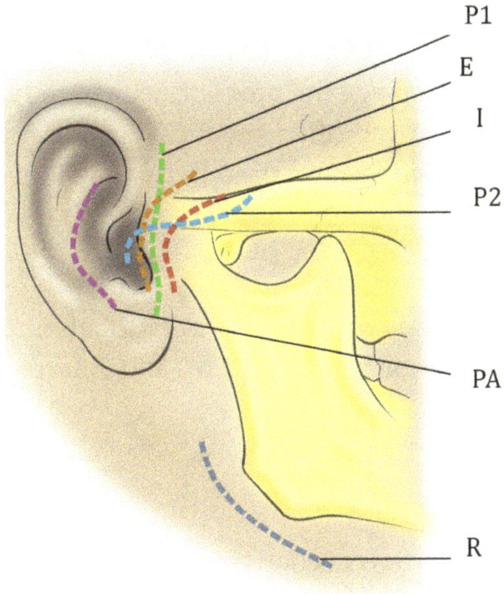

Figure 6. Surgical approaches to the TMJ. P1 and P2—preauricular approaches; PA—postauricular approach; I—inverted hockey stick approach; E—endaural approach. R—retromandibular approach.

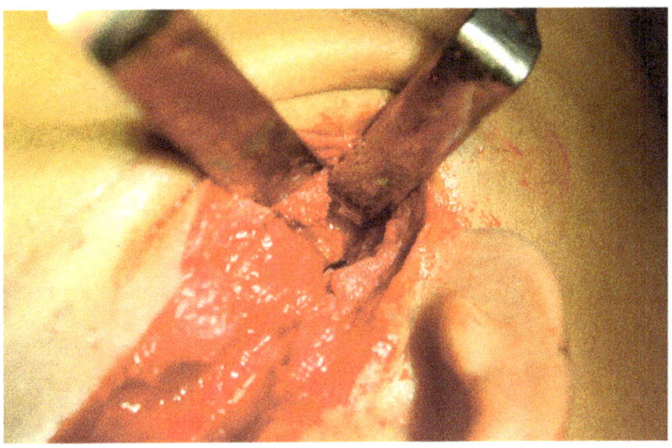

Figure 7. After exposing the articular capsule, it could be incised to reach to the joint spaces.

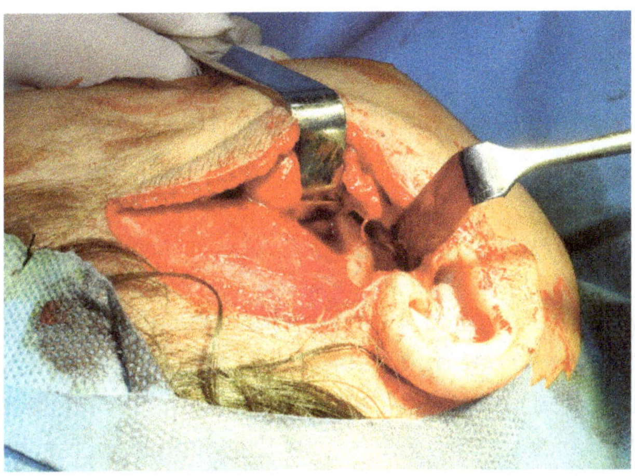

Figure 8. Al-Kayat and Bramley incision to expose the TMJ for condylectomy.

3.1.1. Indications

This approach is ideally used to manage the problems encountered in upper condylar process and TMJ compartments. Al-Kayat modified preauricular incision is routinely used in TMJ ankylosis cases. Preauricular incision is also used in treatment of high condylar fractures.

3.1.2. Advantages

Almost invisible scars are main advantages of a preauricular approach. This surgical technique provides access to the superior part of the TMJ and anteromedially displaced mandibular condyle.

3.1.3. Disadvantages

There is no access to the lower portion of condylar process. Rigid fixation of mandibular condyle fracture is difficult in this approach [7]. The possibility of facial nerve damage is a major disadvantage of this surgical technique.

3.2. Endaural surgical technique

This approach is provided to achieve the benefits of preauricular methods simultaneously with more cosmetic results. The incision is made behind the prominence of the tragus. The skin flap is reflected over the cartilage of the tragus, and then, dissection is continued in the same manner of preauricular approach.

3.2.1. Indications

This technique is indicated when there is the aim to provide the access to the TMJ and fractures of condylar head and neck.

3.2.2. Advantages

The cosmetic result of scar is better than preauricular incision [8].

3.2.3. Disadvantages

Tragus cartilage damage is the main disadvantage of this approach. When the problem happens, poor healing process is expected.

3.3. Postauricular surgical technique

The incision is made 3 mm posterior to the posterior auricular fold and carried to the mastoid fascia (**Figure 9**). Dissection is continued above the mastoid fascia to the external auditory canal which is then transected to retract the pinna anteriorly. Dissection through the superficial layer of temporalis fascia is carried out to the zygomatic arch, and the periosteum is sharply incised to expose the joint. There is no need to suture the cartilage after the surgery, and closing the skin of the ear is enough.

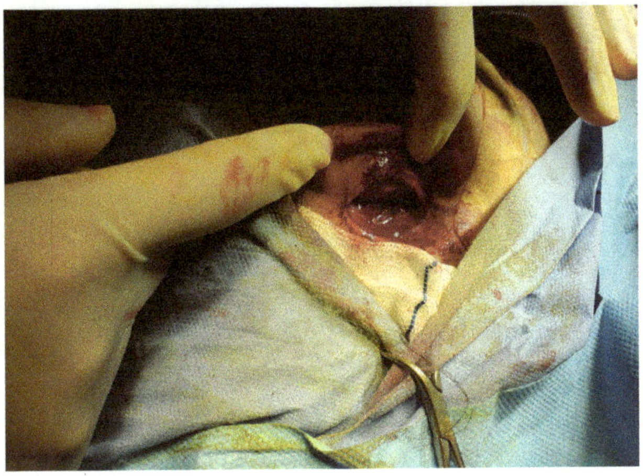

Figure 9. The incision pattern of postauricular approach (Courtesy of Dr. F. Pourdanesh).

3.3.1. Indications

Exposing the entire joint is the main indication of this technique. This approach is also indicated in the patients with the tendency to form keloids who should undergo TMJ surgery.

3.3.2. Advantages

The resulting scar is not very noticeable, and an excellent exposure to the TMJ is provided by this method.

3.3.3. Disadvantages

Auricular stenosis is the main disadvantage of this procedure. External otitis and infection of the TMJ are the contraindications of this approach.

3.4. Submandibular surgical technique

To provide the safety zone of marginal mandibular nerve, the incision is made 2 cm below the inferior border of the mandible (**Figure 10**). The sharp incision is made through the skin and subcutaneous tissue. Then, the platysma is sharply incised to expose the superficial layer of deep cervical fascia. The fascia is incised at the level of the skin incision. The facial artery and vein are retracted or ligated. According to the Hayes-Martin maneuver, ligation and upward retraction of facial vessels protect the marginal mandibular nerve from injury [9]. The dissection is carried to the pterygomasseteric sling. The sling is sharply incised by the blade, and the inferior border of the mandible is exposed (**Figure 11**).

3.4.1. Indications

This approach is usually used for mandibular angle and body fractures and sometimes for low subcondylar factures.

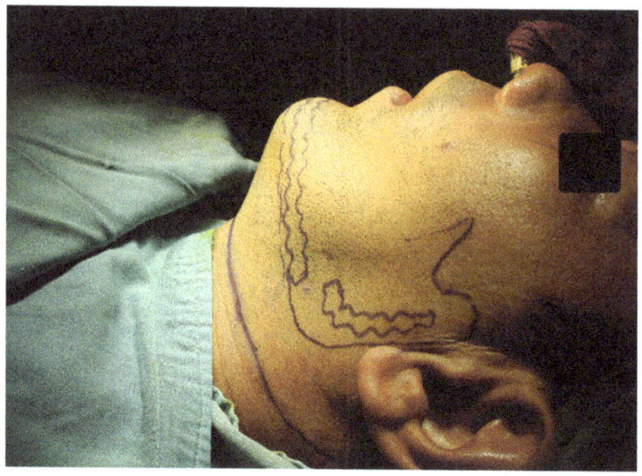

Figure 10. Outline of lateral ramus and submandibular incision. The distance from the inferior border of mandible to the incision should be about 2 cm.

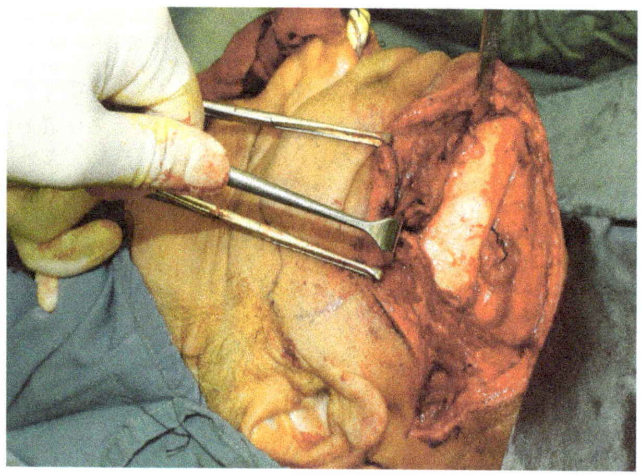

Figure 11. Exposure of mandibular angle, body, and lateral ramus area by submandibular approach.

3.4.2. Advantages

The advantage of this technique is the ability to retract the mandibular angle when the surgeon attempts to reduct the condylar fracture. Also, this method provides good accessibility for anchor screw fixation technique of mandibular subcondyle fractures.

3.4.3. Disadvantages

There is limited access to the high condylar portion and joint spaces.

3.5. Retromandibular surgical technique

The incision is made along the posterior border of mandible 5 mm below the earlobe inferiorly for a distance of about 3 cm. Incision is continued through the skin, subcutaneous tissue, platysma, and superficial musculoaponeuretic system (SMAS). The SMAS layer is undermined, and blunt dissection is continued to the substance of the parotid. The dissection is carried to the periosteum of the posterior border of the mandible. The periosteum is sharply incised, and the access to the lower portion of condylar process is provided.

3.5.1. Indications

This technique is used for internal rigid fixation of low condylar fracture. This approach is also used for fixation of costochondral graft in TMJ region.

3.5.2. Advantages

Good accessibility to the lower portion of condylar fracture and subcondylar area is the main advantage of retromandibular approach. A less noticeable scar in comparison with the submandibular technique is the other advantage of this approach.

3.5.3. Disadvantages

A more visible scar than preauricular incision is the disadvantage of this technique. The access to the joint spaces and anteromedially displaced condyle is limited in this surgical method.

3.6. Rhytidectomy surgical technique

The incision is made in preauricular area and in the neck hairline (**Figure 12**). The skin and subcutaneous tissue are incised, and dissection is carried above the level of SMAS (**Figure 13**).

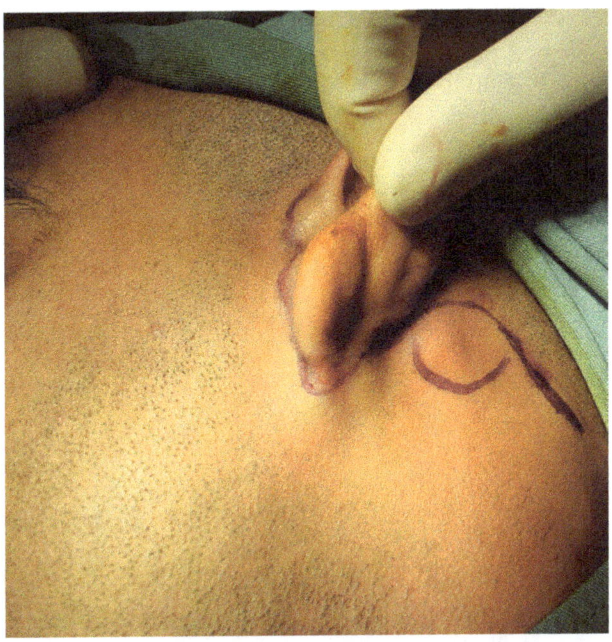

Figure 12. Outline of incision for rhytidectomy approach is combined of preauricular incision and an incision in neck hairline.

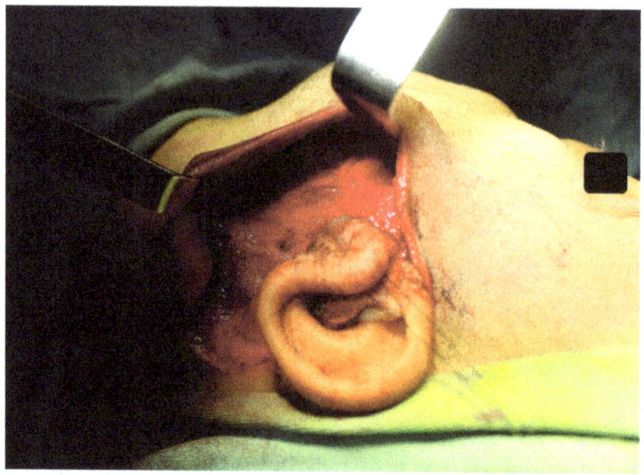

Figure 13. After incising the skin and subcutaneous tissue for rhytidectomy approach, dissection is continued over the SMAS.

A vertical incision is made through the SMAS onto the parotid gland, extending from just below the ear lobe toward the gonial angle. Blunt dissection through the substance of parotid is continued to the posterior border of the mandible. The periosteum is sharply incised, and the entire mandibular ramus is exposed (**Figure 14**).

3.6.1. Indications

This approach is indicated when the accessibility to the lower portion of TMJ is needed similar to the retromandibular technique although its cosmetic results are much beter than the latter technique.

3.6.2. Advantages

Good cosmetic results of the scar and enough access to the condylar process are the most important advantages.

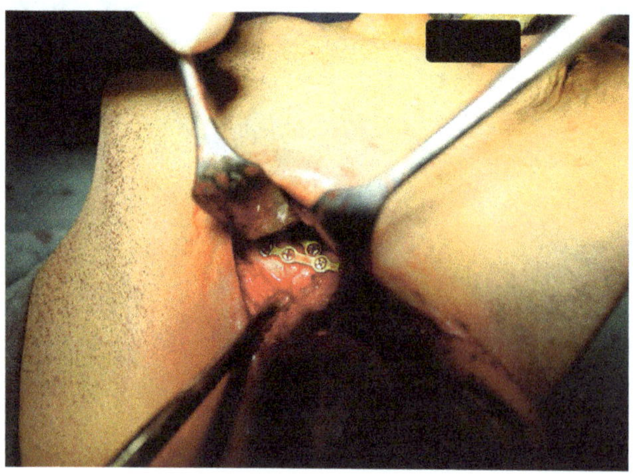

Figure 14. Exposure of condylar neck fracture by rhytidectomy approach. The fracture was reduced and fixed by two miniplates.

3.6.3. Disadvantages

Damage to the branches of facial nerve is the most important disaster that could happen in this method.

3.7. Intraoral approach surgical technique

Incision is made in an external oblique ridge area. Subperiosteal dissection is carried out over the mandibular ramus (**Figure 15**).

3.7.1. Indications

Reduction and fixation of subcondyle fracture are two usual indications of intraoral approach. This method is also used sometimes for condylectomy [10].

3.7.2. Advantages

Invisible scar and preventing from facial nerve damage are the benefits of current approach.

3.7.3. Disadvantages

Limited access to the TMJ is the main problem during this surgical method.

3.8. Endoscopic approach surgical technique

Subperiosteal dissection is performed following the incision of posterior mandibular buccal sulcus. A percutaneous incision is then made perpendicular to the mandibular condyle just to pass the endoscope. Further dissection is then carried under direct vision provided by the endoscope.

3.8.1. Indications

Mandibular condyle fractures are the main indications of this approach.

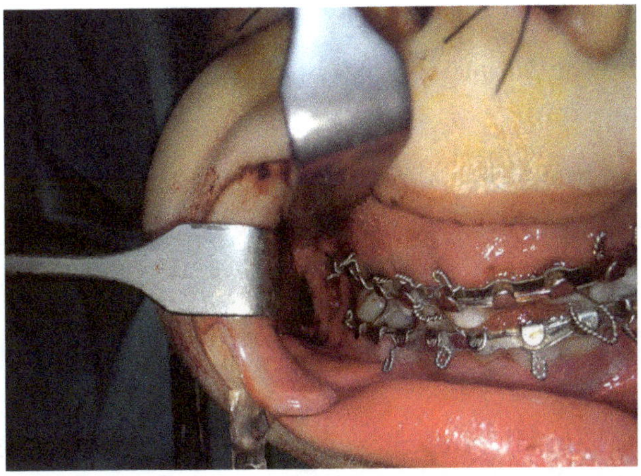

Figure 15. Intraoral approach to manage mandibular subcondyle fracture in a 9-year-old boy.

3.8.2. Advantages

This method is minimally invasive with invisible scars. The possibility of nerve damage during this technique is very low [11].

3.8.3. Disadvantages

Increasing the operation time is a disadvantage of endoscopic technique [12].

4. Conclusion

Deciding on choosing a unique surgical technique for the treatment of all pathologies and diseases of the TMJ is impossible. It is important to understand the pros and cons of all available procedures and choose the best approach with most benefits which provides the best access to the TMJ.

Acknowledgements

We would like to thank Hossein Esmaeelinejad for providing the illustrations of the chapter.

Conflict of interest

The authors declare that they have no conflict of interest.

Author details

Mohammad Esmaeelinejad[1*] and Maryam Sohrabi[2]

*Address all correspondence to: esmaeelnejad@gmail.com

1 Department of Oral and Maxillofacial Surgery, School of Dentistry, Semnan University of Medical Sciences, Semnan, Iran

2 Department of Oral and Maxillofacial Surgery, School of Dentistry, Azad University of Medical Sciences, Tehran, Iran

References

[1] Yang HM, Won SY, Kim HJ, Hu KS. Neurovascular structures of the mandibular angle and condyle: a comprehensive anatomical review. Surgical and Radiologic Anatomy: SRA. 2015;**37**:1109-1118

[2] Al-Kayat A, Bramley P. A modified pre-auricular approach to the temporomandibular joint and malar arch. The British Journal of Oral Surgery. 1979;**17**:91-103

[3] Saylam C, Ucerler H, Orhan M, Ozek C. Anatomic guides to precisely localize the zygomatic branches of the facial nerve. The Journal of Craniofacial Surgery. 2006;**17**:50-53

[4] de Bonnecaze G, Chaput B, Filleron T, Al Hawat A, Vergez S, Chaynes P. The frontal branch of the facial nerve: can we define a safety zone? Surgical and radiologic anatomy: SRA. 2015;**37**:499-506

[5] Pourdanesh F, Esmaeelinejad M, Jafari SM, Nematollahi Z. Facelift: Current Concepts, Techniques, and Principles. In: A Textbook of Advanced Oral and Maxillofacial Surgery Volume 3. InTech; 2016

[6] Saylam C, Ucerler H, Orhan M, Uckan A, Ozek C. Localization of the marginal mandibular branch of the facial nerve. Journal of Craniofacial Surgery. 2007;**18**:137-142

[7] Jayavelu P, Riaz R, Tariq Salam AR, Saravanan B, Karthick R. Difficulties encountered in preauricular approach over retromandibular approach in condylar fracture. Journal of Pharmacy & Bioallied Sciences. 2016;**8**:S175-S1s8

[8] Santos GS, Nogueira LM, Sonoda CK, de Melo WM. Using endaural approach for temporomandibular joint access. The Journal of Craniofacial Surgery. 2014;**25**:1142-1143

[9] Richards AT. Chapter 14 - Surgical Exposures for the Nerves of the Neck A2 - Tubbs, R. Shane. In: Rizk E, Shoja MM, Loukas M, Barbaro N, Spinner RJ, editors. Nerves and Nerve Injuries. San Diego: Academic Press; 2015. p. 201-213

[10] Li B, Sun H, Zhang L, Wang X. Simple way of facilitating intraoral condylectomy and securing the excised condyle: technical note. The British journal of oral & maxillofacial surgery. 2013;**51**:e305-e306

[11] You HJ, Moon KC, Yoon ES, Lee BI, Park SH. Clinical and radiological outcomes of transoral endoscope-assisted treatment of mandibular condylar fractures. International Journal of Oral and Maxillofacial Surgery. 2016;**45**:284-291

[12] Schmelzeisen R, Cienfuegos-Monroy R, Schon R, Chen CT, Cunningham L Jr, Goldhahn S. Patient benefit from endoscopically assisted fixation of condylar neck fractures--a randomized controlled trial. Journal of oral and maxillofacial surgery : Official Journal of the American Association of Oral and Maxillofacial Surgeons. 2009;**67**:147-158

3

Reconstruction of TMJ with Prosthesis Joint

José Thiers Carneiro Junior, Dênis Pimenta e Souza,
Diogo Souza Ferreira Rubim de Assis,
Paulo Hemerson de Moraes and
Francisco de Sousa Neves Filho

Abstract

Temporomandibular joint (TMJ) and the associated muscles turn possible mandibular movements as a complex engineering appliance that may be affected by signs and symptoms such as pain, including in head and neck areas, abnormal jaw movement and clicking or crepitus sounds, classified as temporomandibular disorders (TMD). Some procedures such as discopexy, eminectomy, or arthroplasties, which we consider conservative, can result in ankylosis, even resorption and joint degeneration, limiting surgical options to treat TMJ. The alloplastic prosthesis becomes an option. Total joint reconstruction using prosthesis becomes the treatment choice during the following conditions: previous surgeries including autogenous grafts fail; presence of arthritic diseases; fibrous or bony ankylosis; tumors involving the TMJ; loss of vertical posterior mandible dimension by other TMJ pathologies; and previous prosthetic joint fail. The use of TMJ prosthesis, when compared to other reconstructive procedures, provides immediate function, reducing the duration of surgery and hospitalization time. Disadvantages of the TMJ prosthesis include high cost, prosthesis failure, functional mandibular movements loss, such as protrusion and laterality, and limited fit of stock prosthesis.

Keywords: temporomandibular joint, customized temporomandibular joint prosthesis, prosthesis, prosthetic reconstruction, temporomandibular disorders

1. Introduction

The temporomandibular joint (TMJ) is responsible for the mandibular movements and consists a set of bones, muscles and ligaments. It is subject to various diseases such as congenital, acquired (traumatic), local and systemic diseases and can lead to signs and symptoms such as pain, including in head and neck areas, abnormal jaw movement and clicking or crepitus sounds, classified as temporomandibular disorders (TMD). The complex etiopathogenesis and the variability of symptoms complicate the adoption of standardized diagnostic and therapeutic approaches, as suggested by the number of treatment modalities that have been proposed, such as occlusal splints, physiotherapy, behavioral and physical treatments, drugs and surgery. A surgical approach to the disorders of the TMJ is reserved to a minority of cases who do not respond to traditional and conservative therapies. For these situations, joint reconstructive surgery becomes necessary [1] with autogenous graft bone or alloplastic joint reconstruction, which is a challenge for the maxillo-facial surgeon. We can use autogenous bone for the reconstruction of TMJ and the preferred donor region would be the costal arch. The costochondral graft rib is obtained with an inframammary incision, where it removes part of the 5th, 6th or 7th rib, with about 3–4 cm bone tissue and 5 mm to 1 cm chondral cartilage. These patients may present some complications such as perforation or pleural laceration, resulting in pneumothorax, hemothorax, infection and chronic pain in the donor area. There is also the disadvantage of not having growth potential of the control of this type of graft, occurring overgrowth with mandibular deviation after a few years [2].

TMJ prostheses do not have many complications such as autografts, what qualifies as an alternative to the joint reconstruction. The prostheses are primarily indicated for [3, 4] the following:

- patients who have undergone multiple surgeries TMJ unsuccessfully
- infections with destruction of the mandibular condyle
- chronic inflammation or pathological resorption of TMJ
- autoimmune diseases and collagen diseases (rheumatoid arthritis, psoriatic arthritis, Sjogren's syndrome, lupus, ankylosing spondylitis)
- TMJ ankylosis
- trauma sequelae with severe functional changes
- congenital deformities (hemifacial microsomia)
- tumors in the TMJ area

The advantages for using the TMJ prosthesis are the reduction of surgical time (because there is no need for donor site), shorter hospital stay and immediate function, there is no need for each-jaw blockade postoperatively. As for the disadvantages we can mention the lack of predictability for a revision surgery, the prosthesis size limit (in the case of prefabricated prosthesis or stock), the loss of translational movement causing loss of laterality and protrusion due to detachment of the pterygoid lateral muscle and the high cost [5].

The following are desired characteristics in a joint prosthesis [6]:

- low level of wear and corrosion of materials
- biocompatibility
- low flow and material fatigue
- adaptability anatomical structures and their functions
- stability of the components
- absence of hypersensitivity to materials
- lightness
- functionality

These features do not stop being researched by companies Materials in order to physiologically rebuild the TMJ. Due to the low clinical longevity of these types of prosthesis, a strict follow-up still is needed, for evaluating the anatomical and functional status of patients undergoing this type of treatment. Regardless of whether the TMJ is reconstructed using alloplastic, allogenic or autogenous materials, the following should be the management goals [1]: (1) to improve mandibular function and form; (2) to reduce suffering and disability; (3) to contain excessive treatment and cost; and (4) to prevent morbidity.

2. History

The surgery for TMJ reconstruction began with Risdon, in 1933, inserting gold foil in the articular fossa in an attempt to prevent ankylosis relapse. Eggers in 1946 positioned one tantalum sheet in the pit on the mandibular head after treatment for ankylosis arthroplasty.

In subsequent years, different types of materials and techniques have been developed to repair the TMJ. The first consideration for the use of alloplastic materials has been for treating fibrous and bony ankylosis. Subsequently, they have also been used in attempts to treat osteoarthritis, disc degeneration and loss of articular severe vertical dimension [7].

The history of aloplásticas prostheses has been characterized by failures due to inappropriate designs, inattention to biomechanical principles and ignorance of the already described in the orthopedic literature. Because TMJ is a ginglymus-artrodial articulation and its function is closely associated with occlusion, ATM prosthesis requires features not seen in a conventional orthopedic prosthesis [5].

Nowadays, TMJ prostheses are designed to minimize these failures, using different materials in such different parts or prosthesis components.

3. Indications of prostheses total TMJ [5, 6, 8–10]

- Ankylosis with excessive heterotopic bone formation
- Revision procedures where other treatments have failed (eg. alloplastic reconstruction with Teflon or silastic and autografts)
- Avascular necrosis
- Joints subjected to several previous unsuccessful attempts
- Fractures with extensive destruction
- Important functional deformities
- Benign neoplasms
- Reconstructions post-malignant tumor excision
- Degenerate or resorbed joints with severe anatomical discrepancies
- Development anomalies
- Inflammatory or resorptive disorders locations (osteoarthrosis)
- Autoimmune diseases (rheumatoid arthritis, psoriatic arthritis, ankylosing spondylitis, systemic lupus erythematosus, Sjogren syndrome, scleroderma)
- Severe chronic pain without clinical and surgical resolution of possibilities
- Severe restriction of mouth opening

TMJ prosthesis has special role in bone ankylosis where surgical outcomes cannot be predicted when using other techniques such as autogenous grafts, leading to heterotopic bone growth [11].

4. Advantages of the TMJ implants [12, 13]

- Functionality immediately after surgery
- Symmetry and occlusal stability
- Simpler surgical technique
- Less morbidity (does not require donor area)

5. Contraindications of the prosthesis TMJ [5, 9, 10, 13]

The following are contraindications to placement of ATM protheses:

- Active or chronic infections.

- Patient conditions in which there is no sufficient bone quality or quantity to support the components.
- Systemic diseases with increased susceptibility to infections.
- Patients with extensive drilling on the glenoid fossa or bone defects in the articular eminence or zygomatic arch that could seriously compromise the support of artificial tank.
- Only partial reconstruction of TMJ.
- Allergic reaction to any material used in the prosthesis. Cr-Co-Mo devices should not be used in patients with sensitivity to nickel, as this is also a component of the material.
- Patients with neurological and mental problems who cannot or refuse to follow optimal postoperative care
- Patients with immature skeleton. Do not use in children.
- Patients with marked hyperfunctional habits (ex. dental clenching).
- Patients with foreign body reaction caused by previous implants.
- Patients with high expectation of decreased pain and improved functional activity complete articular.

There is a technical limitation of custom-made prosthesis model on esterolitografia when the patient has a pre-metal prosthesis, as this would need to be removed by additional surgery before the CT scan in order to avoid artifacts produced.

6. Disadvantages of TMJ prosthesis [13, 14]

- The main disadvantage of prostheses is the TMJ loss of translational movement. However, the new biomechanical concept of placing the pivot point inferior to the center of the natural condyle leads to a better translation mouth opening [15], even in patients unable to perform natural protrusive movements. This concept further enhances the mandibular function and would prevent overloads on the natural TMJ contralateral side unilateral prosthesis (**Figure 1**) [16].
- High cost, although the decrease in associated costs, with shorter hospital stay and faster recovery of the patient [13].
- Doubt as the durability of the prosthesis and its possible shortcomings, because among all models of prostheses known there is no giving this predictability. There is much attention as the fixation of the prosthesis to the remaining bone, because over time some screws used to attach can lose efficiency which would lead loss adjustment and lack of component stability [5, 17, 18].

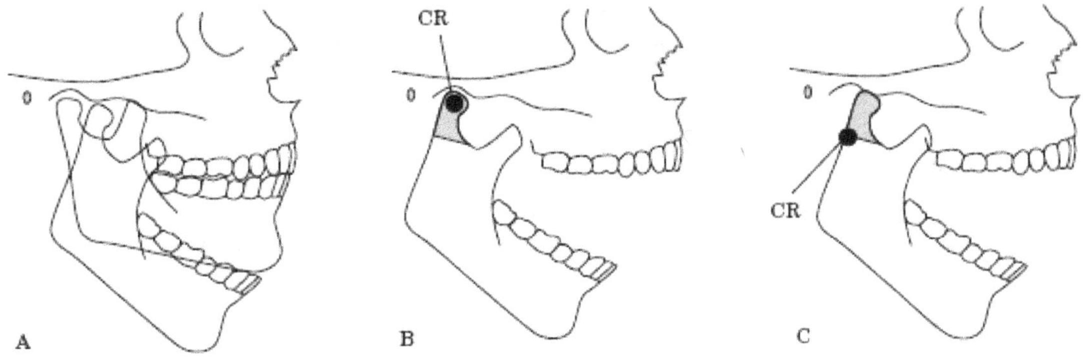

Figure 1. Center of rotation of modern TMJ prosthesis according to concepts of Falkestron (1993). (A) Normal mouth opening; (B) opening mouth rotation center located in the area of the condyle; (C) opening mouth rotation center located 15 mm below the condylar center, imitating the condylar translation [16].

7. Considerations as prothetic TMJ

The success and longevity of the TMJ alloplastic reconstruction are directly attributable to the stability of the prosthesis deployment location, biocompatibility, design, resistance to loads during function over time and correct and aseptic surgical technique [12, 18, 19].

Although the customized prosthesis is considered optimal, the accuracy of computed tomography (CT) used to make the model of the TMJ is of the order of 0.5 mm, resulting in a close fit of the prosthesis. It should also be still considered the dose of radiation while performing the CT scan, the high cost in the manufacture of three-dimensional prototype and the individual adjustment of this type of prosthesis that can consume more time [14].

The stock prosthetics require large number of different anatomical forms because of individual variability of bone structures shapes, mainly for the component of the glenoid fossa. This may hinder a little fit of the prosthesis and choosing the best component [14].

The prostheses of W. Lorenz™ and TMJ™ concepts have similar concepts, but different designs. The materials used in the two prostheses are nowadays the gold standard in orthopedic joint deployment with respect to wear resistance properties and structural stability, showing be reliable materials in prosthetic reconstructions [20, 21].

A major difficulty is knowing the best time to use a denture TMJ, and reconstruction with prosthetic joint should be considered as the final surgical stage and not be used for minor problems [18].

Autogenous grafts have shown better results than the aloplásticas aids in TMJ reconstructions for some authors. This does not mean that autologous grafts and flaps are exempt from complications and sequelae, but these are less frequent and more recoverable than those caused by dentures [22]. On the other hand, it is known that autografts (costochondral, sternoclavicular, myofascial temporal, ear cartilage, dermis or vertical osteotomy of mandibular branch) are used for TMJ reconstruction in similar conditions to the use of hearing aids, which may occur also adverse response and possible failures in its use. There are known factors that contribute to the failure of dentures TMJ, as stated earlier, and success depends on an attempt to minimize these factors [6].

7.1. Stock prostheses

The stock prosthesis, compared to the customized one, requires less time for preoperative preparation. However the disadvantages is need a surgeon with experience because the anatomical variations still a challenge to the prostheses stability. Also the Stock prostheses is not appropriate for some patients with extensive tumors or severe deformities, intraoperative time consume to prepare the mandibular the fossa and mandibular ramus fit with the prosthesis. In contrast, the custom-made prosthesis is more expensive, but it is highly accurate, and it is also considered the prosthesis of choice in patients with major TMJ and mandibular defects [23, 24].

Some stock prostheses are relatively complex and unsuitable with fit and shape. The eminence area irregularities and the fossa bottom with complex depressions result in the instability of the prostheses. Surgeons must take care when removing irregularities by a bone bur and then place the fossa component directly because they got to preserve enough bone to retain the screws on zygomatic arch [24].

The latest inventory prostheses (W. Lorenz™) used nowadays have two components: a condylar composed of cobalt-chromium-molybdenum alloy (Cr-Co-Mo) and titanium alloy coating (Ti-6Al-4V), and a component of the composite cavity of ultra–high molecular weight polyethylene (PUAPM) (**Figure 2**). It also presents evidence of fixtures, with the compound condyle Aluminum and Radel™ plastic tank. Both components are available in various sizes as well as in specific designs for the right and left sides, being fixed to bone by titanium screws [9–21].

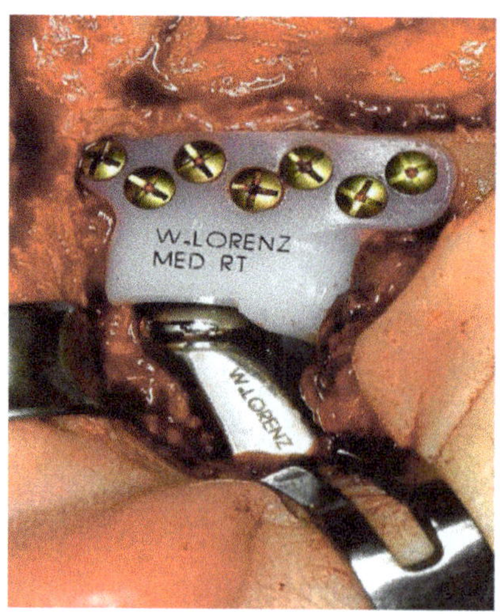

Figure 2. Installed stock prosthesis W. Lorenz. The metallic component of condylar articulating against PUAPM pit fixed with titanium screws is observed [21].

The fossa PUAPM has a minimum of 4 mm thickness in the central region and has a cavity with larger walls to protect the condyle of the heterotopic bone invasion and to prevent its displacement or dislocation. The neck condylar appears as swan neck, avoiding the obstruction problem at the implant-bone interface inherent to the drawing at right angles other condylar prosthesis and is based on the innovation of Falkestrom and Van Loon designs with rotation point lower than that of natural TMJs, resulting in an imitation of translational movement when the mouth opening, which results in 15% interincisal aperture gain [1–21].

The system does not replace normal healthy bone, and chronic pain can continue to exist even after the placement of the prosthesis. The system can also loosen or break due to stress, activity or trauma. The presence of mandibular screws or prior zygomatic arch placement or pre-existing holes may compromise the fixation. Placing the unilateral prosthesis can result in detrimental effects on the contralateral joint. It should also be noted that there may be occlusal changes over time after installation of the prosthesis [9, 10].

The following are cited as adverse effects that may occur after placement of the prosthesis [9, 10]:

1. removal components due to changes caused by overloading or wearing, degenerative changes in the joint surfaces arising from disease or prior implants and corrosion or produce particles of implant material
2. loosening or displacement with or without removal of the implant
3. systemic or superficial infection
4. allergic reaction or foreign body implant components
5. wear fossa
6. edema or facial pain
7. dysfunction of the facial nerve
8. tissue excision
9. heterotopic bone formation
10. training neuroma
11. problems headset
12. dislocation of the prosthesis

The maximum inter-incisor opening ranges from 24.9 mm in the first postoperative month moving up to 36 mm [25], for the second postoperative year, on average, in monitored patients. They are recommended post-surgical care and local measures (surgical wound care and physical therapy), proper diet and medication as well as regular visits to follow-up. The technical scheme of placement of TMJ prostheses can be seen in sequence in **Figure 3** [9, 10].

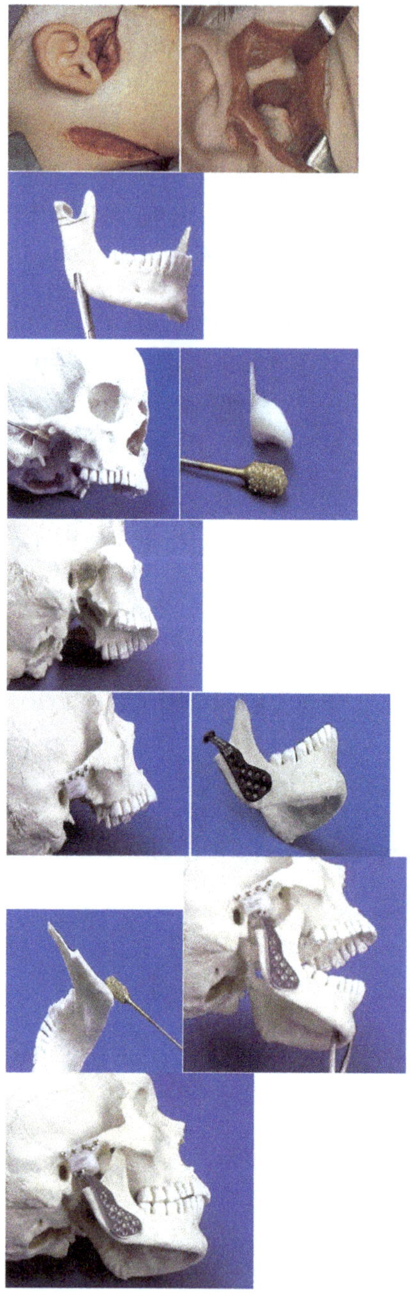

Figure 3. Scheme of surgery and placement of the prosthesis W. Lorenz [9, 10].

The surgical technique for this type of procedure follows the sequence described [25]:

- naso-tracheal intubation directly or assisted by video
- local anesthetic infiltration with vasoconstrictor in pre-auricular region
- pre-auricular incision and dilatation of the tissues in layers
- osteotomy for the removal of the head of ankylosed jaw or mass (in the case of TMJ ankylosis) and realization of the ceiling planing of joint cavity with surgical drills and bone files to adapt the temporal feedback

- feedback fixing the pit/articular eminence with titanium screws, checking the stability and parallel to the zygomatic arch
- conducting submandibular incision (Risdon) with dilatation of the tissue plans for communicating the two surgical approaches
- blocking of patients using screws trans-gingival maxillo-mandibular intercuspidation during surgery not exist occlusal changes
- the condylar component is fixed and the lock to open maxilomandibular mobility check
- if the patient presents the restriction opening movement is carried out a second osteotomy, the coronoidectomy in order to eliminate interference with movement
- the time template is then replaced by the prosthetic fossa component
- sutures were made by planes of the two accesses with vicryl and nylon 5.0 yarn type and curative were kept locally for 48 h
- conducting physiotherapy with isometric exercises and occlusal rehabilitation

7.2. Customized temporomandibular joint prosthesis

Most patients presenting with indications for total TMJ alloplastic reconstruction have distorted anatomy caused by either numerous failed prior surgical interventions/materials or primary or secondary joint disease that compounds the stability problems in the TMJ area. This finding makes it extremely difficult to reconstruct these cases with an off-the-shelf or so-called "stock" device [26]. More recently, with the advent of CT scans with three-dimensional reconstruction (3D-CT) and esterolitografia, it was possible the manufacture of ATM-individualized dentures. This prosthesis (Bioconect Temporomandibular prosthesis design and principles and materials) uses a powerful 3D printing technology to shape the desired metal geometry by melting metal powder layer by layer. The metal used in the creation of the customized implant (temporomandibular joint) is Titanium Ti – 6% Al – 4%, wt% (Ti64 degree 23) with a low oxygen content. An ideal combination is achieved by having a biocompatible metal, titanium, designed at any desired geometric shape for a perfect customized fit. With the advances in heath technology, the work of the Direct Metal Laser Sintering (DMLS) has allowed treatment of clinical cases that were previously practically impossible to treat due to their complexity. With the use of the DMLS technology, the use of various materials and a high range of complexity on the customizations, reduced manufacture time is possible [27].

The fossa component is constructed from two basic materials – Ti64 degree 23 and ultra–high molecular weight polyethylene (UHMWPE). The UHMWPE have a relatively flat functional surface and had a posterior stop to provide a centric relation position for the condylar head of the prosthesis. The customized surgical guides are used specifically for each planning and cutting rails specific to each type of drill, saw or ultrasonic nozzle. Thus, it allows the surgeon to accurately replicate the trans-surgical what was accomplished in planning (**Figure 4**), while other prostheses that are made using plastic prototypes and conventional machining (computer numerical control, CNC) do not allow this essential advantage, thereby causing poor adaptations and failures.

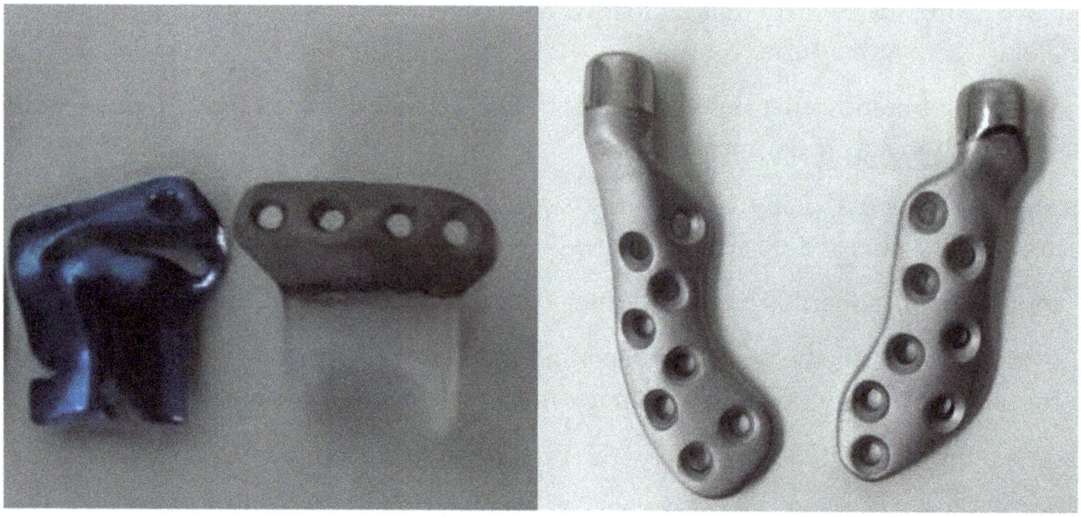

Figure 4. Customized cutting guide; fossa component; mandibular component.

8. Discussion

Treatment with denture TMJ is still a matter of controversy. It is evident that a variety of etiologies and different treatments may be used in the reconstruction, as autogenous and alloplastic grafts, with the indication of TMJ prosthesis based on the surgeon's experience and results described in the literature [5, 6, 8–22, 28].

Previous surgery can be tried, but some patients do not respond satisfactorily to the prosthesis, being an excellent alternative for resolving these cases. One should be aware that the TMJ prosthesis is the final stage in joint reconstruction and should be proposed only for cases where there is no evidence for the possibility of other techniques [16, 29].

The occlusal stability has lead to placement and longevity of the prosthesis. Changes of the occlusal plane, the Z-axis (lateral-lateral), II severe classes, spee curve inversions, overbites or accentuated overjet and multiple missing teeth could compromise the lock stability in trans-operative and post-operative functional balance, causing occlusal and adapting prosthesis overloads, interfering in the right condyle-fossa relationship, which on the long run could interfere with the functional outcome [5, 25].

The commitment of mandibular movements is extremely variable and dependent on the etiology and clinical condition presented. Patients with ankylosis have greater functional impairment mainly due to their severe functional limitation. Also in these patients, both placed prostheses—unilateral and bilateral form—best functional gains are achieved. In cases of patients with idiopathic resorption, trauma sequels and arthrosis of TMJ, the gains are more related to the stability of movement and decrease in symptoms such as headaches, muscle fatigue and local pain [25].

In some cases, there is loss of movement quality, especially the translation of Caused by damage of the lateral pterygoid muscle that was detachment of the site [15, 16]. Furthermore, adaptation and gradient component with respect to the condylar fossa prosthesis cause greater amplitude during translational motion, thereby reducing the limitation of movement that occurred earlier. Note that the maximum opening and also the best efficiency of this type of prosthesis can be achieved by performing coronoidectomy, enabling the mouth opening without interference [5]. Even with the modifications proposed in the most modern prostheses, there are still significant functional loss and functional movement restriction and in particular lateral protrusion, which cannot be measured, and in most cases, values above 6 and 6 mm respectively. In older cases, where the prostheses have not had the spin axis changes, the conditions of laterality and protrusion were even more restricted [16].

Symptomatic conditions such as headaches, muscle fatigue, local pain, swelling and asymmetries can be improved after placement of the prosthesis. However, for all cases there will be some degree of limitation of the excursion of mandible head compared to a normal ATM. Also note that the prosthetic condyle-sump movement occurs across length and the surface thereof, so there is a certain rotation and translation that in cases of Of patients with bony ankylosis can be improved after surgery, since they have no moving none or very limited pre operatively [25].

The movement of the prosthesis occurs because of one's jaw movement, Realized other muscle muscle groups, supra-hyoid, contralateral mandibular elevators, temporal, masseter and medial pterygoid (which keeps some degree functional even after detachment for prosthetic installation). The ability of functional adaptation of the jaw is a decisive factor in the prosthesis-jaw system [5, 11].

Dislocations of the metal component of the polyethylene tank, fixing losses of the prosthesis system to fracture and locoregional bone formation could occur, but there are frequent complications. Some case reports of these complication It has been caused to failure of the surgical technique, both the component adjustment, in osteotomies and wear bone, the choice of location of bone resection, the lack of stability of the components and their attachment to the bone and also in Setup component in improper angles [5, 6, 8–25, 30].

A good surgical technique combined with postoperative physiotherapy and functional with adequate maintenance, proper fixation and favorable angle means that there is clinical success [25]. Modern custom-made prostheses have a pit format that allows great adaptation to the temporal bone and are placed parallel to the zygomatic arch Restricting several movements. The component thickness is a decisive factor that hinders exaggerated bone formations and local ankylosis [21].

The behavior of the TMJ contralateral to the prosthesis, in cases of execution of unilateral prosthesis, requires particular attention, because the functional balance achieved in short time is great, but the behavior of the anatomical structures is somewhat uncertain way, and condylar resorption, disc dislocations, muscle aches, some functional restriction by anatomical limitation of the contra-lateral prosthesis, chewing functional changes, periodontal and progressive joint degeneration may occur [25].

9. Conclusion

In conclusion, the TMJ prostheses have the reconstruction order to articulate and fulfill this role satisfactorily. Due to developments over time, Their biomechanical principles and biocompatibility have made TMJ prostheses reliable and a safe alternative for the reconstruction of the joint. Long-term studies are needed, because clinical longevity of patients undergoing this type of prosthesis is still less [5, 12–25, 30].

10. Case report of alloplastic temporomandibular joint W. Lorenz

Case report orthognatic with alloplastic temporomandibular joint W. Lorenz.

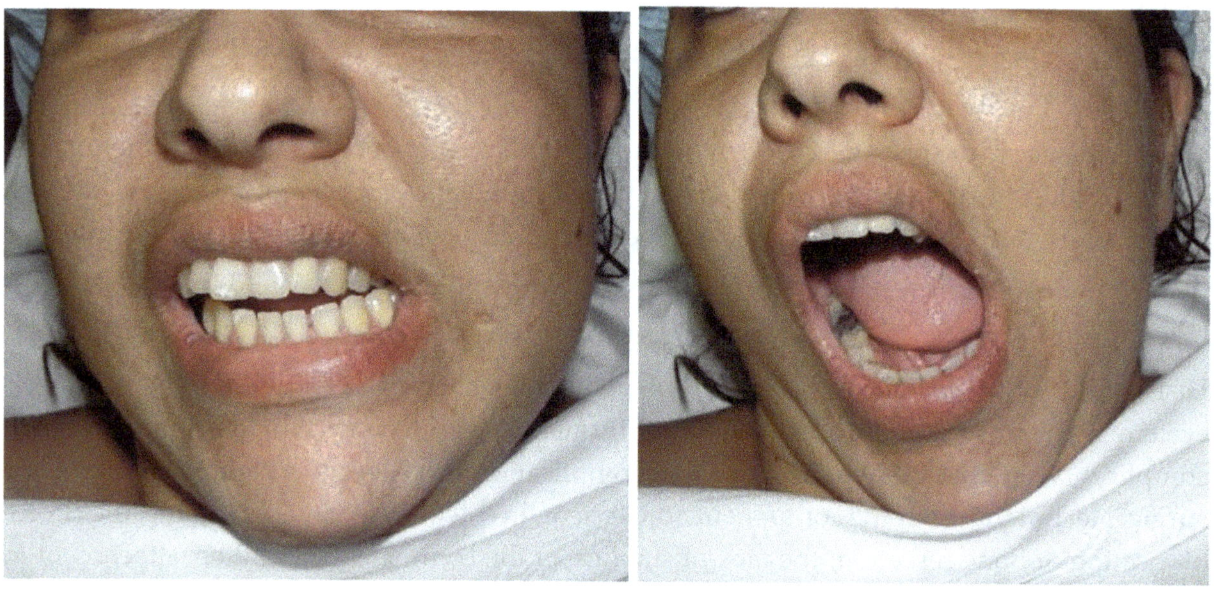

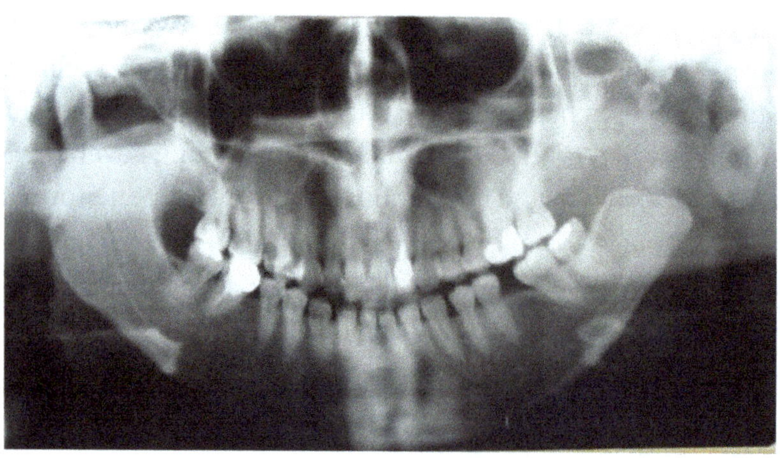

Patient with mandibular defect after remove Aneurysmal bone cyst deviation of the mandible.

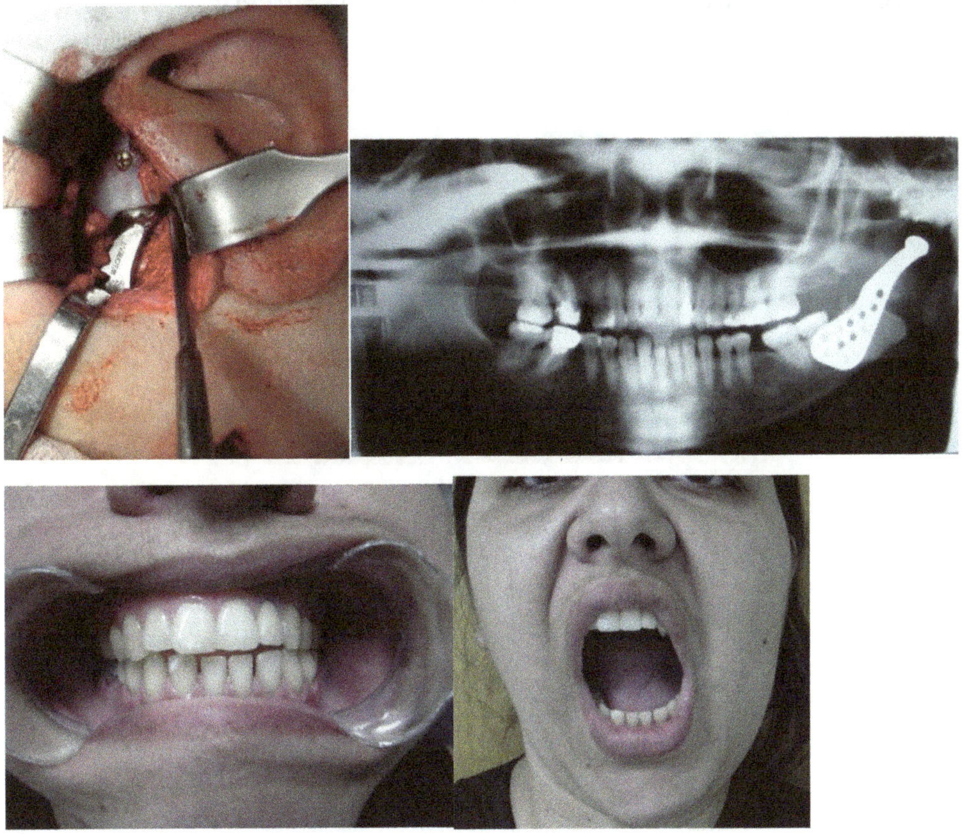

Provide adequate stability of occlusal bite. Decrease the deviation of the mandible.

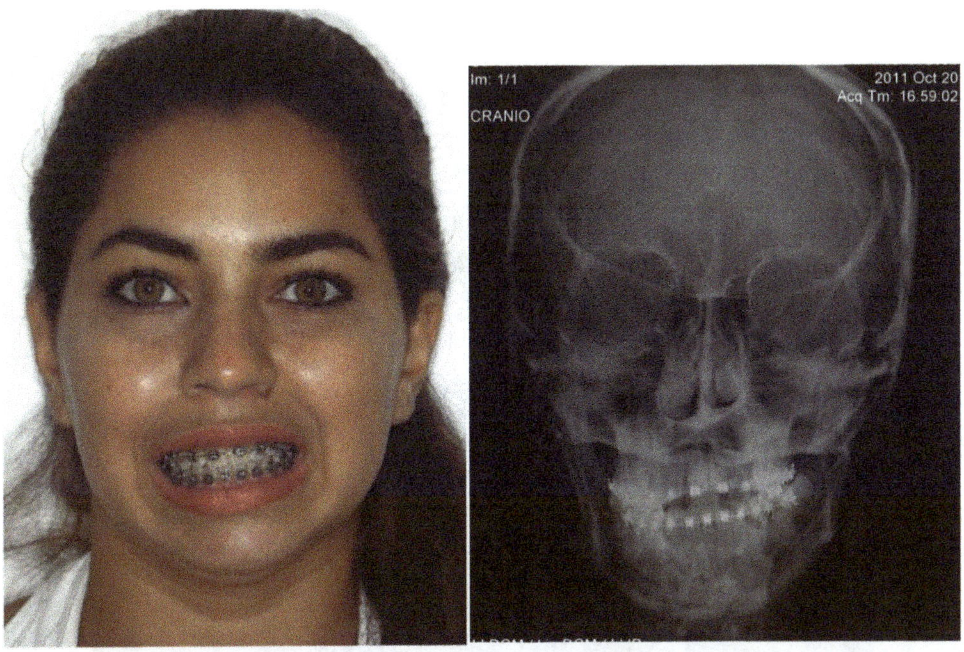

Patient with condylar resorption after trauma Occlusal plane alteration facial symmetry occlusal relationship before treatment.

Concomitant Temporomandibular Joint and Orthognathic Surgery.

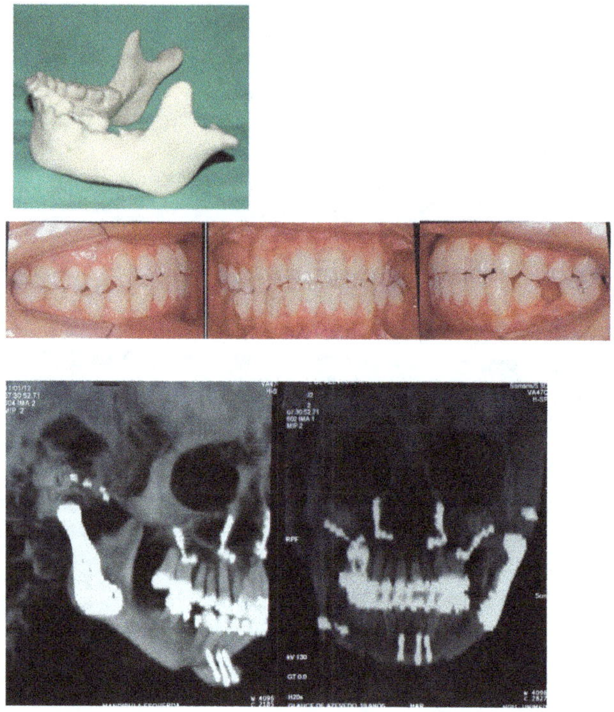

Correction of Facial Asymmetry and occlusal bite.

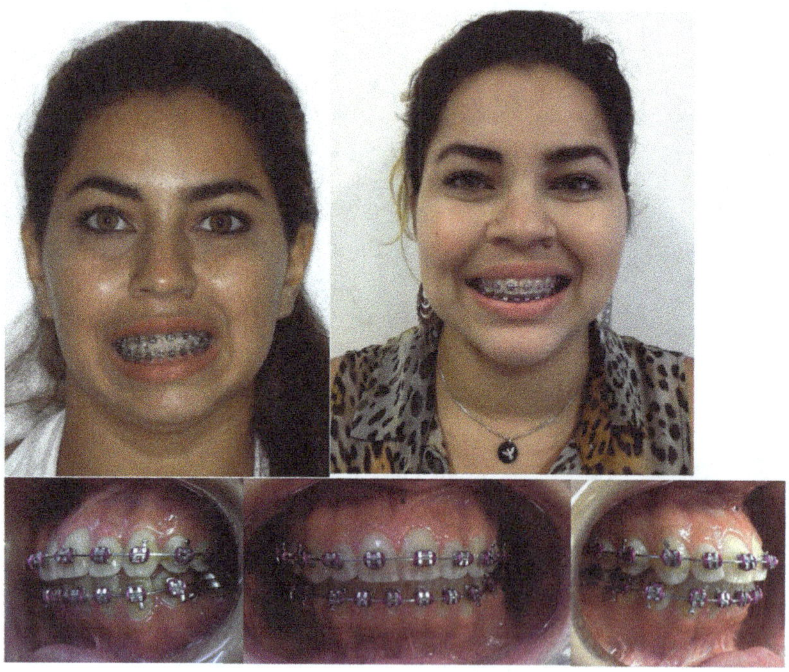

Author details

José Thiers Carneiro Junior[1*], Dênis Pimenta e Souza[2], Diogo Souza Ferreira Rubim de Assis[3], Paulo Hemerson de Moraes[4] and Francisco de Sousa Neves Filho[1]

*Address all correspondence to: jthiers53@uol.com.br

1 Federal University of Pará (UFPA), Belém, Brazil

2 University of São Paulo (USP), São Paulo, Brazil

3 Federal University of Maranhão (UFMA), Brazil

4 University of Campinas (UNICAM), Brazil

References

[1] Guarda-Nardini L, Manfredini D, Berrone S, Ferronato G. Total temporomandibular joint prosthesis as a surgical option for severe mouth opening restriction. A case report of a bilateral intervention. Reumatismo 2007;59: 322–7.

[2] Politis C, Fossion E, Bossuyt M. The use of costochondral grafts in arthroplasty of the temporomandibular joint. J Cranio Maxillofac Surg 1987;15(6):345-54.

[3] Kieh CL, DesPrez JD, Converse CF. Total prothetic replacement of the temporomandibular joint. Ann Plast Surg 1979;(2):5-15.

[4] Ko EWC, Huang CS, Chen YR. Temporomandibular joint reconstruction in children using costochondral grafts. J Oral Maxillofac Surg 1999;57(7):789-98; discussion 799-800.

[5] Quinn P. Alloplastic reconstruction of the Temporomandibular Joint. In: Fonseca RJ. Oral and Maxillofacial Surgery: Temporomandibular Disorders, Philadelphia: WB Saunders Company; 2000. cap.17, p. 316-32.

[6] Wolford LM, Pitta MC, Reichel-Fischel O, Franco PF. TMJ concepts/techmedica custom made TMJ total prothesis: 5-year follow-up study. Int J Oral Maxillofac Surg 2003;32:268-74.

[7] Morgan DH. Development of alloplastic materials for temporomandibular joint prothesis: a historical perspective with clinical illustration. Cranio 1992;10(3):192-204

[8] Saeed NR, Hensher R, McLeod NMH, Kent JN. Reconstruction of the temporomandibular joint autogenous compared with alloplastic. Br J Oral Maxillofac Surg 2002;(40): 296-9.

[9] W. Lorenz Surgical. Total TMJ replacement system patient information. Jacksonville: W Lorenz; 2005. Folheto informative

[10] W. Lorenz Surgical. Total TMJ replacement system interactive Cd-Rom. Dordrecht: W.Lorenz Surgical; 2005.

[11] Guven O. Treatment of temporomandibular joint ankylosis by modified fossa prosthesis. J Craniomaxillofac Surg 2004;(32):236–42.

[12] Adame CG. Temporomandibular reconstruction : alloplastic prostheses. Rev Esp Cir Oral Maxillofacial 2005;27(1):7–14.

[13] Mercuri LG, Use of alloplastic protheses for TMJ reconstruction. J.Oral Maxillofac Surg 2000;(58):70-5.

[14] Van Loon JP, DeBont LGM, Boering G. Evaluation of Temporomandibular joint prostheses: review of the literature from 1946 to 1994 and implications for future prothesis designs. J Oral Maxillofac Surg 1995;53:984-96.

[15] Falkestrom CH. Biomechanical design of total temporomandibular joint replacement [thesis]. University of Groningen; 1993.

[16] Van Loon JP, De Bont LGM, Stegenga B, Spijkervet FKL, Verkerke GJ. Groningen Temporomandibular joint prosthesis. Development and first clinical application. Int J Oral Maxillofac Surg. 2002;31:44-52.

[17] Wolford LM. Temporomandibular joint devices: treatment factors and outcomes. Oral Surg Oral Med Oral Pathol Oral Radiol Endod 1997;83:143-9.

[18] Wolford LM. Factors to consider in joint prothesis systems. Proc (Bayl Univ Med Cent). 2006;19(3):232-8

[19] Mercuri LG, Wolford LM, Sanders B, White RD, Giobbie-Hurder A. Long-term follow-up of the CAD/CAM patient fitted total temporomandibular joint reconstruction system. J Oral Maxillofac Surg 2002;(60):1440-8.

[20] Curry JT, Alexander R. Comparison of 2 temporomandibular joint total joint prosthesis systems. J Oral Maxillofac Surg 2004;62(2):261.

[21] Westermark A, Koppel D, Leiggener C. Condylar replacement alone is not sufficient for prosthetic reconstruction of the temporomandibular joint. Int J Oral Maxillofac Surg 2006;35:488-92.

[22] Gonzalez GR. Temporomandibular reconstruction :autologous graft. Rev Esp Cir Oral Maxillofac 2005;27(1):15–28.

[23] Westermark A, Heden P, Aagaard E, Cornelius CP. The use of TMJ concepts prostheses to reconstruct patients with major temporomandibular joint and mandibular defects. Int J Oral Maxillofac Surg 2011;40:487–496.

[24] ShanYong Z, Liu H, Yang C, Zhang X, Abdelrehem A, Zheng J, Jiao Z, Chen M, Qiu Y. Modified surgical techniques for total alloplastic temporomandibular joint replacement: One institution's experience. J Cranio-Maxillo-Facial Surg 2015;43:934–939.

[25] Souza DP, Temprano AB, Shinohara EH, Lobo LF, Falchet PF. Clinical evaluation of patients with total temporomandibular joint replacement. Rev Esp Cir Oral Maxilofac. 2013;35(3):107–115.

[26] De Moraes PH; Pozzer L, Olate S, Sato FRL, Moreira RWF. TMJ total joint prosthesis for condylar fracture malunion. Int J Odontostomat,2012;6(2):241–244

[27] De Moraes PH, Olate S, Cantin M, Assis AF, Santos E, Silva FO, Silva LO. Anatomical reproducibility through 3D printing in cranio-maxillo-facial defects. Int J Morphol, 2015;33(3):826–830

[28] Capote A, Rodriguez-Campo FJ, Escorial V, Munoz-Guerra M. Total tempomandibular joint reconstruction with alloplastic prothesis. Review our experience. J Cranio Maxillofac Surg 2006;34(6 Suppl):S1.

[29] Mercuri LG, Anspach, WE. Principles for the revision of failed TMJ protheses. Int J Oral Maxillofac Surg 2003;(32):353–9.

[30] Wolford LM., Dingwerth DJ, Talwar RM., Pitta MC. Comparison of 2 temporomandibular joint total joint prothesis systems. J Oral Maxillofac Surg 2003a;61:685–90.

4

Benign Tumors of Temporomandibular Joint

Mehmet Emre Yurttutan,
Ayşegül Tüzüner Öncül and Hakan Alpay Karasu

Abstract

The temporomandibular joint (TMJ) forms a complex functional system with teeth, bones, connected muscles and ligaments. Any discomfort in any of these structures directly affects the joint. The complaints are mostly pain, malocclusion and swelling. Temporomandibular joint tumors are very uncommon but show symptoms similar to intra-articular disorders that make up most of these disorders. The most common TMJ-specific benign tumors are classified after a brief literature review. Our classification also includes the osteoma of the TMJ, other than World Health Organization's (WHO) classification of soft tissue and bone tumors. This benign tumor was also included in the classification because of its higher frequency in the literature. The treatment of these neoplasms may be conservative or radical surgery.

Keywords: cartilage tumors, temporomandibular joint tumors, cartilage tumors, osteogenic tumors, osteochondroma, chondroma, chondroblastoma, pigmented villonodular synovitis, synovial chondromatosis, osteoma, juxta-articular myxoma

1. Introduction

Primary neoplasms of the bones are rare, amounting to only 0.2% of the overall human tumor. Primary neoplasms originating in the temporomandibular joint (TMJ) are extremely rare. Their clinical manifestations are usually related to the temporomandibular dysfunction (TMD) and include pre-auricular swelling, pain, trismus, deviation of mandibular movement and malocclusion. Such symptoms should not be neglected and advanced imaging methods should be used with the thought that it may be neoplasia. Also the clinical symptoms and radiological appearance of many tumors are similar. Therefore, the differential diagnosis must be made carefully [1].

TMJ-specific benign tumors		
Bone tumors	1. Cartilage tumors	Osteochondroma
		Chondroma
		Chondroblastoma
		Synovial chondromatosis
	2. Osteogenic tumors	Osteoma
		Osteoid osteoma
		Ostaoblastoma
	3. Giant cell tumors	Giant cell tumor
	4. Vascular tumors	Hemangioma
	5. Lipogenic tumors	Lipoma
	6. Bone-related odontogenic tumors	Ossifying fibroma
Soft tissue tumors	1. Fibrohistiocytic tumors	Pigmented villonodular synovitis
	2. Tumors of uncertain differentiation	Juxta-articular myxoma

Table 1. Benign temporomandibular joint tumors.

Temporomandibular joint consists of bone structures and soft tissues such as temporal bone, mandibular condyle, articular disc, articular capsule and ligaments. The tumors that will be formed in this region will also develop from bone and soft tissue origin.

The most common TMJ-specific benign tumors are classified after a brief literature review. Our classification also includes the osteoma of the TMJ, other than World Health Organization's (WHO) classification of soft tissue and bone tumors [2]. This benign tumor also included in the classification because of its higher frequency in the literature (**Table 1**).

Table 1 represents benign TMJ tumors. These tumors are classified under two section.

2. Cartilage tumors

Tumors producing a chondroid matrix will be described in this group. Many benign cartilage tumors are asymptomatic. Radiographic findings are critical to diagnosis of cartilaginous tumors.

2.1. Osteochondroma

Osteochondroma is a common slow-growing tumor that cartilage-capped bony projection arising from the outside surface of bone containing a marrow cavity that is continuous with that of the underlying bone appears close to the growth plate at the end of long bones [3]. In very few cases of temporomandibular joint, osteochondroma have been reported [4]. Osteochondroma is usually located at the medial surface of mandibular condyle [5]. The average age of occurrence is 16.5 and males are affected 3 times as often as females [6].

The most common clinical symptoms are malocclusion, with unilateral posterior open bite on the affected side and a crossbite on the contralateral side, and progressive facial asymmetry, limited and often painful mandibular movements and clicking [7, 8].

The reason for osteochondroma is uncertain, but traumatic, developmental, neoplastic and reparative occasions have been considered as possible factors [6, 9]. The most commonly accepted view is a metaplastic change of the periosteum and/or the osteochondral layer in the condyle, leading to the production of cartilage, which subsequently ossifies [8]. Complications of OC are osseous deformity, fracture, vascular compromise, bursa generation and malignant transformation [6]. CT can provide excellent anatomy of the lesion and demonstrate calcification in the cartilage cap whereas MRI confirms the diagnosis by demonstrating the cartilaginous cap [4].

The differential diagnosis of benign neoplasms known to involve the mandibular condyle includes osteoma, osteoblastoma, chondroma, chondroblastoma and osteochondroma. Osteomas are benign tumors that consist primarily of mature, compact, cancellous bone [9]. Chondromas consist of well-defined lobules of mature hyaline cartilage that may contain areas of calcification. Chondroblastomas consist of a proliferation of immature cartilage cells, with focal production of a variably differentiated cartilaginous matrix [10]. Osteochondroma is presumed to arise from herniation of cartilage through the epiphyseal plate in the formative years. Radiographically, the lesion is easily differentiated from chondroma because it is most frequently an extraneous appendage, rather than a rarefaction within the normal jaw confines, and is more radiopaque, which represents its true ossification [11].

Osteochondromas can be treated by total condylectomy or local resection of the lesion and condylar replacement if the tumor involves the mandibular condyle. On the other hand, if the tumor affects limited part of the condylar surface, preservation of the remaining part of the condyle and reshaping can be done [6, 12].

In the case of an osteochondroma of the author of this chapter, Dr Karasu, the tumor was removed under general anesthesia. On a panoramic radiograph, a well-defined, bone-like, radiopaque mass was seen in the left condylar head (**Figure 1**). Axial and coronal computed tomographic (CT) scans revealed an opaque mass around the mandibular condyle (**Figures 2** and **3**). The patient's three-dimensional CT image showed a large mass in the anteromedial region of the left condyle (**Figure 4**). The tumor was excised under general anesthesia. The upper and lower compartments of the temporomandibular joint were accessed through an auriculotemporal approach. The surgical field was expanded with retraction along the masseter muscle downward. The disc, which adhered to the lesion at the anterior aspect of the condyle, was resected. The tumor was resected en bloc. The lesion could be easily separated from the surrounding tissues (**Figure 5**). Histologically, it was noted that the nodular mass was covered with a proliferative cap of cartilage with underlying zones of cancellous bone and irregular calcified cartilage. The osteocytes and chondrocytes were individually housed in a lacuna with a single nucleus (**Figure 6**). Sixteen-year follow-up assessments revealed satisfactory function and occlusion. There was no evidence of recurrence [11].

2.2. Chondroma

Chondroma is a rare, benign tumor of mature hyaline cartilage of mesenchymal origin [13]. Chondromas, are common in the small bones of the hands and feet, but are extremely rare in the TMJ area [14, 15]. Chondromas are classified into three types as (a) enchondroma that arises from medullary cavity, (b) juxtacortical that originate adjacent to the periosteum below

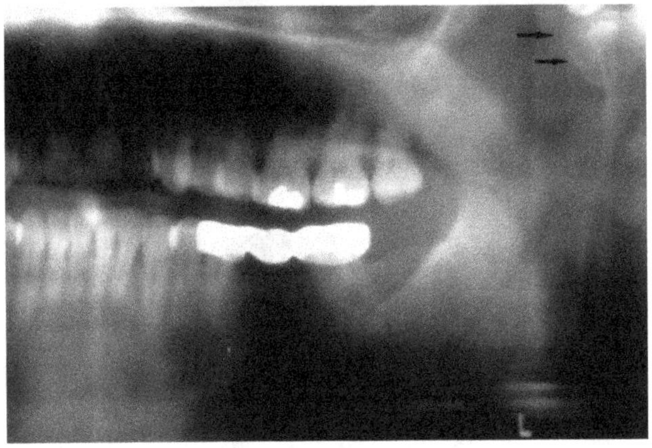

Figure 1. Panoramic radiograph, showing a bone-like, radiopaque mass in the left condylar head.

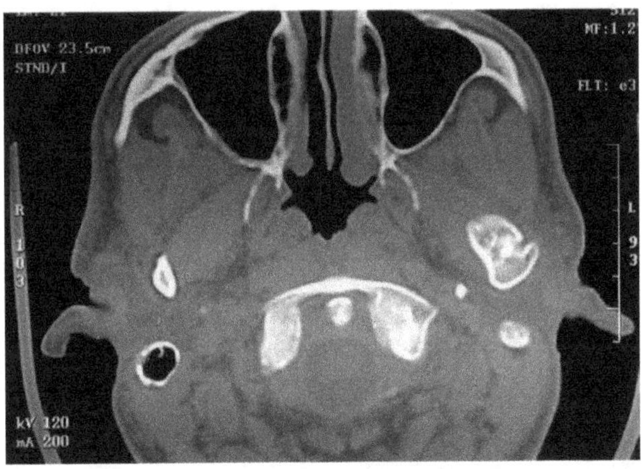

Figure 2. Axial CT scan, showing a well-defined, opaque mass.

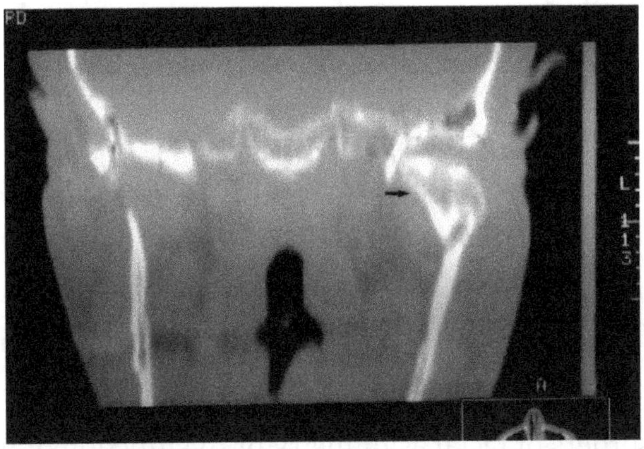

Figure 3. Coronal CT scan, showing localization of the osteochondroma.

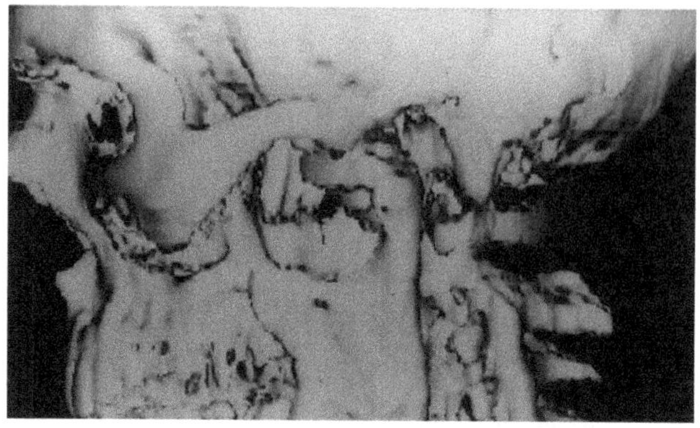

Figure 4. Three-dimensional CT view of the osteochondroma.

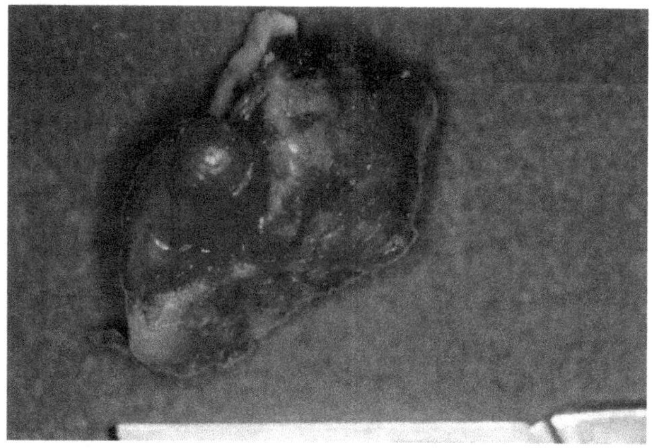

Figure 5. Mass resected from the left condyle.

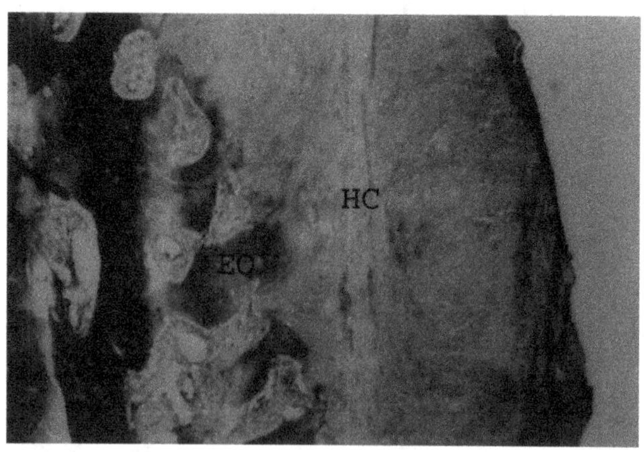

Figure 6. Histopathological aspect of the osteochondroma. The cancellous bone is surfaced by a cap of hyaline cartilage (HC). A zone of endochondral ossification (EO) appears between the cartilaginous cap and underlying cancellous bone (hematoxylin and eosin; magnification, 200).

the cortical face and (c) extra-skeletal that can be seen in the tongue and buccal mucosa [16, 17]. Chondromas are equally seen in men and women and most patients are 30–40 years old [14].

Chondromas are generally asymptomatic. Its signs and symptoms can mimic those of patients with more common disorders of facial asymmetry or dysfunction of the temporomandibular joint as clicking, limited mouth opening and deviation [18].

Radiographically, chondromas are irregular radiolucent or mottled region of the bone. There may be some calcification foci ranging from powder like to dense aggregates [19].

The differential diagnosis for bony or cartilaginous hyperplastic lesion of the temporomandibular joint may include condylar hyperplasia, osteochondroma, osteoma, chondroma, osteoblastoma, fibrous dysplasia, ossifying fibroma (OF), chondromyxoid fibromas, synovial chondromatosis, chondroblastoma, chondrosarcoma and osteosarcoma [20, 21].

Chondromas can be treated as low-grade chondrosarcomas by surgical treatment of mandibular condyle to avoid recurrence [13].

2.3. Chondroblastoma

Chondroblastoma is a rare benign, cartilaginous, destructive tumor derived from immature cartilage cells which occurs infrequently in the head and neck area [22, 23]. Most chondroblastoma cases arise in the epiphysis of long bones such as distal femur, proximal tibia and proximal humerus [24]. It is more common in women [25].

Chondroblastoma shows similar clinical symptoms associated with temporomandibular disorders such as sound in the joint, decreased range of motion, swelling, pain, trismus and changing occlusion. If chondroblastoma occurs at the temporal bone, additional symptoms such as otalgia, paresthesia, hearing loss, ear noise and facial nerve weakness may be seen [26].

Computerized imaging (CT) and magnetic resonance imaging (MRI) are the most common diagnostic imaging techniques to identify chondroblastoma. On imaging, round radiolucent lesions with sharp bony edges are found in bone [27].

Differential diagnosis should be done with chondrosarcoma, chondromyxoid fibroma, synovial sarcoma, synovial chondromatosis and aneurysmal bone cyst. Biopsy is necessary for the definite diagnosis [28, 29].

Treatment alternatives are curettage, resection and excision. Chondroblastoma can be treated by conservative curettage when infiltration of bone has not occurred or is limited. Complete excision of the tumor reduces recurrence [30].

In the case of a chondroblastoma of the authors of this chapter, Dr Oncul and Dr Yurttutan, the tumor was removed under general anesthesia. A 35-year-old female patient had complaint of pain and asymmetry. The patient's three-dimensional CT image showed a large mass in the anteromedial region of the left condyle (**Figure 7**). The tumor was resected via a pre-auricular access (**Figures 8** and **9**), the mass was removed by performing condylectomy (**Figure 10**).

2.4. Synovial chondromatosis

Synovial chondromatosis (SC) is a rare benign nodular cartilaginous proliferative non-neoplastic lesion arising from the synovial membrane or the fibro-cartilaginous disc of the joints becoming loose bodies within the joint space [3, 31]. The first report of SC of the temporomandibular joint (TMJ) was in 1776 [32].

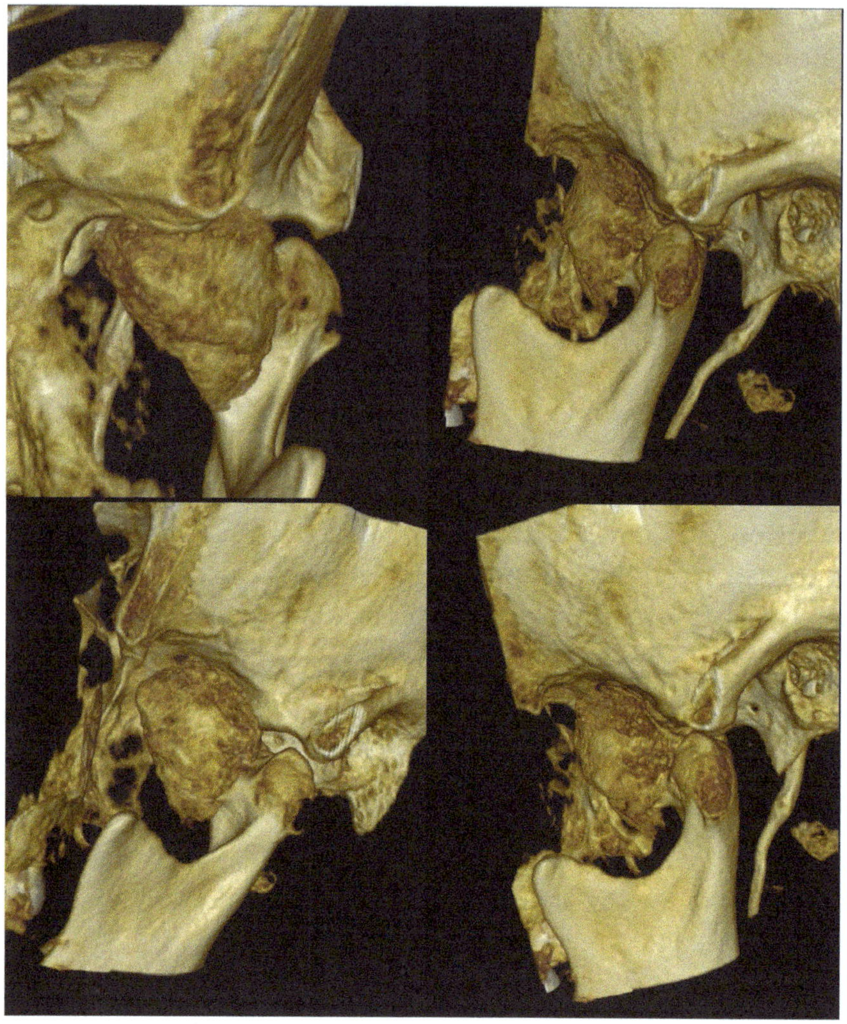

Figure 7. Three-dimensional CT view of the chondroblastoma.

The etiology of SC is unclear but it is thought to be a trauma history, occlusal disorders, bruxism and degenerative arthritis [33]. SC of TMJ is 2.5 times more common in females, mainly between 30 and 50 years old [34].

SC has three histological stages:

1. metaplasia found in the synovial membrane without the presence of detached particles.
2. metaplasia found in the synovial membrane with the presence of detached particles.
3. presence of detached particles which may vary in size [3].

Clinical signs and symptoms of SC is local diffuse pain, pre-auricular swelling, limitation of mandibular movement, joint sounds, tenderness, deviation of mouth opening [35].

Computerized imaging (CT), magnetic resonance imaging (MRI) and orthopantomography are the most common diagnostic imaging techniques. The main findings are widening of the joint space, changes in bone surface of joint and calcified loose bodies [36].

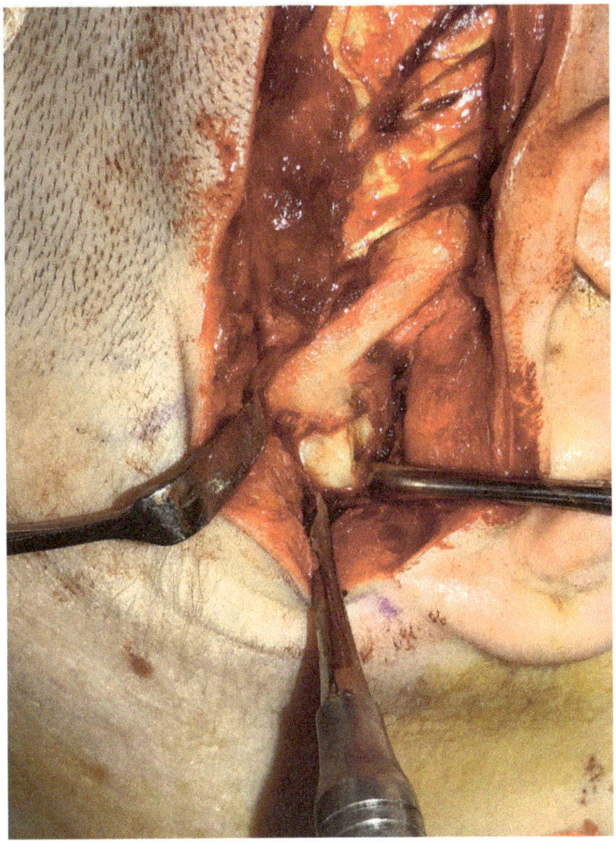

Figure 8. Intraoperative view of the condyle with the chondroblastoma.

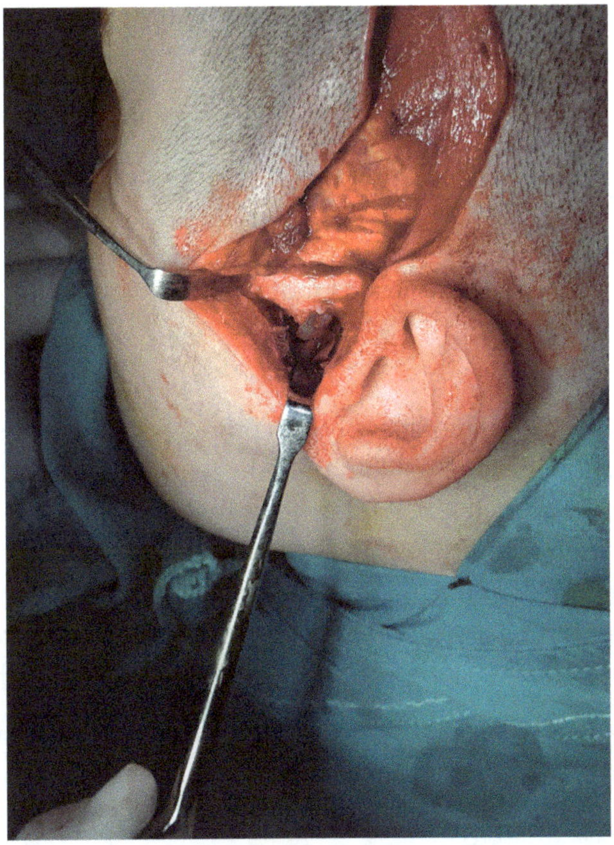

Figure 9. Intraoperative view after the excision of chondroblastoma.

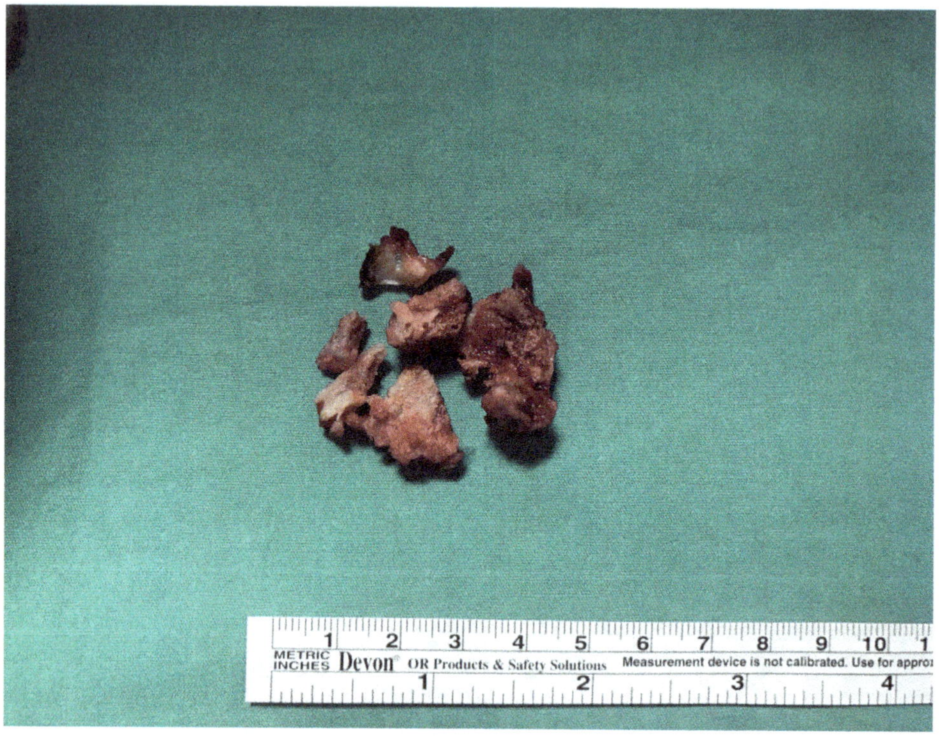

Figure 10. Macroscopic view of the pathology.

Differential diagnosis should be done with internal derangements, osteoarthritis, osteochondromas, villonodular synovitis, chondroblastoma and focal osteochondritis [37].

Synovectomy with removal of loose body from the joint space is the most preferred procedure. It can be applied in combination with discectomy or condylectomy. No recurrence when loose bodies are removed [38].

3. Osteogenic tumors

Osteogenic tumors are defined as neoplasms that produce an osteoid or bony matrix.

3.1. Osteoma

Osteomas are benign osteogenic tumors involving compact or cancellous bone proliferation and arising from periosteum (peripheral osteoma), endosteum (central osteoma) and even extra-skeletal soft tissue, but they are actually hamartomas that can be seen in membranous bone [39, 40]. Most osteomas of the maxillofacial region occur in the mandible. Peripheral osteomas typically arise at the inferior border of the mandibular body [41, 42]. Only a few cases involving the temporomandibular joint have been reported [43]. Men seem to be more affected than women. The exact cause is unknown, whereas belief in reactive and neoplastic theories maintains [1].

Histologically, compact type osteomas (ivory) consist primarily of dense lamellar bone, and cancellous type osteomas have an abundance of bone marrow [42].

The growth of osteomas occurring in TMJ may result in morphologic and functional disturbances, including facial asymmetry, malocclusion and limited mouth opening [44].

Radiographically, osteoma appears as a well-defined uniform radiopacity or as well-defined radiopacity with evidence of internal trabecular structure. In their centers such masses may exhibit a mixed radiolucent-radiopaque appearance depending on the amount of marrow tissues present [39, 45]. Panoramic radiography, CT, MRI and radionuclide scanning (scintigraphy) have been utilized for imaging of osteomas of the TMJ region [46].

The differential diagnosis is established with exostoses, osteoid osteoma and osteoblastoma [46]. Osteomas of the condyle are lobulated; conversely, hyperplasia results in enlargement of the condyle that retains in its inventive form [47]. Osteoid osteoma and osteoblastoma are frequently painful and grow more rapidly than peripheral osteoma [1].

Large osteomas at TMJ can be treated by condylectomy and tumor resection. No recurrence is reported after surgery [43].

In the case of an osteoma of the author of this chapter, Dr Oncul, the tumor was removed under general anesthesia. A 45-year-old male patient had complaint of habitual luxation which had been present for 5 years and asymmetry (**Figure 11**). The tumor was resected via a pre-auricular access (**Figure 12**), the mass was removed by performing a condylectomy, preserving the articular meniscus (**Figure 13**). Microscopic examination showed a central nidus surrounded by a layer of dense cortical bone. The nidus consisted inconsiderable amount of interstitial connective tissue. No abnormal mitosis or malignancy findings were seen (**Figure 14**) [48].

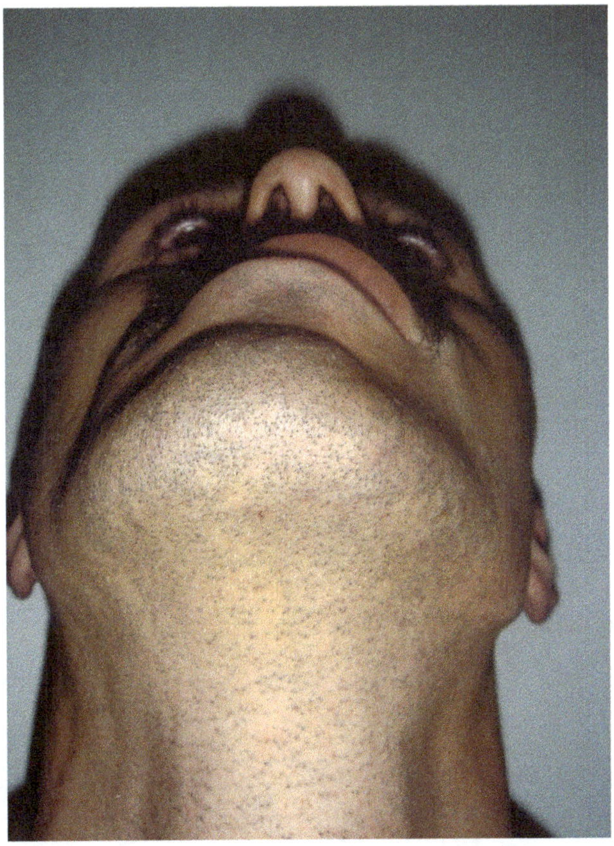

Figure 11. Preoperative frontal view of the mandibular asymmetry.

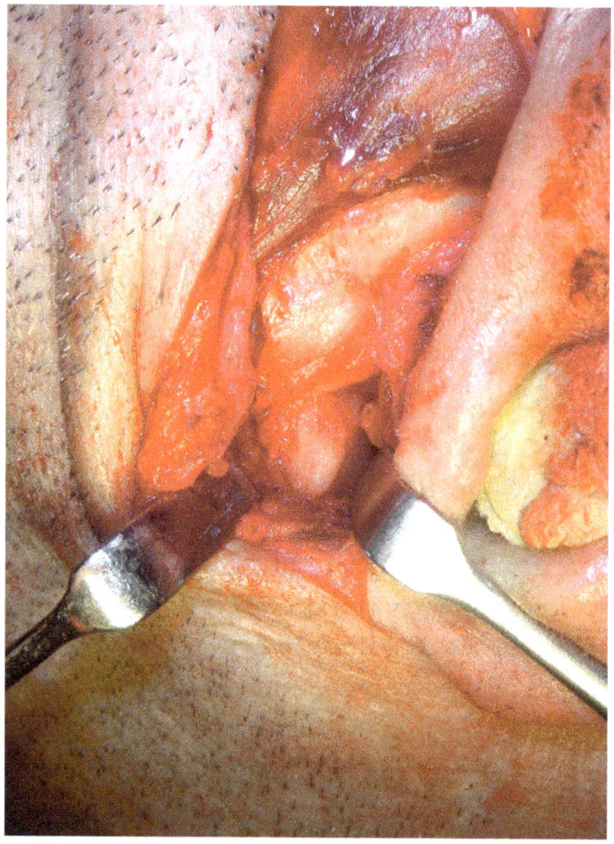

Figure 12. Intraoperative view of the condyle with the osteoma.

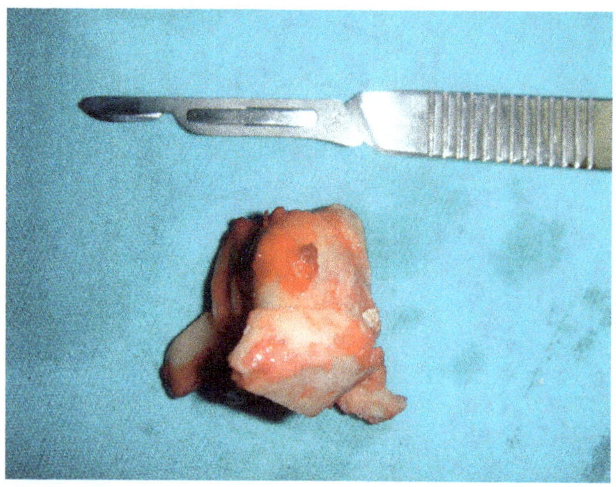

Figure 13. Macroscopic view of the pathology.

3.2. Osteoid osteoma

Osteoid osteoma is a benign bone-forming tumor characterized by small size, limited growth potential and disproportionate pain. Osteoid osteoma usually affects children and adolescents, although it is occasionally seen in older individuals. It is more common in males [2]. Osteoid osteoma is rarely described in TMJ [49].

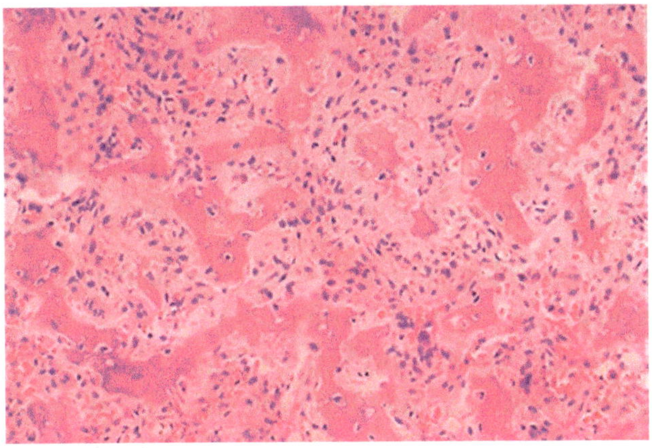

Figure 14. Histopathological aspect of the osteoma.

The trio of complaints for osteoid osteoma of the jaw is pain, swelling and tenderness [50].

The most typical symptom of osteoid osteoma is spontaneous pain, usually responsive to non-steroidal anti-inflammatory drugs (NSAIDs). At first, the pain is light and discontinuous, but later becomes severe and constant [51].

A characteristic radiographic finding is 'nidus', which represents a small, round, clear, non-calcified, well-demarcated radiolucency in the subjacent cortex surrounded by sclerotic bone, not larger than 2 cm [3]. CT and cone beam computed tomography (CBCT) are superior to MRI in diagnosing and precisely localizing these bone tumors in TMJ [46, 50].

The differential diagnosis of osteoid osteoma is established which includes bone island/solitary enostosis, intracortical bone abscess (Brodie abscess), sclerosing forms of osteomyelitis and early diagnosis of osteosarcoma or osteoblastoma, fibroma or fibrous dysplasia [14, 51].

However, the sequestrum of osteomyelitis is irregular rather than a well-demarcated round lesion and is usually located in the bone marrow, not in the cortical plate [50].

The most important criterion to distinguish osteoid osteoma from osteoblastoma: osteoid osteomas are typically <1 cm in size, whereas osteoblast [52] stomas are generally >2 cm. An osteoid osteoma usually contains only a single calcification, whereas an osteoblastoma contains multiple calcifications. However, the osteoblastoma differs from the osteoid osteoma in that it has a greater growth potential, is frequently painless, and becomes heavily calcified when subjected to radiological examination [51].

Surgical removal of the osteoid osteoma is the most advised treatment option if the pain is not relieved by NSAIDs. En bloc excision or cortical shaving and curettage of the nidus are sufficient and can provide immediate relief of symptoms. After the nidus is removed, all symptoms eventually disappear [46, 50, 53].

3.3. Osteoblastoma

Osteoblastoma is a rare benign bone-forming neoplasm which produces woven bone spicules, which are bordered by prominent osteoblasts. Osteoblastoma is uncommon, accounting for about 1% of all bone tumors and is more common in women and affects patients in the age range of 10–30 years [2]. The tumor normally involves the long bones, spine and sacrum. Less than 10% of osteoblastomas are located in the maxillofacial region [54, 55]. Osteoblastoma involving the TMJ is very rare [56].

Complaints for osteoblastoma are dull persistent pain and swelling [57]. Even if NSAIDs is used, the pain will not decrease in contrast to osteoid osteoma [56].

Osteoblastoma has identical histological features to osteoid osteoma [2]. Osteoblastomas are characterized by numerous plump osteoblastic cells producing and lining the haphazardly arranged lesional trabeculae of osteoid and woven bone. Numerous blood vessels are often seen in the osteoblastic and fibrous stroma filling the lesional inter-trabecular areas. Five scattered multinucleated giant cells resembling osteoclasts are also generally seen. Mitotic figures may be seen, but these are usually sparse and have a normal configuration [58]. Osteoblastoma and osteoid osteoma are histopathologically very similar, and diagnosis is often based on the size of the lesion, with an osteoid osteoma being less than 1 cm in diameter and an osteoblastoma being larger than 2 cm [59].

The radiographic features are well-defined expansile lesions contain small scattered calcifications [59]. Radiographic differential diagnosis of osteoblastoma should include osteogenic sarcoma, chondrosarcoma, osteoid osteoma and aneurysmal bone cyst [3].

The treatment choice of osteoblastoma for TMJ is conservative surgery. Recurrences after complete excision are uncommon [55].

4. Giant cell tumors

Almost every lesion in the bone can contain giant cells, sometimes a large number. To be characterized as a giant cell tumor (GCT), the neoplasm must have oval mononuclear cells and more or less evenly distributed giant cells.

4.1. Giant cell tumor

Giant cell tumors (GCTs) are a benign, locally aggressive neoplasm which is composed of sheets of neoplastic ovoid mononuclear cells interspersed with uniformly distributed large, osteoclast-like giant cells. GCT is classified as an "intermediate locally aggressive, rarely metastasizing" bone tumor by World Health Organization (WHO) [2]. The prevalence of GCTs peaks in adults in their 30s or 40s [60, 61]. GCTs are frequently identified at the epiphyses of long bones, particularly in the proximal tibia, distal femur and distal radius [62]. Craniofacial bone involvement is rare but has been reported to occur in the mandible, temporal bone, maxilla, occipital and sphenoid [63]. Less than 30 cases of GCT in the TMJ have been reported. Patients with GCTs at TMJ are presented with progressive pain and swelling. Due to compression or local invasion, hearing impairment, facial nerve paralysis, headache, visual area defects, double vision, visual loss, tinnitus, otalgia, vertigo and trismus can occur [64]. Discomforts as jaw locking, mandibular deviation and clicking can also be seen. These three symptoms and signs are also common with temporomandibular disorders [65].

Recent experiments have characterized GCTs as consisting of three cell types: (1) osteoclast-like, multinucleated giant cells; (2) round mononuclear cells resembling monocytes and (3) spindle-shaped, fibroblast-like stromal cells [66].

GCTs appear lytic, subarticular, eccentrically located and usually lack a sclerotic rim on radiographs. Local bony destruction, cortical breakthrough and soft tissue expansion may also be seen [67]. MRI is the preferred imaging modality for GCTs, as the diagnostic accuracy of MRI is high and it can detect soft tissue and intra-articular extension [68].

Important differential diagnoses of GCTs are giant cell reparative granuloma, hyperparathyroidism, non-ossifying fibroma, chondroblastoma, solid areas of aneurysmal bone cyst, malignant fibrous histiocytoma and osteogenic sarcoma [69].

Various modalities have been used in the treatment of GCTs including surgery, cryotherapy, radiotherapy, calcitonin, corticosteroids, a interferon and recently, the monoclonal antibody against receptor activator of nuclear factor kappa-B ligand (RANKL) denosumab [70, 71]. Intralesional curettage is not recommended for GCTs in the skull base because recurrence in this location would complicate further treatment and make it unresectable for reoperation [72]. However, because of the complexity of the craniofacial anatomy, wide excisions or en bloc resections for head and neck GCTs should be attempted. Radiotherapy can be applied for cases where wide excision cannot be achieved or for patients who are not fit for surgery [73]. But radiotherapy as a sole treatment modality is not recommended due to high (60–70%) recurrence rates [74]. Denosumab, a receptor activator of nuclear factor kappa-B ligand (RANKL) inhibitor can be used in recurrent and unresectable GCTs [75]. Denosumab specifically inhibits osteoclast-mediated bone destruction by GCTs [76]. Denosumab can be used to reduce the tumor size preoperatively [74].

5. Vascular tumors

Primary vascular tumors are rare in bone. Hemangiomas occur as coincidental findings in the skull or spine. X-ray features are almost always diagnostic. They rarely cause clinical symptoms.

5.1. Hemangioma

Intraosseous hemangiomas are benign vasoformative neoplasm or developmental condition of endothelial origin tumors occurring most often in the maxilla and mandible after the skull and vertebrae [2]. Clinically, hemangiomas of the mandible are often presented as slow-growing expansile lesions. They occur twice as often in women. Hemangiomas present as radiolucent lesions, which may have a unicystic- or multicystic-like "soap bubbly," "honeycomb" or "trabeculated" appearance [77]. The differential diagnosis for this radiographic appearance must also include: ameloblastoma, odontogenic keratocyst, central giant cell granulomata, giant cell tumor of hyperparathyroidism, aneurysmal bone cyst and metastatic lesions [78]. Treatment may include embolization, sclerosing agents and surgery [79].

6. Lipogenic tumors

Lipomas are rare in the bones and are found incidentally in the X-rays and contain calcaneus. Radiography shows a well-defined area of lucency with a central calcification area.

6.1. Intraosseous lipoma

Lipoma of bone is a benign neoplasm of adipocytes that arises within the medullary cavity, cortex or on the surface of bone. Lipoma of bone is rare and accounts for less than 0.1% of primary bone tumors [2]. The jaw is its most uncommon bone location.

Etiology of lipoma is not clear but possible etiological factors may be dental trauma, disruption of the post-extraction healing process, retention of radicular remains, medullary bone infarction (common in elderly) or osteoporotic bones [80–82]. They are generally asymptomatic, being diagnosed by chance during a radiographic examination. Symptoms depend on its size, location, time of evolution and growth rate. Pain, swelling and numbness may occur [83, 84]. Radiological appearance of intraosseous lipoma is well-circumscribed radiolucent unilocular or multilocular lesion. Treatment involves curettage of the lesion, with or without grafting the cavity [85].

7. Bone-related odontogenic tumors

Odontogenic tumors are rare, some of them very rare, but they can be an important diagnostic and therapeutic problem.

7.1. Ossifying fibroma

Ossifying fibroma (OF) is a well-demarcated lesion composed of fibrocellular tissue and mineralized material of varying appearances [86]. The mandible (especially the molar region) is affected more often than the maxilla [87]. Ossifying fibroma is mainly diagnosed between the second and fourth decades of life, with women being affected more frequently than men [88, 89]. Ossifying fibroma of craniofacial bones is composed of two components: fibrous stroma and bone elements that show various degrees of maturation [90]. The treatment of choice is surgical excision. Enucleation and curettage could be suitable for small and well-defined lesions; however, larger masses require radical surgery [91]. Condylectomy may be performed with an immediate TMJ reconstruction [92].

8. Fibrohistiocytic tumors

Diffuse and localized forms of the giant cell tumor of the tendon sheath are more common with the descriptive category of fibrohistiocytic lesions.

8.1. Pigmented villonodular synovitis

Pigmented villonodular synovitis (PVNS) is a rare, benign tumor but is a locally aggressive tumor of the synovial membrane with an annual incidence [93]. Lesions originate from the joint capsule, tendon sheath or bursae and occur most commonly in the knee, hip and ankle [94]. The etiology of PVNS is not clear and may result from chronic inflammation, trauma or represent a distinct neoplastic process [95–97]. It is considered as fibrohistiocytic tumor by the World Health Organization classification of bone and soft tissue tumors. Tenosynovial giant cell tumor, diffuse-type giant cell tumor, villonodular synovitis, giant cell tumor of the tendon sheath and nodular tenosynovitis are the synonyms of that tumor [2]. PVNS of the temporomandibular joint (TMJ) is a rare variant with less than 80 cases reported in the literature [98]. This slow-growing tumor may be seen in all age groups. The peak age of occurrence is between 30 and 50 ages [99]. PVNS has been shown to have a synovial cell origin immunophenotypically and is reported to involve myofibroblastic differentiation [100, 101]. The tumor is composed of monocyte, multinucleated giant cells and foam cells distributing in a fibrous stroma, presenting hemosiderin deposition [102]. It has a higher gender predilection in females [103].

PVNS can enlarge into the middle cranial fossa, displacing the temporal lobe and invading the dura mater. Patients are generally present with an enlarging pre-auricular mass, pain, trismus or hearing loss [104]. The radiological appearance of PVNS on CT is a contrast-enhancing intra-articular lesion originating in the glenoid fossa, with focal areas of hyperdensity or cysts. It produces variable bony remodeling or erosion of the adjacent bone [105]. On MRI, the most characteristic finding is a mass with low signal intensity on T1 and GRE-T2 weighted sequences, reflecting the deposition of blood degradation products. Occasionally, hyperintense areas on T1 or GRE-T2 sequences may appear due to the presence of lipids or cysts, respectively [106].

The differential diagnosis is established with osteoarthritic change, chondroblastoma, chondrosarcoma, aneurysmal bone cyst, rhabdomyosarcoma, plasmacytoma, cholesteatoma, intraosseous meningioma, reparative granuloma, tumoral calcium pyrophosphate dihydrate crystal deposition disease, chondroma of the tendon sheath, synovial chondromatosis, tendon sheath fibroma, synovial hemangioma, synovial sarcoma, embryonal rhabdomyosarcoma, giant cell granuloma, brown tumor and malignant fibrous histiocytoma [107, 108].

Therapy for PVNS of the TMJ and temporal bone remains surgical. PVNS of the temporal bone most commonly acquires the diffuse form of disease involving the contiguous synovial space with extension into adjacent structures. Accordingly, limited resection or curettage carries a high rate of recurrence, whereas wide local resection, when feasible, is usually curative [104, 109]. The surgical approach must be carefully planned to allow for a complete removal of the tumor while minimizing surgical trauma [110].

9. Tumors of uncertain differentiation

For tumors in this category, in most cases, there is no clear idea on the differentiation line (or normal cellular counterpart) that these lesions repeat.

9.1. Juxta-articular myxoma

Juxta-articular myxoma is a rare, benign soft tissue tumor that usually arises in the vicinity of a large joint, has histological features resembling a cellular myxoma [2]. There are reported cases involving myxomas of the knee, shoulder, elbow, wrist and hip. To our knowledge, however, there is just one reported cases of juxta-articular myxomas of the temporomandibular joint (TMJ) [111]. The juxta-articular myxoma resembles the common myxoma, however, it is distinguished by its association with the underlying connective tissue components of the joint. These include the associated tendons, joint capsule, meniscus and synovium [112]. Palpable swelling is occasionally associated with pain, tenderness or a functional limitation may occur [113, 114]. Like the common myxoma, the treatment of choice for the juxta-articular myxomas is complete local excision [115]. Tumors extending into the infratemporal fossa are notoriously difficult to resect [116].

Author details

Mehmet Emre Yurttutan*, Ayşegül Tüzüner Öncül and Hakan Alpay Karasu

*Address all correspondence to: yurttutan@ankara.edu.tr

Faculty of Dentistry, Department of Oral and Maxillofacial Surgery, Ankara University, Ankara, Turkey

References

[1] Fonseca RJ. Oral and Maxillofacial Surgery: Temporomandibular Disorders. USA: Saunders; 2000

[2] Flecther CDM, Unni KK, Mertens F. World Health Organization Classification of Tumours of Soft Tissue and Bone. IARC: Lyon; 2002

[3] Robert EM, Stern D. Oral and Maxillofacial Pathology, A Rationale for Diagnosis and Treatment. India: Quintessence; 2003

[4] Andrade NN, Gandhewar TM, Kapoor P, Thomas R. Osteochondroma of the mandibular condyle – Report of an atypical case and the importance of computed tomography. Journal of oral Biology and Craniofacial Research. 2014;**4**(3):208-213

[5] Kurita K, Ogi N, Echiverre NV, Yoshida K. Osteochondroma of the mandibular condyle. A case report. International Journal of Oral and Maxillofacial Surgery. 1999;**28**(5):380-382

[6] Murphey MD, Choi JJ, Kransdorf MJ, Flemming DJ, Gannon FH. Imaging of osteochondroma: Variants and complications with radiologic-pathologic correlation. Radiographics: A Review Publication of the Radiological Society of North America, Inc. 2000;**20**(5):1407-1434

[7] Gaines RE Jr, Lee MB, Crocker DJ. Osteochondroma of the mandibular condyle: Case report and review of the literature. Journal of Oral and Maxillofacial Surgery: Official Journal of the American Association of Oral and Maxillofacial Surgeons. 1992;**50**(8):899-903

[8] Koole R, Steenks MH, Witkamp TD, Slootweg PJ, Shaefer J. Osteochondroma of the mandibular condyle. A case report. International Journal of Oral and Maxillofacial Surgery. 1996;**25**(3):203-205

[9] Henry CH, Granite EL, Rafetto LK. Osteochondroma of the mandibular condyle: Report of a case and review of the literature. Journal of Oral and Maxillofacial Surgery: Official Journal of the American Association of Oral and Maxillofacial Surgeons. 1992;**50**(10):1102-1108

[10] Spahr J, Elzay RP, Kay S, Frable WJ. Chondroblastoma of the temporomandibular joint arising from articular cartilage: A previously unreported presentation of an uncommon neoplasm. Oral Surgery, Oral Medicine, and Oral Pathology. 1982;**54**(4):430-435

[11] Karasu HA, Ortakoglu K, Okcu KM, Gunhan O. Osteochondroma of the mandibular condyle: Report of a case and review of the literature. Military Medicine. 2005;**170**(9):797-801

[12] Utumi ER, Pedron IG, Perrella A, Zambon CE, Ceccheti MM, Cavalcanti MG. Osteochondroma of the temporomandibular joint: A case report. Brazilian Dental Journal. 2010;**21**(3):253-258

[13] Marchetti C, Mazzoni S, Bertoni F. Chondroma of the mandibular condyle-relapse of a rare benign chondroid tumour after 5 years' follow-up: Case report. The British Journal of Oral & Maxillofacial Surgery. 2012;**50**(5):e69-e71

[14] do Egito Vasconcelos BC, Porto GG, Bessa-Nogueira RV. Rare benign tumors of the mandibular condyle: Report of 2 cases and literature review. Journal of Oral and Maxillofacial Surgery: Official Journal of the American Association of Oral and Maxillofacial Surgeons. 2007;**65**(9):1830-1835

[15] Heitz C, Vogt BF, Bergoli RD, Hirsch WD, de Souza CE, Silva DN. Chondroma in temporomandibular region – Case report and therapeutic considerations. Oral and Maxillofacial Surgery. 2012;**16**(1):75-78

[16] Chandu A, Spencer JA, Dyson DP. Chondroma of the mandibular condyle: An example of a rare tumour. Dento Maxillo Facial Radiology. 1997;**26**(4):242-245

[17] Chang SE, Lee MW, Choi JH, Sung KJ, Moon KC, Koh JKA. Case of lingual chondroma. The British Journal of Dermatology. 1999;**141**(4):773-774

[18] Dhirawani RB, Anand K, Lalwani G, Pathak S, Thakkar B. True chondroma of the mandibular condyle: A rare case. Annals of Maxillofacial Surgery. 2014;**4**(2):220-223

[19] Fechner RE, Mills SE. Atlas of Tumor Pathology – Tumors of the Bones and Joints. Armed Forces Institute of Pathology: Washington, DC; 1993

[20] Shintaku WH, Venturin JS, Langlais RP, Clark GT. Imaging modalities to access bony tumors and hyperplasic reactions of the temporomandibular joint. Journal of Oral and Maxillofacial Surgery: Official Journal of the American Association of Oral and Maxillofacial Surgeons. 2010;**68**(8):1911-1921

[21] Lazow SK, Pihlstrom RT, Solomon MP, Berger JR. Condylar chondroma: Report of a case. Journal of Oral and Maxillofacial Surgery: Official Journal of the American Association of Oral and Maxillofacial Surgeons. 1998;**56**(3):373-378

[22] Payne M, Yusuf H. Benign chondroblastoma involving the mandibular condyle. The British Journal of Oral & Maxillofacial Surgery. 1987;**25**(3):250-255

[23] Jaffe HL, Lichtenstein L. Benign chondroblastoma of bone: A reinterpretation of the so-called calcifying or chondromatous giant cell tumor. The American Journal of Pathology. 1942;**18**(6):969-991

[24] Varvares MA, Cheney ML, Goodman ML, Ceisler E, Montgomery WW. Chondroblastoma of the temporal bone. Case report and literature review. The Annals of Otology, Rhinology, and Laryngology. 1992;**101**(9):763-769

[25] Bui P, Ivan D, Oliver D, Busaidy KF, Wilson J. Chondroblastoma of the temporomandibular joint: Report of a case and literature review. Journal of Oral and Maxillofacial Surgery: Official Journal of the American Association of Oral and Maxillofacial Surgeons. 2009;**67**(2):405-409

[26] Moon IS, Kim J, Lee HK, Lee WS. Surgical treatment and outcomes of temporal bone chondroblastoma. European Archives of Oto-Rhino-Laryngology: Official Journal of the European Federation of Oto-Rhino-Laryngological Societies (EUFOS): Affiliated with the German Society for Oto-Rhino-Laryngology – Head and Neck Surgery. 2008;**265**(12):1447-1454

[27] Bloem JL, Mulder JD. Chondroblastoma: A clinical and radiological study of 104 cases. Skeletal Radiology. 1985;**14**(1):1-9

[28] Warner BF, Luna MA, Robert Newland T. Temporomandibular joint neoplasms and pseudotumors. Advances in Anatomic Pathology. 2000;**7**(6):365-381

[29] Kondoh T, Hamada Y, Kamei K, Seto K. Chondroblastoma of the mandibular condyle: Report of a case. Journal of Oral and Maxillofacial Surgery: Official Journal of the American Association of Oral and Maxillofacial Surgeons. 2002;**60**(2):198-203

[30] Kim SM, Hong SW, Ryu DJ, Huh JK. Chondroblastoma of the temporomandibular joint lateral capsule: A case report. Cranio: The Journal of Craniomandibular Practice. 2015;**33**(4):306-311

[31] Milgram JW. The classification of loose bodies in human joints. Clinical Orthopaedics and Related Research. 1977;**124**:282-291

[32] Yokota N, Inenaga C, Tokuyama T, Nishizawa S, Miura K, Namba H. Synovial chondromatosis of the temporomandibular joint with intracranial extension. Neurologia Medico-Chirurgica. 2008;**48**(6):266-270

[33] Holmlund AB, Eriksson L, Reinholt FP. Synovial chondromatosis of the temporomandibular joint: Clinical, surgical and histological aspects. International Journal of Oral and Maxillofacial Surgery. 2003;**32**(2):143-147

[34] Mankin HJ, editor. Synovial Chondromatosis in Pathophysiology of Orthopaedic Diseases. Rosemont, IL: American Academy Orthopaedic Surgeons; 2006

[35] Petito AR, Bennett J, Assael LA, Carlotti AE Jr. Synovial chondromatosis of the temporomandibular joint: Varying presentation in 4 cases. Oral Surgery, Oral Medicine, Oral Pathology, Oral Radiology, and Endodontics. 2000;**90**(6):758-764

[36] Guarda-Nardini L, Piccotti F, Ferronato G, Manfredini D. Synovial chondromatosis of the temporomandibular joint: A case description with systematic literature review. International Journal of Oral and Maxillofacial Surgery. 2010;**39**(8):745-755

[37] Pinto AA, Jr, Ferreira e Costa R, de Sousa SF, Chagas MR, do Carmo MA, de Lacerda JC. Synovial chondromatosis of the temporomandibular joint successfully treated by surgery. Head and Neck Pathology. 2015;**9**(4):525-529

[38] Ionna F, Amantea M, Mastrangelo F, Ballini A, Maglione MG, Aversa C, et al. Innovative surgical management of the synovial chondromatosis of temporo-mandibular joints: Highly conservative surgical technique. The Journal of Craniofacial Surgery. 2016;**27**(5):1197-1201

[39] Yonezu H, Wakoh M, Otonari T, Sano T, Hashimoto S, Uchiyama T. Osteoma of mandibular condyle as cause of acute pain and limited-mouth-opening: Case report. The Bulletin of Tokyo Dental College. 2007;**48**(4):193-197

[40] Yang C, Qiu WL. Osteoid osteoma of the eminence of the temporomandibular joint. The British Journal of Oral & Maxillofacial Surgery. 2001;**39**(5):404-406

[41] Schneider LC, Dolinsky HB, Grodjesk JE. Solitary peripheral osteoma of the jaws: Report of case and review of literature. Journal of Oral Surgery (American Dental Association: 1965). 1980;**38**(6):452-455

[42] Kaplan I, Calderon S, Buchner A. Peripheral osteoma of the mandible: A study of 10 new cases and analysis of the literature. Journal of Oral and Maxillofacial Surgery: Official Journal of the American Association of Oral and Maxillofacial Surgeons. 1994;**52**(5):467-470

[43] Kondoh T, Seto K, Kobayashi K. Osteoma of the mandibular condyle: Report of a case with a review of the literature. Journal of Oral and Maxillofacial Surgery: Official Journal of the American Association of Oral and Maxillofacial Surgeons. 1998;**56**(8):972-979

[44] Bulut E, Acikgoz A, Ozan B, Gunhan O. Large peripheral osteoma of the mandible: A case report. International Journal of Dentistry. 2010;**2010**:834761

[45] Siar CH, Jalil AA, Ram S, Ng KH. Osteoma of the condyle as the cause of limited-mouth opening: A case report. Journal of Oral Science. 2004;**46**(1):51-53

[46] Misra N, Srivastava S, Bodade PR, Rastogi V. Osteoma of temporomandibular joint: a rarity. BMJ case reports. 2013;**2013**:1-5

[47] Thoma KH. Tumors of the condyle and temporomandibular joint. Oral Surgery, Oral Medicine, and Oral Pathology. 1954;**7**(10):1091-1107

[48] Tuzuner Oncul AM, Turalı S, Kadıoglu MN, Ergul KC, Arpacı H, Karasu HA. Benign Tumoral Growths of the Mandibular Condyle. XXI Congress of the European Association for Cranio-Maxillo-Facial Surgery; Dubrovnik, Crotia. Dubrovnik: European Association for Cranio-Maxillo-Facial Surgery; 2012. p. 369-370

[49] Deferm JT, Steens SCA, Vriens D, Bekers EM, Kalaykova SI, Borstlap WA. Chronic temporomandibular joint pain: Two cases of osteoid osteoma and a review of the literature. International Journal of Oral and Maxillofacial Surgery. 2017;**46**(9):1130-1137

[50] An SY, Shin HI, Choi KS, Park JW, Kim YG, Benavides E, et al. Unusual osteoid osteoma of the mandible: Report of case and review of the literature. Oral Surgery, Oral Medicine, Oral Pathology and Oral Radiology. 2013;**116**(2):e134-e140

[51] Tochihara S, Sato T, Yamamoto H, Asada K, Ishibashi K. Osteoid osteoma in mandibular condyle. International Journal of Oral and Maxillofacial Surgery. 2001;**30**(5):455-457

[52] Kroon HM, Schurmans J. Osteoblastoma: Clinical and radiologic findings in 98 new cases. Radiology. 1990;**175**(3):783-790

[53] Goto T, Shinoda Y, Okuma T, Ogura K, Tsuda Y, Yamakawa K, et al. Administration of nonsteroidal anti-inflammatory drugs accelerates spontaneous healing of osteoid osteoma. Archives of Orthopaedic and Trauma Surgery. 2011;**131**(5):619-625

[54] Ohkawa M, Fujiwara N, Tanabe M, Takashima H, Satoh K, Mori Y, et al. Benign osteoblastoma of the temporal bone. AJNR – American Journal of Neuroradiology. 1997;**18**(2):324-326

[55] Wozniak AW, Nowaczyk MT, Osmola K, Golusinski W. Malignant transformation of an osteoblastoma of the mandible: Case report and review of the literature. European Archives of Oto-Rhino-Laryngology: Official Journal of the European Federation of Oto-Rhino-Laryngological Societies (EUFOS): Affiliated with the German Society for Oto-Rhino-Laryngology – Head and Neck Surgery. 2010;**267**(6):845-849

[56] Jones AC, Prihoda TJ, Kacher JE, Odingo NA, Freedman PD. Osteoblastoma of the maxilla and mandible: A report of 24 cases, review of the literature, and discussion of its relationship to osteoid osteoma of the jaws. Oral Surgery, Oral Medicine, Oral Pathology, Oral Radiology, and Endodontics. 2006;**102**(5):639-650

[57] Rawal YB, Angiero F, Allen CM, Kalmar JR, Sedghizadeh PP, Steinhilber AM. Gnathic osteoblastoma: Clinicopathologic review of seven cases with long-term follow-up. Oral Oncology. 2006;**42**(2):123-130

[58] Neville B, Damm DD, Allen C, Chi A. Oral and Maxillofacial Pathology. 4 ed. Missouri: Elsevier; 2016

[59] Emanuelsson J, Allen CM, Rydin K, Sjostrom M. Osteoblastoma of the temporal articular tubercle misdiagnosed as a temporomandibular joint disorder. International Journal of Oral and Maxillofacial Surgery. 2017;**46**(5):610-613

[60] Nishimura K, Satoh T, Maesawa C, Ishijima K, Sato H. Giant cell tumor of the larynx: A case report and review of the literature. American Journal of Otolaryngology. 2007;**28**(6):436-440

[61] van der Heijden L, Dijkstra PD, van de Sande MA, Kroep JR, Nout RA, van Rijswijk CS, et al. The clinical approach toward giant cell tumor of bone. The Oncologist. 2014;**19**(5):550-561

[62] Bibas-Bonet H, Fauze RA, Lavado MG, Paez RO, Nieman J. Garcin syndrome resulting from a giant cell tumor of the skull base in a child. Pediatric Neurology. 2003;**28**(5):392-395

[63] Bertoni F, Unni KK, Beabout JW, Ebersold MJ. Giant cell tumor of the skull. Cancer. 1992;**70**(5):1124-1132

[64] Findlay JM, Chiasson D, Hudson AR, Chui M. Giant-cell tumor of the middle cranial fossa. Case report. Journal of Neurosurgery. 1987;**66**(6):924-928

[65] Manfredini D, Guarda-Nardini L, Winocur E, Piccotti F, Ahlberg J, Lobbezoo F. Research diagnostic criteria for temporomandibular disorders: A systematic review of axis I epidemiologic findings. Oral Surgery, Oral Medicine, Oral Pathology, Oral Radiology, and Endodontics. 2011;**112**(4):453-462

[66] Wulling M, Engels C, Jesse N, Werner M, Delling G, Kaiser E. The nature of giant cell tumor of bone. Journal of Cancer Research and Clinical Oncology. 2001;**127**(8):467-474

[67] Wang CS, Lou JH, Liao JS, Ding XY, LJ D, Lu Y, et al. Recurrence in giant cell tumour of bone: Imaging features and risk factors. La Radiologia Medica. 2013;**118**(3):456-464

[68] Purohit S, Pardiwala DN. Imaging of giant cell tumor of bone. Indian Journal of Orthopaedics. 2007;**41**(2):91-96

[69] Zheng MH, Robbins P, Xu J, Huang L, Wood DJ, Papadimitriou JM. The histogenesis of giant cell tumour of bone: A model of interaction between neoplastic cells and osteoclasts. Histology and Histopathology. 2001;**16**(1):297-307

[70] Lopez-Pousa A, Martin Broto J, Garrido T, Vazquez J. Giant cell tumour of bone: New treatments in development. Clinical & Translational Oncology: Official Publication of the Federation of Spanish Oncology Societies and of the National Cancer Institute of Mexico. 2015;**17**(6):419-430

[71] Xu SF, Adams B, Yu XC, Xu M. Denosumab and giant cell tumour of bone-a review and future management considerations. Current Oncology (Toronto, Ont). 2013;**20**(5):e442-e447

[72] Prasad SC, Piccirillo E, Nuseir A, Sequino G, De Donato G, Paties CT, et al. Giant cell tumors of the skull base: Case series and current concepts. Audiology & Neuro-Otology. 2014;**19**(1):12-21

[73] Chen ZX, DZ G, ZH Y, Qian TN, Huang YR, YH H, et al. Radiation therapy of giant cell tumor of bone: Analysis of 35 patients. International Journal of Radiation Oncology, Biology, Physics. 1986;**12**(3):329-334

[74] Nicoli TK, Saat R, Kontio R, Piippo A, Tarkkanen M, Tarkkanen J, et al. Multidisciplinary approach to management of temporal bone giant cell tumor. Journal of Neurological Surgery Reports. 2016;**77**(3):e144-e149

[75] Branstetter DG, Nelson SD, Manivel JC, Blay JY, Chawla S, Thomas DM, et al. Denosumab induces tumor reduction and bone formation in patients with giant-cell tumor of bone. Clinical Cancer Research: An Official Journal of the American Association for Cancer Research. 2012;**18**(16):4415-4424

[76] Chawla S, Henshaw R, Seeger L, Choy E, Blay JY, Ferrari S, et al. Safety and efficacy of denosumab for adults and skeletally mature adolescents with giant cell tumour of bone: Interim analysis of an open-label, parallel-group, phase 2 study. The Lancet Oncology. 2013;**14**(9):901-908

[77] DelBalso AM, Banyas JB, Wild LM. Hemangioma of the mandibular condyle and ramus. AJNR – American Journal of Neuroradiology. 1994;**15**(9):1703-1705

[78] Lund BA, Dahlin DC. Hemangiomas of the mandible and maxilla. Journal of Oral Surgery, Anesthesia, and Hospital Dental Service. 1964;22:234-242

[79] Guibert-Tranier F, Piton J, Riche MC, Merland JJ, Caille JM. Vascular malformations of the mandible (intraosseous haemangiomas). The importance of preoperative embolization. A study of 9 cases. European Journal of Radiology. 1982;**2**(4):257-272

[80] Barker GR, Sloan P. Intraosseous lipomas: Clinical features of a mandibular case with possible aetiology. The British Journal of Oral & Maxillofacial Surgery. 1986;**24**(6):459-463

[81] Basheer S, Abraham J, Shameena P, Balan A. Intraosseous lipoma of mandible presenting as a swelling. Journal of Oral and Maxillofacial Pathology: JOMFP. 2013;**17**(1):126-128

[82] Hemavathy S, Roy S, Kiresur A. Intraosseous angiolipoma of the mandible. Journal of Oral and Maxillofacial Pathology: JOMFP. 2012;**16**(2):283-287

[83] Buric N, Krasic D, Visnjic M, Katic V. Intraosseous mandibular lipoma: A case report and review of the literature. Journal of Oral and Maxillofacial Surgery: Official Journal of the American Association of Oral and Maxillofacial Surgeons. 2001;**59**(11):1367-1371

[84] Gonzalez-Perez LM, Perez-Ceballos JL, Carranza-Carranza A. Mandibular intraosseous lipoma: Clinical features of a condylar location. International Journal of Oral and Maxillofacial Surgery. 2010;**39**(6):617-620

[85] Sanjuan A, Dean A, Garcia B, Alamillos F, Roldan E, Blanco A. Condylar intramedullary intraosseous lipoma: Contribution of a new case and review of the literature. Journal of Clinical and Experimental Dentistry. 2017;**9**(3):e498-e502

[86] Barnes L, Eveson JW, Reichart P, Sidransky D. World Health Organization Classification of Tumours. Pathology and Genetics of Head and Neck Tumours. IARC: Lyon; 2005

[87] Vegas Bustamante E, Gargallo Albiol J, Berini Aytes L, Gay Escoda C. Benign fibro-osseous lesions of the maxillas: Analysis of 11 cases. Medicina oral, patologia oral y cirugia bucal. 2008;**13**(10):E653-E656

[88] Speight PM, Carlos R. Maxillofacial fibro-osseous lesions. Current Diagnostic Pathology 2006;**12**:1-10

[89] Eversole R, Su L, ElMofty S. Benign fibro-osseous lesions of the craniofacial complex. A review. Head and Neck Pathology. 2008;**2**(3):177-202

[90] YS F, Perzin KH. Non-epithelial tumors of the nasal cavity, paranasal sinuses, and nasopharynx. A clinicopathologic study. II. Osseous and fibro-osseous lesions, including osteoma, fibrous dysplasia, ossifying fibroma, osteoblastoma, giant cell tumor, and osteosarcoma. Cancer. 1974;**33**(5):1289-1305

[91] Chang CC, Hung HY, Chang JY, CH Y, Wang YP, Liu BY, et al. Central ossifying fibroma: A clinicopathologic study of 28 cases. Journal of the Formosan Medical Association = Taiwan yi zhi. 2008;**107**(4):288-294

[92] Zavattero E, Garzino-Demo P, Berrone S. Ossifying fibroma affecting the mandibular condyle: Report of an uncommon case. The Journal of Craniofacial Surgery. 2013;**24**(4):e351-e353

[93] Myers BW, Masi AT. Pigmented villonodular synovitis and tenosynovitis: A clinical epidemiologic study of 166 cases and literature review. Medicine. 1980;**59**(3):223-238

[94] Granowitz SP, D'Antonio J, Mankin HL. The pathogenesis and long-term end results of pigmented villonodular synovitis. Clinical Orthopaedics and Related Research. 1976;**114**:335-351

[95] Oehler S, Fassbender HG, Neureiter D, Meyer-Scholten C, Kirchner T, Aigner T. Cell populations involved in pigmented villonodular synovitis of the knee. The Journal of Rheumatology. 2000;**27**(2):463-470

[96] Choong PF, Willen H, Nilbert M, Mertens F, Mandahl N, Carlen B, et al. Pigmented villonodular synovitis. Monoclonality and metastasis – A case for neoplastic origin? Acta Orthopaedica Scandinavica. 1995;**66**(1):64-68

[97] Vandeweyer E, Somerhausen ND, Andry G. Guess what! clinical course of the patient and histological findings. European Journal of Dermatology: EJD. 2000;**10**(8):639-640

[98] Joshi K, Huang B, Scanga L, Buchman C, Chera BS. Postoperative radiotherapy for diffuse pigmented villonodular synovitis of the temporomandibular joint. American Journal of Otolaryngology. 2015;**36**(1):106-113

[99] Vogrincic GS, O'Connell JX, Gilks CB. Giant cell tumor of tendon sheath is a polyclonal cellular proliferation. Human Pathology. 1997;**28**(7):815-819

[100] Cavaliere A, Sidoni A, Bucciarelli E. Giant cell tumor of tendon sheath: Immunohistochemical study of 20 cases. Tumori. 1997;**83**(5):841-846

[101] Carlson ML, Osetinsky LM, Alon EE, Inwards CY, Lane JI, Moore EJ. Tenosynovial giant cell tumors of the temporomandibular joint and lateral skull base: Review of 11 cases. The Laryngoscope. 2017;**127**(10):2340-2346

[102] Somerhausen NS, Fletcher CD. Diffuse-type giant cell tumor: Clinicopathologic and immunohistochemical analysis of 50 cases with extraarticular disease. The American Journal of Surgical Pathology. 2000;**24**(4):479-492

[103] Kisnisci RS, Tuz HH, Gunhan O, Onder E. Villonodular synovitis of the temporomandibular joint: Case report. Journal of Oral and Maxillofacial Surgery: Official Journal of the American Association of Oral and Maxillofacial Surgeons. 2001;**59**(12):1482-1484

[104] Safaee M, Oh T, Sun MZ, Parsa AT, McDermott MW, El-Sayed IH, et al. Pigmented villonodular synovitis of the temporomandibular joint with intracranial extension: A case series and systematic review. Head & Neck. 2015;**37**(8):1213-1224

[105] Le WJ, Li MH, Yu Q, Shi HM. Pigmented villonodular synovitis of the temporomandibular joint: CT imaging findings. Clinical Imaging. 2014;**38**(1):6-10

[106] Kim KW, Han MH, Park SW, Kim SH, Lee HJ, Jae HJ, et al. Pigmented villonodular synovitis of the temporomandibular joint: MR findings in four cases. European Journal of Radiology. 2004;**49**(3):229-234

[107] Stojadinovic S, Reinert S, Wildforster U, Jundt G. Destruction of the glenoid joint fossa by a tenosynovial giant-cell tumour of the skull base: A case report. International Journal of Oral and Maxillofacial Surgery. 1999;**28**(2):132-134

[108] Rustin MH, Robinson TW. Giant-cell tumour of the tendon sheath – An uncommon tumour presenting to dermatologists. Clinical and Experimental Dermatology. 1989;**14**(6):466-468

[109] Damodar D, Chan N, Kokot N. Pigmented villonodular synovitis of the temporomandibular joint: Case report and review of the literature. Head & Neck. 2015;**37**(12):E194-E199

[110] Carlson ML, Osetinsky LM, Alon EE, Inwards CY, Lane JI, Moore EJ. Tenosynovial giant cell tumors of the temporomandibular joint and lateral skull base: Review of 11 cases. The Laryngoscope. 2016

[111] Ye ZX, Yang C, Chen MJ, Wilson JJ. Juxta-articular Myxoma of the temporomandibular joint. The Journal of Craniofacial Surgery. 2015;**26**(8):e695-e696

[112] Allen PW. Myxoma is not a single entity: A review of the concept of myxoma. Annals of Diagnostic Pathology. 2000;**4**(2):99-123

[113] Somford MP, de Vries JS, Dingemans W, de Jonge M, Maas M, Schaap GR, et al. Juxta-articular myxoma of the knee. The Journal of Knee Surgery. 2011;**24**(4):299-301

[114] Korver RJ, Theunissen PH, van de Kreeke WT, van der Linde MJ, Heyligers IC. Juxta-articular myxoma of the knee in a 5-year-old boy: A case report and review of the literature (2009: 12b). European Radiology. 2010;**20**(3):764-768

[115] Tse JJ, Vander S. The soft tissue myxoma of the head and neck region – Report of a case and literature review. Head & Neck Surgery. 1985;**7**(6):479-483

[116] Mansour OI, Carrau RL, Snyderman CH, Kassam AB. Preauricular infratemporal fossa surgical approach: Modifications of the technique and surgical indications. Skull Base: Official Journal of North American Skull Base Society. 2004;**14**(3):143-151 discussion 51

5

Myofascial Pain Dysfunction Syndrome: Etiology, Diagnosis, and Treatment

Serdar Gözler

Abstract

Myofascial pain dysfunction syndrome (MPDS) is a stomatognathic system disturbance, which consists of pain, jaw movement irregularities, and muscle spasm. Hyperexcitation of peripheral sensory neurons causes a reaction of induction in the motor neuron and then spasms of the masticatory muscles follow. Long-term spasm causes muscular pain and irregular mandibular motion. Pain is the most important inducer and therefore must be managed firstly in order to manage the muscle spasms. Symptomatic treatment approaches may be useful, but after symptom elimination, etiologically based treatment must be provided to the patient. The neurophysiology of the stomatognathic system must be well understood to determine a proper treatment for the MPDS condition. Both symptomatic and etiological treatment methods have been proposed by differing authors as potential solutions for MPDS. Occlusal splints are a commonly used treatment for relieving MPDS symptoms. Alternatively, some forms of occlusal adjustment (not all) have been shown to be an effective, permanent treatment course for myofascial pain dysfunction syndrome. This chapter describes the neural controls over the stomatognathic system and how that system can neurologically promote the MPDS disease state. It then details the computer-guided MPDS occlusal adjustment treatment known as disclusion time reduction that has been shown in many published studies to be a highly effective myofascial pain dysfunction syndrome (MPDS) therapy.

Keywords: MPDS, muscle pain dysfunction syndrome, TMD, stomatognathic system problems, masticatory muscle problems

1. Introduction

In the year 1996, the National institute of Health (NIH, USA) held a conference from which the NIH issued a pamphlet of clinical guidelines regarding temporomandibular disorders (TMD).

In the NIH report as well as from the National Institute of Dental Research (NIDR) (NIH publication no. 94-3487), no distinction was made between temporomandibular disorders and myofascial pain dysfunction syndrome (MPDS). All potential etiological factors, clinical symptoms, the diagnoses and the treatment recommendations fell under the single term, "Temporomandibular Disorders" [1]. There was no clear distinction made between TMJ internal derangements and myofascial pain dysfunction syndrome. Additionally, the final report did not recommend any definitive treatment for temporomandibular disorders. Although the NIH meeting attendees claimed to have solved the "TMJ problem," no consensus was reached making the conference a complete disappointment. However, later in 1999, Dr. Peter Dawson opposed the conference results in an article that was cosponsored by American Equilibration Society (AES, Chicago, IL, USA) [2]. After further numerous arguments, no consensus was found regarding the etiology or treatments that should be applied in TMD cases.

Of note is that 4 years before the release of the NIH report in 1991, Dr. Robert Barry Kerstein from Tufts University School of Dental Medicine in Boston Massachusetts had developed a T-Scan I time-based coronoplasty procedure, which focused on reducing excursive movement disclusion times [3]. According to this study, the length of disclusion time was correlated to high levels of masseter and temporalis excursive muscle activity levels [3] that were of diagnostic importance when evaluating differing etiologic factors of chronic MPDS [2]. These early studies were the beginning of a series of studies about this topic [3, 4]. As Dawson noted in his article, there had been found an evidence-based relationship between occlusion and MPDS. Often MPDS symptoms affected the chewing system mechanics because the symptoms had a close association with the dental occlusion and its relationship to the central nervous system (CNS).

Myofascial pain dysfunction syndrome is a common term that is used in other medical branches outside of Dentistry [5–7]. But in the last few decades, this term has been used in Dental Medicine to describe orofacial chronic pain [8, 9], often abbreviated in the literature as MPDS [3]. MPDS is a functional disease related to the masticatory muscles, the neural structures and the temporomandibular joint structures. MPDS syndrome can be a very uncomfortable condition for a patient. The patient can barely move their mandible, and often there is pain in the face and head area. Sometimes, the pain may extend to neck and dorsal area. Most typical symptoms are acute hypercontraction (spasm) of the muscles, and laxity of the TM joint ligaments. The symptoms of the MPDS are explained in detail later in this chapter [5, 10–12].

Etiologically, the MPDS muscle and TM joint symptoms have been linked primarily to the occlusion [2, 3, 13, 14]. Muscle spasm is caused by occlusal surface friction and prolonged disclusion time overcompressing the posterior tooth PDLs causing hyperfunction and ischemia in the muscles. This leads to muscle fatigue and then poor mandibular movements. This is what leads to deterioration of the movements.

Muscle spasm is usually caused by occlusal surface friction and prolonged disclusion time [15] overcompressing the posterior tooth periodontal ligament mechanoreceptors causing hyperfunction and ischemia in the muscles. This leads to muscle fatigue and then poor mandibular movements [16].

The deterioration of mandibular movements can be accelerated by deterioration of the occlusion. A filling, crown, or a bridge will always cause the occlusion to deteriorate. Alternatively, ligament laxity affects the movements of the joint structures in the glenoid fossa and often occurs without patient awareness of the problem's existence.

Myofascial pain dysfunction syndrome (MPDS) is one particular type of temporomandibular disorder (TMD) [12]. Historically, clinicians and researchers have subclassified TMDs into either intracapsular disorders or masticatory muscle disorders (such as local myalgia, myofascial pain, centrally mediated myalgia, myospasm, myositis, myofibrotic contracture, and masticatory muscle neoplastic disease). TMJ internal derangement may not be involved with MPDS. However, when a temporomandibular joint irregularity occurs along with the symptoms of MPDS, the complete problematic condition should be considered as temporomandibular joint disease [17, 18]. All masticatory organs participating in oral function may or may not be involved in MPDS.

Before discussing about the etiologic factors and treatment techniques related to MPDS, it is necessary to properly understand the neural mechanisms of masticatory system.

Muscular pain is a typical and a decisive symptom of MPDS. Functional disorders that occur in the stomatognathic system are a cause of pain. If the functional disorders are not successfully treated, pain may be present for years. Pain minimization during function is the result of the protective mechanisms within the stomatognathic system.

The most important stomatognathic function is chewing. There is a great relationship between impairment of chewing function and painful muscle problems [13, 16, 17, 19–24]. During the chewing function, tooth contact occurs at the extreme end of the chewing cycle when occlusal force is applied to crush the food bolus. In this way, the resultant chewed food is readied for swallowing. For the chewed food product to be effectively prepared for swallowing, all related functions must occur in a harmonious order. Hence, the duration of chewing, the control of the mandibular movements, the masticatory muscle contractions, the level of force applied during the bolus crush, temporomandibular joint movements, the tooth-tooth interactions, and the neural feedback mechanisms all must interact synergistically (**Figure 1**).

The relationship between muscle malfunction and MPDS is a two-sided problem, where each affects the other. Muscle malfunction triggers MPDS, while MPDS causes impairment of masticatory movements. Stomatognathic system functions are the best diagnostic indicator of dysfunction. The main purpose of the stomatognathic system is to perform the best chewing possible, which requires a very well-coordinated system. As proper chewing evolves within the developmental period of human growth, it becomes optimal during the adult years. Deciduous, mixed, and permanent dentitions have their own chewing patterns [25], with the chewing pattern being closely linked to a person's dental condition [24]. However, corruption of the chewing pattern indicates the beginnings of myofascial distortion [26, 27].

As is the case with other body functions, the chewing pattern results from a complex integration of the neural and the myofascial structures. The resultant product of chewing is chewed food that is readied for swallowing. The most effective determining factor of a good chewing pattern is the dental occlusion [28], whereby the structural posture, the stretching of muscles and the chewing process itself are improved by upper and lower tooth contact. However, changes to the dental occlusion from tooth loss, orthodontic tooth movement, restorative dentistry, or mechanical trauma, all of which can alter the neurologic input significantly, may be the most important etiological factor leading to the impairment of chewing mechanism [19].

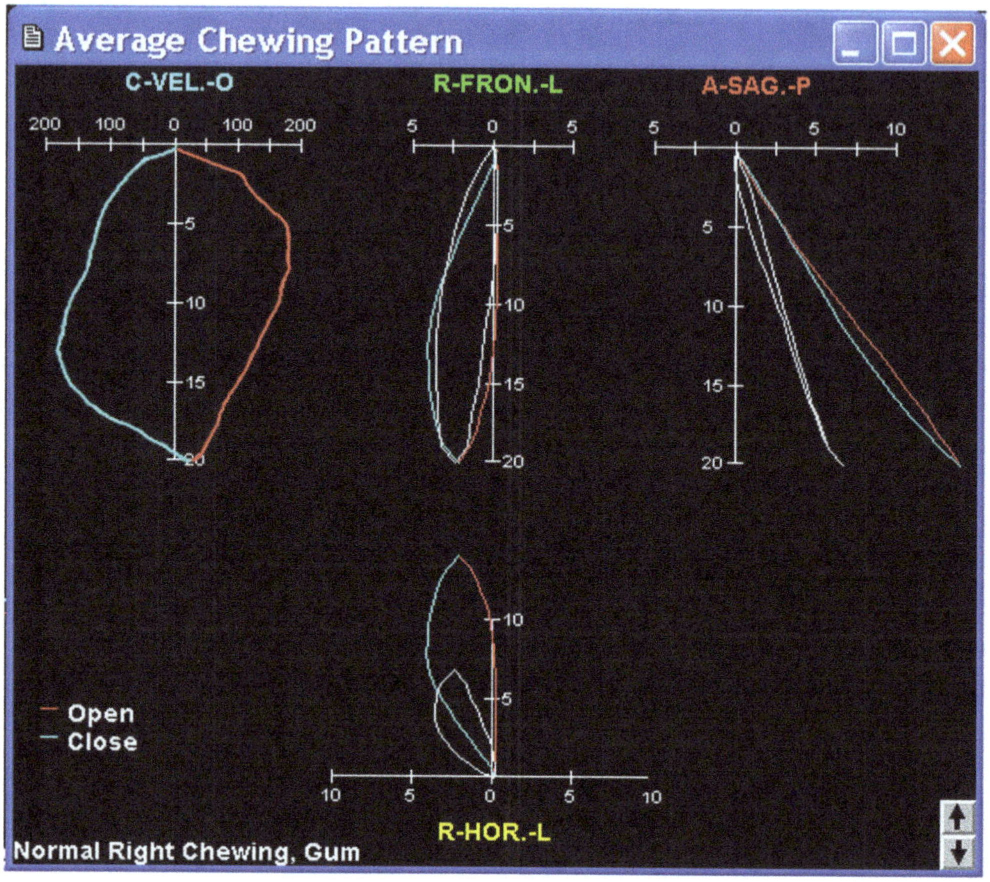

Figure 1. A normal mastication pattern in three planes as recorded by a Jaw Tracker (3-D Electrognathograph, BioResearch Assoc., Milwaukee, WI, USA). Excellent chewing ability evolves in the developing human from youth into the adult years. An ideal chewing pattern requires harmony between all the masticatory functional organs.

Nervous system mechanoreceptors in and around the teeth transmit neural information to the central nervous system (CNS) regarding the nature of the masticatory function. This neural feedback mechanism is designed to protect the physiologic borders of the chewing pattern and controls the masticatory system mechanics. Neural sensors collect all the necessary neural input during chewing function as it is a sensory process. However, the mandibular functional and parafunctional movements are controlled by the motor function of the neural system. The neuromuscular mechanism of stomatognathic system collects the neural input that controls mandibular motion [29, 30].

2. Neuronal mechanism of masticatory system

Myofascial pain dysfunction syndrome (MPDS) can be used as general definition for one type musculoskeletal human disease state that consists of specific muscular symptoms. In a patient with temporomandibular disorders, MPDS often results from the hypercontraction of the masticatory elevator muscles. Spasm of one or more elevator muscles is a serious problem, which may cause pain, muscle tenderness, limitation of mandibular movements, and induce changes in the temporomandibular joint structural alignment. Muscle spasm usually emanates through the central nervous system (CNS) from the neural mechanoreceptors located in and around the teeth that hypercontract the elevator muscles. Along with muscle spasm, painful trigger points can also be a component of the MPDS condition. Some trigger points may be classified as latent [5, 6, 31, 32], in that they only occur when a muscle is pressed upon.

The neuronal mechanism is a determining factor in the development of MPDS. The central nervous system (CNS) controls all activities of the masticatory system including the contraction of masticatory muscles, the sequence of contractions, the level of contraction, the posture of mandible, the mandibular movements, and the resultant occlusal force, all of which are influenced by the occlusal relationship of upper and lower teeth [33]. The control mechanism of the nervous system is based on environmental neural data input. Every function of the masticatory system has a characteristic pattern that occurs within certain physiologic limits. Any overreaching from a physiologic limit can lead to a symptom of a particular problem. For example, any deviation in the opening (or closing) movement of the mandible is often the result of a muscle spasm that occurs during the opening movement. Limited mouth opening mouth (or S-shaped masticatory movement) is also an indication there is a problem within the stomatognathic system. Functional movements that designed by central nervous system (CNS) are outside of their physiologic limits. Many pathological conditions can also be produced by the central nervous system (CNS). If there is a strong but problematic feedback mechanism present in stomatognathic system, certain pathological conditions may increase in frequency and intensity, unless the pathology is not removed. Every type of nonphysiological movement has its own specific characteristics.

3. Central nervous system and the stomatognathic system

The neural system mechanics must be very well understood to ascertain the etiology of a stomatognathic system pathology.

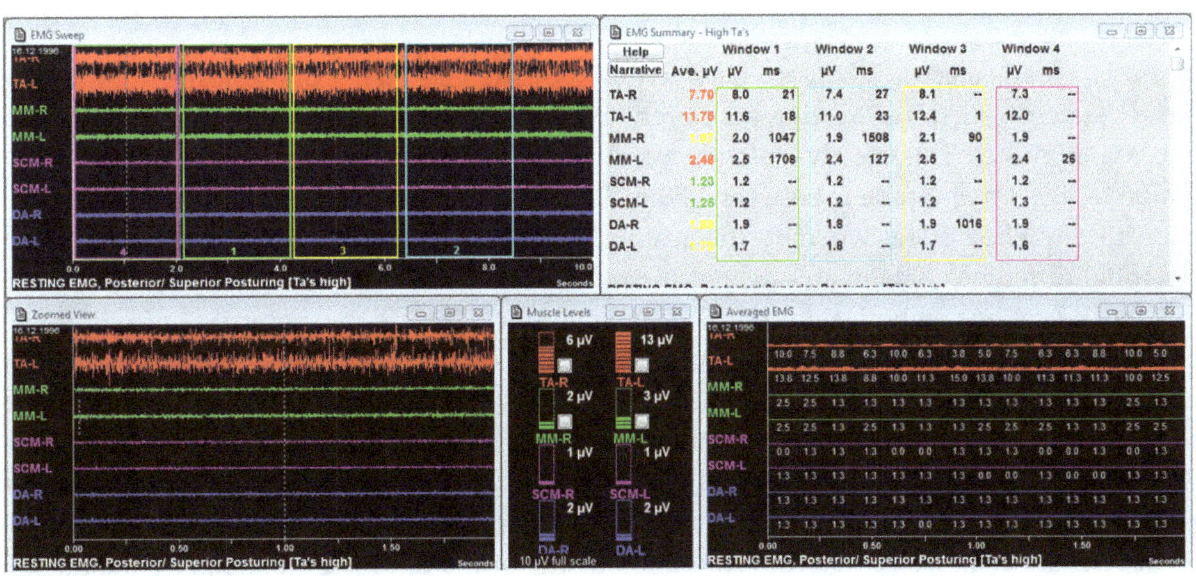

Figure 2. A resting EMG recording of the masseter and temporalis muscles. Note, there is slight electrical activity providing tension to these muscles when holding the mandible in the rest position.

The stomatognathic system neural network is comprised of three basic parts:

1. Perception of the sensory inputs.
2. Evaluation of the gathered inputs.
3. Reaction to the inputs.

Sensory input collection is an ongoing function of the neural system that can be conscious or unconscious. There is a continuous data stream entering the CNS from the peripheral nervous system (PNS), which gathers environmental data that send impulses to the masticatory muscle fibers to establish postural tonus activity. This occurs even when there is no function, such that there is a slight tension in the muscles when at rest (**Figure 2**).

4. Neurons and myocites (muscle cells)

The human body consists of billions of similarly constructed cells that contain the cytoplasm, a nucleus, some chromosomes, some mitochondria, and some ribosomes. But some cells are different from the ordinary cells, despite that they also have cytoplasm, a nucleus, and ribosomes, but also contain neurons. Neurons and muscle cells are an excitable type of cell because they can receive electrical impulses and transfer the environmental neurologic data biochemically. These special cells are known as inducible cells.

The functional unit of the motor system, the motor unit, is composed of a motor neuron and a group of muscle fibers with similar, if not identical, structural and functional properties. These are inducible cells known as neurons and myocites (muscle cell).

5. Membrane potential difference and the firing of a neuron

There is a static electrical balance between the outside and inside of a cell membrane. This steady state is called the "resting membrane potential," which does not change unless there exists a stimulus. This steady-state electrical potential difference between the outside and inside of a cell membrane is between −50 mV and −100 mV. A stimulus changes this steady state to an action state, whereby the resting potential difference is turned into an action potential difference. The main cause of the potential difference results from the existence of anions and cations on both sides of the cell membrane. Outside the membrane are positively charged natrium cations. Positively charged natrium ions attach to negatively charged chlorine ions (Cl−) that are outside of the membrane. However, despite the presence of negative ions (such as chlorine and HCO_3), the outer side of the membrane remains positively charged. Alternatively, the inside of the membrane is negatively charged because positively charged potassium (K+) ions diffuse "down" its steep concentration gradient to move out of a cell via leakage channels. This K+ ion movement to outside of the cell membrane makes the outside more positively charged than inside the cell membrane. Outside the positive ions side at the edge of the membrane, with the inside negative ions located at the inner edge of the membrane.

Therefore, the electrical potential difference exists on both sides of the membrane. A change in the electrical activity within the cell membrane plays an important role in the character of sensory conduction.

6. Neural receptors in the stomatognathic area: the collection of peripheral data and the neural response

All masticatory system functions are governed by the central nervous system (CNS). In order to coordinate what function occurs, and when, how much, and how it should occur physiologically, the CNS gathers information about the environment in which the function is to take place. There is a continuous flow of information between the sensory and motor neurons within the stomatognathic system and the central nervous system (CNS). Physiologically, proper oral functions like mastication, swallowing, and speaking need a rhythmic process whereby all parts of the masticatory system are coordinated so that the activity of the jaw muscles, the tongue, the cheeks, and the lips work synergistically to achieve correct function.

There are two basic neurologic components of mastication:

- the central pattern generator (and the)
- the peripheral control mechanisms

For controlling and managing oral function, the central nervous system (CNS) must initially sense the environmental data. This data collection process is provided to the CNS by the mechano and sensory receptors of the peripheral nervous structures (PNS). Data collected from these receptors are transferred to the other levels of central nervous system (CNS). These receptors are specialized neurons for gathering the environmental sensory data related to the many sensorimotor functions, involving the coordinated contraction and inhibition of the musculature located around the mouth, at the tongue, larynx, pharynx, and esophagus bilaterally [34]. Moreover, according to the localization of the function, there are many differing types of receptors present in the mouth. The data received from receptors are transferred electrochemically to differing levels of the central nervous system (CNS). In this way, the peripheral neural control modulates the output of the central pattern generator and associated motor neurons, so that most effective occlusal forces are developed during chewing, without overly damaging the masticatory organs.

Transmission of the peripheral neural data is provided to the CNS by a neuron's axons and dendrites. Dendrites receive the potential from the previous neuron. If a nerve cell is stimulated, the transmembrane voltage is necessarily changed. The stimulation may be excitatory or inhibitory. If the membrane stimulus is insufficient to cause the transmembrane potential to reach the threshold, then the membrane will not activate. If the excitatory stimulus is strong enough, the transmembrane potential reaches the threshold, and the membrane produces a characteristic electric impulse, known as the *nerve impulse*. This is the basic principle of the stimulus and transmission of a neuron.

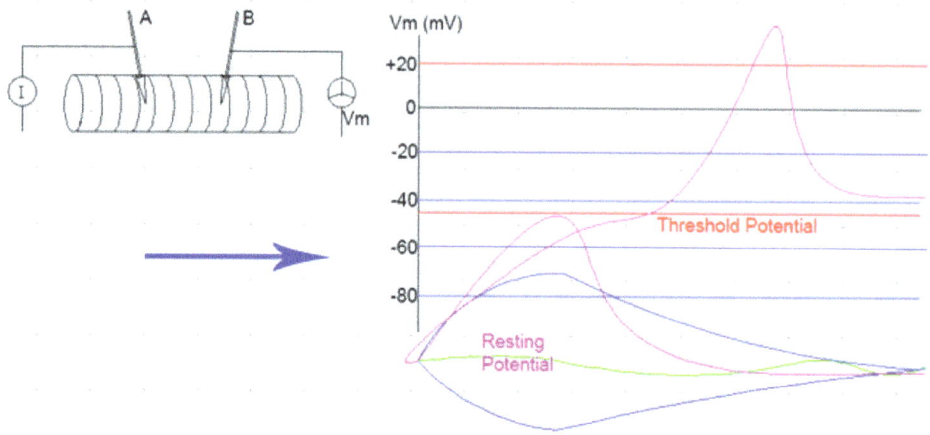

Figure 3. A very tiny premature contact that is not removed for a long time will have a sufficient excitatory level for instigating a nerve impulse. When the total sum level of stimulus reaches the threshold level, an action potential can emerge. This is known as the All-or-None principle.

The membrane potential may reach the threshold by a short, strong stimulus, or by *a longer, weaker stimulus*. A very tiny premature contact that is not removed and is clinically present for a long time will have a sufficient excitatory level for starting a nerve impulse (**Figure 3**). This is the result of nerve cell's All-or-None principle. Premature contacts can lead to pain, which then leads to the formation of a stronger stimulus. The CNS sends a nociceptive warning to the muscles to move the mandible toward the opposite arch side as a reflex action to lessen the pain. If the premature contact on one side was not removed, spasm on the other side tends to persist. Aggregating stimuli will increase the spasms, which may be a major etiological cause of myofascial pain dysfunction syndrome [14] (**Figure 3**).

A sudden nociceptive stimulus can cause a special type escape reflex known as the "jaw jerk reflex." The jaw-jerk myotatic reflex is activated by the sudden stretching of the jaw-closing muscles spindles. The jaw jerk reflex is one of the most important neuronal patterns as it may or may not be nociceptive. The repetition of nociceptive stimuli that causes a reflex action early on during the development of dysfunction may after awhile cease to exist. This adaptation to the stimulus initiates the failure of the CNS to continue to respond to the stimulus. With the jaw jerk mechanism reflex over time, this insensitivity to further immediate noxious stimulation develops irritated neural tissue, which worsens from the intense and prolonged stimulation [7]. This worsening can lead to reduced mandibular vertical opening (**Figure 4**).

Information from the peripheral nervous system (PNS) tissues outside the CNS is continuously transferred into the CNS onto higher centers in the brain stem and cortex for interpretation and evaluation. All human functional and parafunctional movements are based on five major sensory systems:

- Olfaction
- Taste
- Vision
- Hearing
- Touch

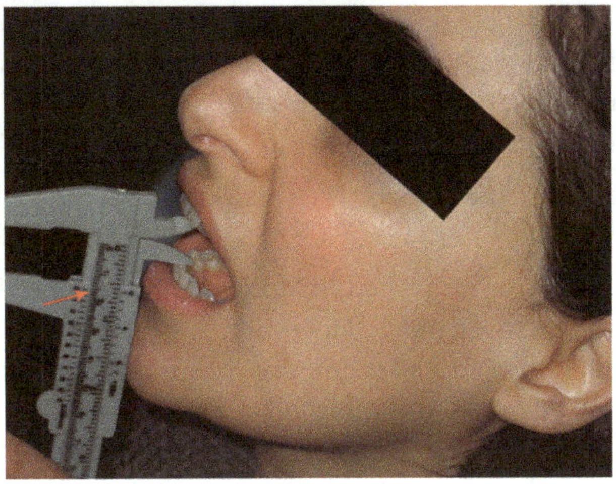

Figure 4. Spasm of the elevator muscles and limited maximum mouth opening of less than 25 mm indicates this women exhibits significant muscular dysfunction. This critical distance of healthy limited opening in men is 35–40 mm.

Touch sensory activity (Touch) is the critical neurologic control for the stomatognathic system's functional and parafunctional movements.

Neural receptors perform two important tasks:

- The gathering of sensory information
- The transfer of the sensory response into the CNS and then back out to the muscles.

Mandibular functional movement sensory detection and the associated reflex responses are shaped by information gathered from the periodontal ligament mechanoreceptors in response to tooth compressions during chewing and from the temperature and touch receptors present in the pulp, the gingival tissues, and the mucobuccal tissues. One of the most important neural receptors is the pulpal mechanoreceptors, which together with periodontal mechanoreceptors carry tooth loading information to the CNS. These receptors transmit the intensity of force acting on a tooth as it contacts its opposing tooth counterpart, the changes of the force velocity at occlusal impact, a tooth's movement direction during chewing, and the hardness of the food bolus. Moreover, the periodontal ligaments are also extremely important structures because their mechanoreceptors within the PDL are highly concentrated [34–38]. Receptors in the periodontal ligaments control and guide all functional and parafunctional movements because they relay information about the magnitude of tooth loads, which is described by the mean firing rate response of loaded periodontal receptors [34].

Several studies have indicated that the extracellular matrix collagens of the periodontal ligament have a high turnover and remodeling rate that are much higher than collagen turnover observed in the gingiva, skin, and bone [39]. The periodontal ligaments themselves are basically striated muscles with muscle spindles located within the fibers of the ligaments. These ligament fiber muscle spindles gather stretching and compression information when teeth are under tooth movement within the PDL space.

Periodontal mechanoreceptors respond to the forces that are applied to teeth. They have been studied in histological and electrophysiological investigations that illustrated periodontal mechanoreceptors signal information about the degree of tooth loads because they have special force-encoding properties, which provides for functional control of human mastication. Microneurography recordings from single nerve fibers revealed that human periodontal receptors adapt slowly to maintained tooth loads. Most receptors are broadly tuned to the direction of force application, while about half respond to forces that are applied to more than one tooth at a time. Populations of periodontal receptors reliably encode information about both how the teeth are stimulated, and the direction that forces are applied to the individual teeth.

Another important receptor type is "periodontal ligament integrins" [40], which are cell-surface receptors that connect cells to the collagen-rich and mechanically stressed periodontal ligament microenvironment. Mutations in integrin subunits have been found to cause clinical disorders in man that correlate well with mice, in which the same integrins are deleted [40]. Integrins are able to transduce signals intracellularly following ligand binding ("outside-in" signaling). However, unlike most other cell receptors, integrins can shift between high- and low-affinity conformations for ligand binding, whereby the signal direction is reversed ("inside-out" signaling). Depending on the cell type, integrins can be either basally activated, as is the case with most adherent cells that are attached to a basement membrane, or they can be basally inactive, like platelets or leukocytes that freely circulate until activated to undergo platelet aggregation or mediate an inflammatory response [41].

Ultimately, all the collected load data from the pulp, the periodontal ligament receptors, and the mucosa are transmitted to the CNS via the trigeminal nerve (V) ganglions. Ganglions are the neurologic distribution center for both the afferent and efferent neural pathways.

Basically, there are two important ganglions involved in craniofacial area with neuroanatomic ties to the stomatognathic system:

- Trigeminal ganglion
- Mesencephalic nucleus

6.1. Pain: an alarm system for protection of the body

Living organisms need to be able to sense their immediate environment if they are to withdraw from or avoid potentially hazardous situations. One of the most typical examples of this protective mechanism is jaw jerk reflex. Sudden, strange matter that is perceived during chewing leads to the formation of this reflex. However, shortly after the identification of a hard substance, the central nervous system (CNS) reduces the reflex level to normal levels. Sometimes, the jaw jerk reflex may occur as a nociceptive reaction. For example, touching the pulp meter to the tooth surface can lead to a typical jaw jerk reflex.

Reflexes are involuntary and relatively stereotyped responses to specific stimuli. Stimulated receptors send afferent impulses to the central nervous system (CNS), which are then transmitted through efferent nerve fibers to the cells, muscles, and organs that carry out the *reflex response*. The entire pathway is known as the *reflex arc* [42]. The afferent impulses generated at the receptors are conveyed via fast-twitch Ia fibers to the spinal alpha motor neuron. Their α_1 process impulses excite the agonistic muscle of an opposing muscle pair. Despite the monosynaptic nature of intrinsic reflexes, extrinsic reflexes are polysynaptic, where there are both afferent and efferent arms within the chain of spinal interneurons.

A protective reflex is not continuous because the reflex stimulus is defined in the memory, and after few cycles, it does not cause the repeated reflex. Development of the multicellular structures in the nervous system evolves a specialized apparatus that detects and reacts to external stimuli, when combined together with the evolution of specific transduction proteins, and enables the CNS to accurately differentiate between innocuous and noxious stimuli. This early warning system, which is further elaborated, develops the capacity to increase its sensitivity following an exposure to an injurious stimulus, which is known as nociceptive sensitization. In mammals, the early warning protective pain that occurs in response to noxious stimuli (nociceptive pain) is mediated by specialized, high-threshold primary sensory neurons (nociceptors) [43].

Pain management is one of the most important therapeutic interventions. Chronic pain is the main reason that patients seek out health care, while also being the most common reason for disability and addiction, and being the highest driver of health care costs. Most often, myopain conditions are the pain source. As such, it has been reported that in the United States, more than 100 million adults suffer from myofascial pain dysfunction syndrome. In dentistry, MPDS is defined as one type of masticatory system problem [32]. However, myofascial pain (MFP) is the most common cause of persistent regional back pain, headaches, and facial pain [10].

Myofascial pain is pain that arises from the muscles or the related fascia. The trigger point concept has been a widely studied aspect of myofascial pain dysfunction syndrome. Many hypotheses of how trigger points evolve are based on the opinions of experienced clinicians who treat and research trigger points. Trigger points are most often discussed as a component of myofascial pain syndromes where widespread or regional muscular pain is associated with hyperalgesia, psychological disturbance, and significant restriction of daily function [44]. Trigger points are 2–5 mm diameter points of increased hypersensitivity in palpable bands of the skeletal muscle, tendons, and ligaments with decreasing hypersensitivity as one palpates the band further away from the trigger point. As stated before, trigger points may be active or latent. An active trigger point causes spontaneous pain at rest, with an increase in pain on contraction or stretching of the involved muscle. There is often restricted muscular range of motion. Any pain on motion may cause "pseudo-muscle weakness" due to pin reflex inhibition. A latent trigger point is a focal area of tenderness and tightness in a muscle that does not result in spontaneous pain, but must be palpated to elicit the pain. However, a latent trigger point may restrict the range of motion and result in weakness of the muscle involved.

The characteristic symptoms of a myofascial pain dysfunction syndrome trigger points have been previously described by R. Bennett as follows [5]:

1. A focal point of tenderness to palpation of the muscle involved,
2. Patient complaint from trigger point palpation,
3. Palpation reveals an induration of the adjacent muscle (the "taut band"),
4. A restricted range of motion in the muscle involved,
5. Pain is accompanied by pseudo-weakness of the muscle involved,
6. Referred pain can result with continuous applied pressure on the trigger point that lasts approximately 5 s in duration.

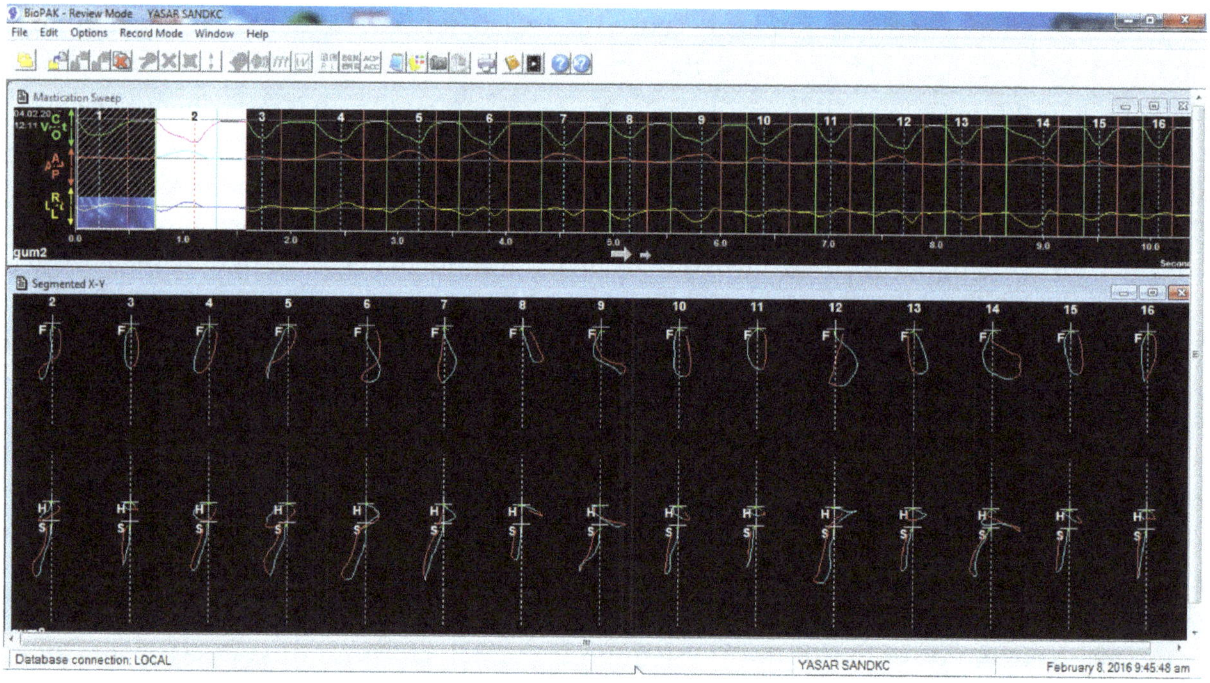

Figure 5. Irregular masticatory pattern of a patient with new denture while the CNS tries to develop a new chewing pattern to accommodate the new denture. Chewing patterns are not similar to each other and irregular.

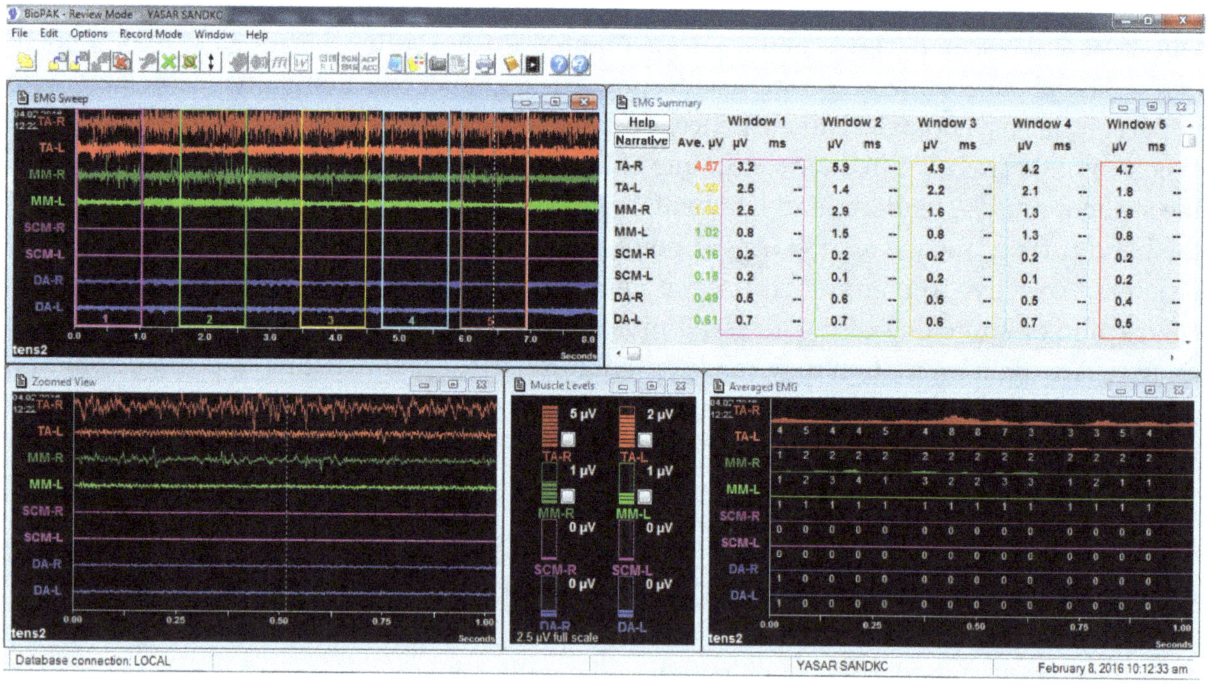

Figure 6. Both the temporalis and masseter muscle electrical activity levels are higher than the physiological average resting values. This is not unexpected during the development of new prosthesis adaptation.

Pain perception is not simply determined by the intensity of nociceptive stimulation but also depends upon psychological factors such as the emotional and motivational state of the patient. The chronic pain threshold is divergent from the patient's level of fear and/or anxiety [45]. Memory and pain, though two richly diverse fields, have many underlying commonalities. Both, for example, contain conscious and unconscious processes that allow for the acquisition of altered behavior in response to environmental stimuli [46]. After a very hot liquid is brought into the mouth, this warm sensation will be placed in the permanent memory to be remembered easily in later scenarios where the patient will drink a very hot liquid once again. However, if a new hot liquid experience is repeated a number of times over a long time frame, the patient's reflex response to hot liquid will slowly disappear. As a learned function repeats, it becomes a reflex state.

A new complete denture adaptation process a patient must go through when receiving a different prosthesis than they are physically used to involves the development of a new denture chewing model. If the new prosthesis causes pain, the pain will be perceived as more prominent in the patients' psyche, compared to the known chewing pattern of the old denture that was saved in the patient's memory. The central nervous system (CNS) will develop a reflex protective mechanism against the pain, such that the protected pattern of chewing will take a very different shape from a healthy average chewing pattern (**Figure 5**).

The electromyographic record of the same patient with the new denture shows that all four elevator muscles are in hyperactivity, exhibiting higher than the average values (**Figure 6**).

7. The importance of breaking the pain cycle in treatment of MPDS; the role of occlusal splints

Chronic pain is a habitual pattern generated by the central nervous system (CNS) that must be broken before trying to treat myofascial pain dysfunction syndrome.

Chronic pain is a nonphysiologic and extraordinary somatosensory process that can take place either in the peripheral or central nervous systems that is sustained beyond the normally expected time frame relative to the existence of a stimulus. This scenario, although somewhat explanatory, only provides for part of the story. Chronic pain is often clandestinely ambiguous and can be difficult to pinpoint its primary causative location. The perception of pain results from the summation and culmination of the nerve transduction process that arises from temporarily stimulated and affected peripheral nociceptors. Nociceptors may be specific for painful stimuli or they may be generally responsive to a wide range of mechanical, thermal, chemical, and/or electrical stimuli. Nociceptive responses are transmitted from peripheral sites into the CNS via myelinated (type A-delta) or unmyelinated (type C) nerve fibers [47].

Masticatory system myofascial pain constitutes one of the most important chronic problems that is encountered in clinical dental practice. Pain is a critical factor in evolving this chronic problem because pain increases muscle contraction, and more spasms from the excess contractions increase the level of pain. Elongation of the contraction time leads to the formation of trigger points.

Within the literature, dental occlusion appears to be a key causative agent for MPDS because all kinds of treatment suggestions for MPDS are targeted on changing the occlusion in some way. In a study by Laskin et al. [48], the authors remarked that although many aspects of the MPDS are either controversial or unexplored, most investigators and clinicians seem to agree that the majority of patients with MPDS report relatively rapid improvement or symptom disappearances with splint therapy [48]. Splint therapy is a very effective occlusion determinant because when splint is placed between occluding teeth, the occlusion changes dramatically which can quickly break the pain generating pattern. However, all researchers agree that a splint therapy protocol must be provided by only skilled clinicians.

There are many types of splints in dentistry such as custom splints, prefabric splints, posterior splints, anterior jig, hard splints, soft splints, etc. Each splint is described in detail by its advocate. The following factors should be taken into account during splint construction [44, 49]:

1. The treatment protocol must be provided by skilled clinicians
2. All masticatory activities can be changed by changing the occlusion
3. Splint therapy changes the tooth-to-tooth occlusal relationships, which then changes the neuromuscular activity accordingly
4. Prolonged hyperactivity of muscles can cause heightened synaptic transmission. Consequently, long contraction durations decrease action potential threshold levels and decrease the patient's pain threshold.
5. During the use of a splint, there must be careful follow-up; if complications occur from splint treatment, the therapy should be terminated immediately.
6. If the splint is only used for a temporary occlusal correction, a 3–4 day use period should be sufficient. The best splints to be used for this purpose are either hydrostatic splints or hard splints because the surface of these designs does not allow teeth to engage and clash, which allows the masticatory muscles to freely exist in a harmonic balance.
7. After acquiring muscle balance and improved physiologic muscle contraction reestablishment, splint therapy must be stopped and an etiological treatment must be initiated.

Basically, splints are applied for a specific purpose [48, 50–52]. Therefore, it is very important to determine the type of splint, application period, and schedule, if applicable (**Figure 7**). Using a proper splint for a longer period of time may cause the patient to worsen in a variety of ways (worsening of MPDS symptoms; creating an open occlusion, intruding of teeth out of occlusal contact). Hence, splint treatment duration and its daily schedule are important to manage properly.

7.1. Occlusal analysis and occlusal adjustments

Removing of premature contacts with occlusal adjustment is one of the most important methods for breaking the neuromuscular cycle in myofascial pain dysfunction syndrome [53]. Changing the occlusal scheme and balancing of the occlusion are very effective methods for pinpointing and eliminating extraordinary neural firings. Hence, an occlusal analysis has always been an important diagnostic component of the treatment efforts to resolve MPDS symptoms. Several decades ago, dentists were performing occlusal analysis solely with mounted casts on semi-adjustable or fully adjustable dental articulators. There was no scientific method for performing intraoral occlusal analysis, and no real effective way to measure occlusal forces between all the contacting teeth.

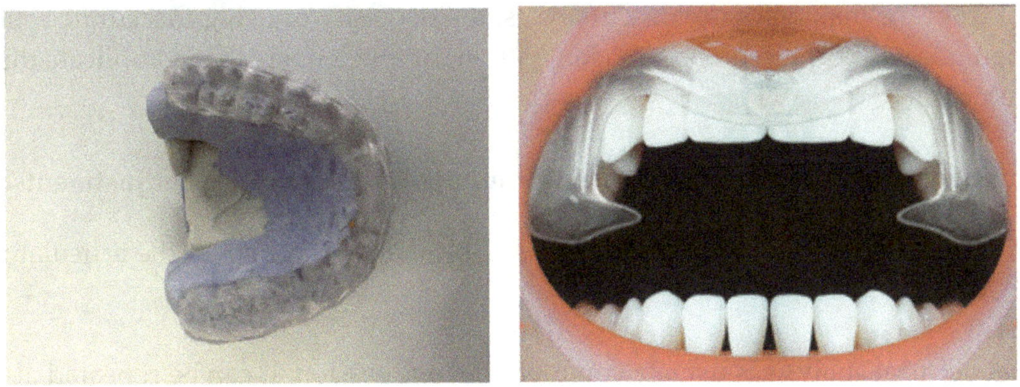

(a) (b)

Figure 7. Splint therapy must be performed by a skilled clinician. Hard splints are very effective for changing the occlusal relationship between upper and lower jaws (maxillary splint; left pane). Hydrostatic soft splints (right pane) are helpful in creating muscular balance and physiologic harmonization. An etiologically based treatment for MPDS can be instituted after 3–5 days of successful splint therapy.

The very simple principal rule that was widely believed, purported is that proper occlusal function resulted from the close relationship between condylar movements and the occlusal contact relationships. To utilize this thinking clinically, most articulator systems were designed with the following requirements:

1. Some special equipment was built to detect condylar movements. The Lauritzen Hinge Axis Locator [54, 55] or Condylator Joint Tracer [56, 57] are examples of these types of condylar movement analysis tools. However, these devices are not easy to manage, often require repeated and difficult-to-make registrations, both intra- and extra-orally [58].

2. Completion of the condylar tracing procedure usually requests more than one visit.

3. Registration of centric relation location needs special devices and careful working.

4. Articulator-based diagnostic work is not repeatable and cannot be digitally stored. It is difficult to compare two different analyses on the same articulator, as one must be removed to mount another set of casts.

5. Two different registrations may be quite different, spatially. This difference can arise from making registrations at different times of the day for both the operator and the patient, from impression material setting distortion, registration material setting distortion, and from differing degress of poured stone setting contraction. Because many variables come into play with the articulating of dental casts, precision levels of the differing analyses may be quite inconsistent from one analysis to another.

Therefore, occlusal analysis performed on articulators for occlusal adjustment can be difficult and time-consuming; and once completed, it is not necessarily reliably to be accurate for diagnosis and treatment.

The development of the computerized occlusal analysis method (T-Scan 9, with the Novus Recording Handle, and the HD Recording Sensor, Tekscan, Inc. S. Boston, MA, USA) has been removed from the making of occlusal analyses, the necessity of using inaccurate articulator-based methods, which present the clinician with many challengers that complicate their clinical usefulness.

7.2. Computer-based occlusal analyses and computer-guided occlusal adjustments

Computer-based occlusal analyses have many clinical advantages over the articulator-based method:

1. Digital occlusal analysis is usually completed in one session. It can be repeated at another session, if there is a need.
2. Digital occlusal analysis data can be stored and recalled easily, so that many analyses of a single patient can be compared with each other, over time, to observe changes in the occlusal status as the patient ages.
3. The recording and data acquisition is quick to accomplish chairside, so that many occlusal analyses and corrective adjustments can be performed in same treatment session.
4. Adjustment results can be compared with the preoperative status of the occlusion to observe that occlusal force and timing improvements have been therapeutically obtained.
5. The cost of performing the occlusal analysis has decreased sharply.

As with every new method, the earliest T-Scan computer-based occlusal analyzing systems (T-Scan I, II, III; Tekscan Inc. S. Boston, MA, USA) were questioned as to their clinical reliability [59, 60]. However, the modern The T-Scan HD recording sensor (**Figure 8a**) has been shown to accurately measure 256 differing relative occlusal force levels [3–6, 55, 61] with 95% of force reproduction capability [4]. Other recent T-Scan studies show the T-Scan accurately records occlusal contact time sequencing [62, 63]. Today's T-Scan Novus System with the version 9 software is a highly advanced digital occlusal force and timing analyzer that can be used

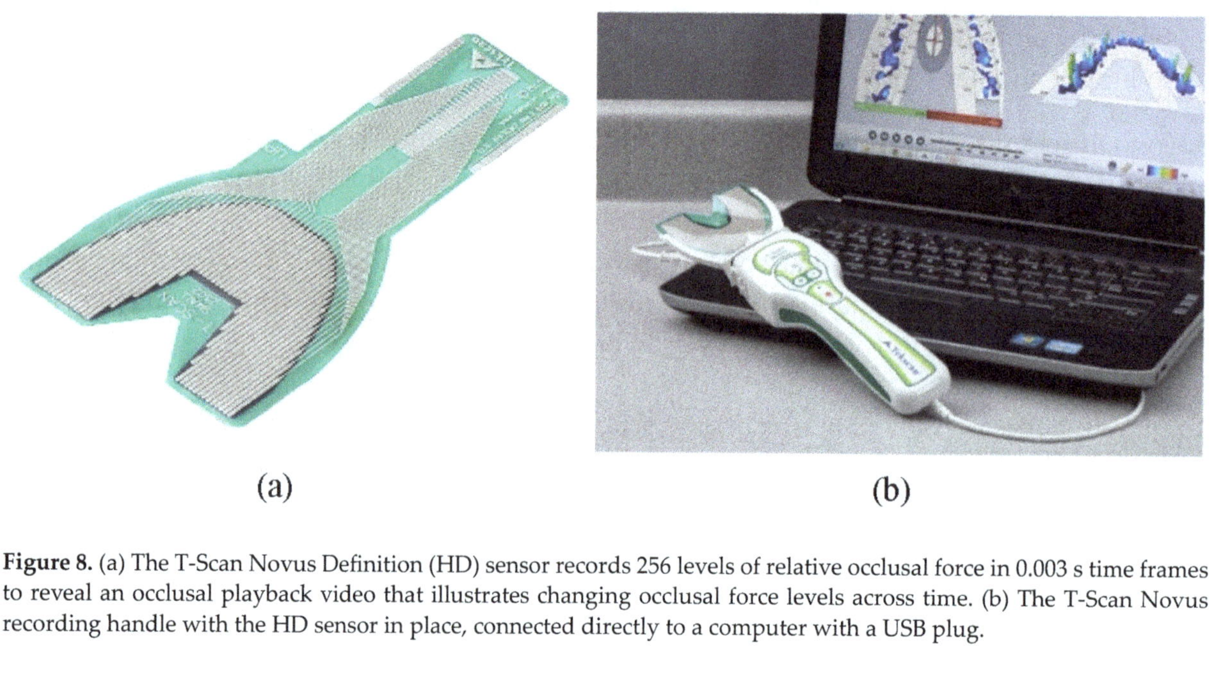

(a) (b)

Figure 8. (a) The T-Scan Novus Definition (HD) sensor records 256 levels of relative occlusal force in 0.003 s time frames to reveal an occlusal playback video that illustrates changing occlusal force levels across time. (b) The T-Scan Novus recording handle with the HD sensor in place, connected directly to a computer with a USB plug.

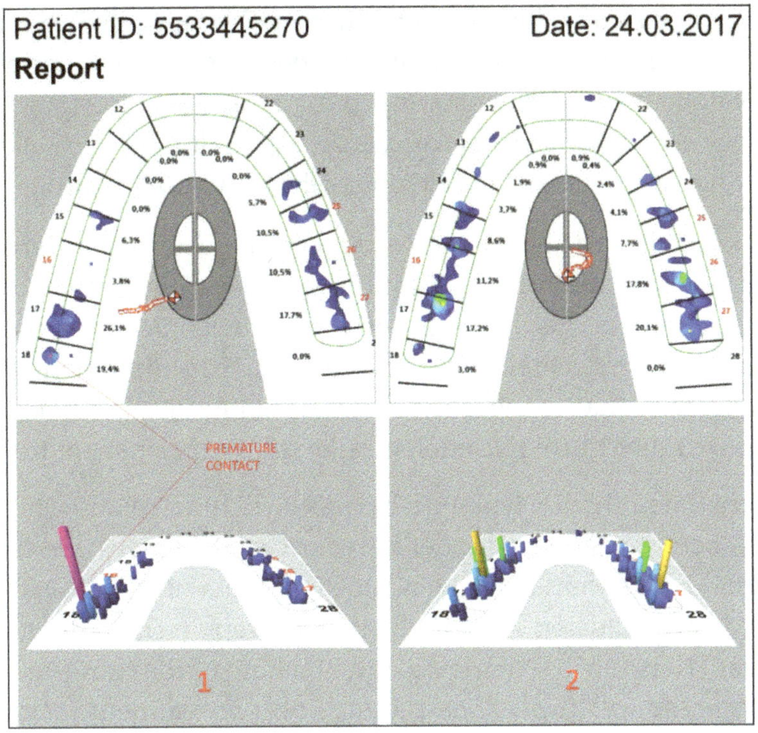

Figure 9. Premature contacts are contacts that rise to very high force well before the maximum intercuspal position (MIP) (pane 1) are visible with the T-Scan occlusal analysis system. Tooth #18 rises quickly to high occlusal force (tall pink column; left pane #1), as other closure contacts are low force (dark blue columns; left pane #1). Then later in the same T-Scan recording (pane 2), the #18 forceful contact lessens to low force while other occluding teeth increased in force bilaterally (pane #2).

chairside to treat a wide range of commonly encountered occlusal force problems. Moreover, additional research and clinical publications have illustrated how the T-Scan occlusal analysis method can be used in many dental medicine disciplines (**Figure 8a** and **b**) [64–67].

The correction of orthodontic and prosthodontic occlusal problems has become much easier for clinicians who use computerized occlusal analysis. Prior to the development of the T-Scan, dentists could only "look at" the occlusion, and now with T-Scan sensor interposed between occluding teeth during mandibular functional movements, dentists are able to see occlusal force changes over time as occlusal contacts on opposing teeth engage and interact frictionally (**Figure 9**). Note in **Figure 9** how during the early part of a patient self-closure into MIP, tooth #18 rises quickly to high occlusal force (tall pink column; left pane #1), as all the other closure tooth contacts maintain a low force state (dark blue columns; left pane#1). Then later in the same T-Scan recording, when more of the patient's teeth fully interdigitate closer to complete intercuspation, the #18 premature forceful contact lessens to a low force state, while other occluding teeth increased in force bilaterally (light green and yellow columns: right pane #2).

7.3. Disclusion time reduction therapy with the immediate complete anterior guidance development coronoplasty

Changing occlusal relationships between the upper and lower teeth breaks sharply the neuromuscular loop that causes acute muscle spasm. There are many studies that have shown the effect periodontal receptors have on functional and parafunctional occlusal excursions [34–38, 68]. An occlusal movement is modeled within the central nervous system (CNS), but the main trigger of action potential firing is the excitation of peripheral neurons from the peripheral nervous system (PNS) [33]. Continuous peripheral neuronal firing causes ongoing muscle contractions that lead to muscle fatigue and ischemia from toxic lactic acid buildup, which all ultimately leads to muscle spasms that rise and repeatedly peak, unless the continuous neuronal firing stopped.

This neurologic mechanism is the main reason why adjusting the dental occlusion with T-Scan time-based occlusal surface modifications has been highly effective MPDS therapy [4–38, 59, 69–71]. Applying occlusal splints, local anesthetic injections, botox injections, and similar nonocclusal treatment methods are temporary and symptomatic. Orthodontic treatment, restorative dentistry that changes the occlusal relationship, and occlusal coronoplasty are treatments aimed at the neurologic etiologically and are permanent treatment methods.

It has long been advocated that to achieve a balanced occlusal relationship, the acute spasm must be eliminated before commencing definitive occlusal changes. Occlusal splints are the most common method for eliminating the acute symptoms of MPDS. However, since 1991, a new T-Scan-based "Disocclusion Time Reduction Therapy (DTR)" method has been developed by Dr. Robert B. Kerstein, for changing and breaking of the firing-reaction-spasm in the neuromuscular loop. The treatment itself requires no pretreatment splint therapy and has been shown in multiple studies performed over the past 26 years to rapidly lessen muscle activity levels and improve human chewing function in 7 days following initial treatment because the therapy works from within the CNS [69, 70, 72–74]. According to Dr. Kerstein, "Disocclusion Time Reduction Therapy" reduces the Disocclusion Time [15], which lessens the time posterior teeth frictionally engage during excursions, which thereby stops the neuronal action potentials from hyperfunctioning the masticatory muscles. To accomplish this, the Disocclusion time must be less than 0.4 s per excursion. However, this particular time of 0.4 s cannot be accurately calculated without using the T-Scan occlusal analysis system. Disocclusion time reduction therapy is one of the most important, etiologically directed treatment methods available because it drastically lessens the volume of PDL mechanoreceptor compressions thereby disrupting the neuronal trigger for occlusally induced MPDS symptoms. However, there are still many disagreements on the reliability of the "Disocclusion Time Reduction Therapy", despite it being repeatedly shown in multiple studies to affect positive physiologic changes within the stomatognathic system. As DTR is usually performed as a coronoplasty (known as immediate complete anterior guidance development (ICAGD)), [9] these disagreements about DTR's patient benefits are founded in that prior, unmeasured occlusal adjustment studies where no T-Scan measurements of the occlusion were involved in the rendered treatment have shown limited occlusal equilibration effectiveness in treating MPDS symptoms. Occlusal equilibration procedurally lacks precision and treats positionally eliminating the prematurity from CR-CO, while only adjusting nonworking side interferences [75–78]. Periodontal neuronal mechanoreceptors surround all teeth on all sides of the roots. By leaving the working side teeth untreated meant occlusal equilibration to CR did not alter the CNS input enough to obtain predictable therapeutic MPDS results.

ICAGD is very different occlusal adjustment procedure from occlusal equilibration [79], in that ICAGD is an excursively focused coronoplasty performed from the maximum intercuspal position (MIP) without mandibular manipulation to centric relation. ICAGD is a measurement-driven, computer-guided occlusal adjustment procedure that shortens prolonged excursive movement occlusal surface contact frictional durations. The main objective of ICAGD is to shorten the posterior disclusion time to ≤0.5 s per excursion because 0.41 was the first studied, physiologic mean disclusion time. ICAGD is always performed today with the T-Scan synchronized to the BioEMG III Electromyography system (T-Scan 9/BioEMG III, Tekscan Inc. S. Boston, MA, USA; Bioresearch Assoc., Milwaukee, WI, USA). The patient wears electromyography electrodes upon the masseter and temporalis muscles throughout the entire occlusal adjustment process to ensure that changes in muscle hyperactivity can be properly observed post treatment.

Most importantly, ICAGD treats both the working and nonworking sides including all premolars involved in excursive contacts, thereby greatly reducing the PDL and pulpal mechanoreceptor CNS input from all fictionally engaged posterior occlusal surfaces. All these procedural differences are published in occlusal adjustment studies, ICAGD has been shown to be far more effective than Occlusal Equilibration in treating MPDS.

8. Disclusion time reduction case example

An example of disocclusion time reduction therapy performed with the immediate complete anterior guidance development coronoplasty is presented below.

8.1. Patient description

A 30-year-old female airline flight attendant presented with a Class I anterior relationship post orthodontics that was completed in her teenage years. A number of posterior teeth demonstrated cuspal wear and appear slightly sanded away. All third molars were previously extracted (**Figures 10** and **11a**, **b**).

8.2. History and presentation of occlusal disease

For 1.5 years before consultation, the patient had experienced chronic bilateral masseter tension, with regular morning jaw soreness that worsened during stressful periods. The patient reported clenching during the day and bruxing to some degree during the nighttime. Most of her discomfort was in the masseter region bilaterally, with some temporal headache

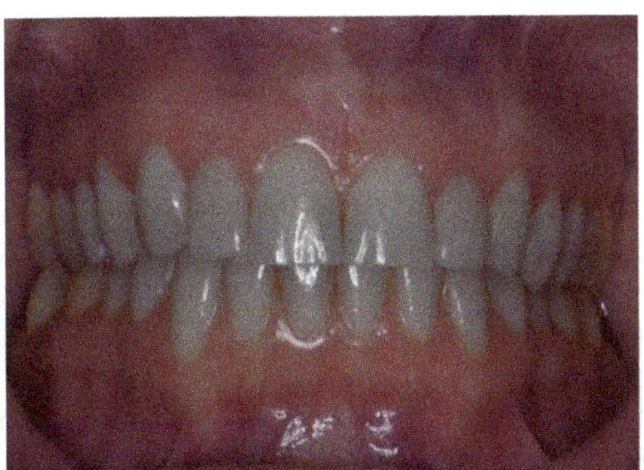

Figure 10. Frontal view of an MPDS female patient showing a Class I anterior relationship with average vertical overlap and available canine guidance contacts bilaterally.

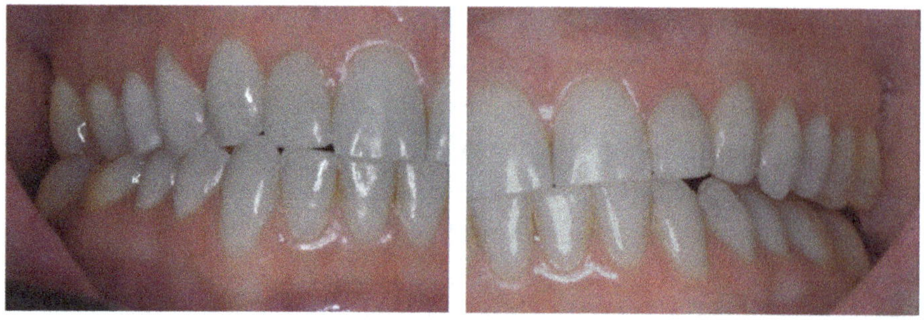

(a) (b)

Figure 11. (a) 1 mm into the right excursion as the canine teeth began to engage. Note the complete buccal posterior group function and excursive friction visible. (b) Early in the left lateral movement, opposing posterior teeth frictionally engage both buccally and lingually (unseen). The posterior group function visible is worsened by the nonvertical opposing tooth orientation.

(a)

(b)

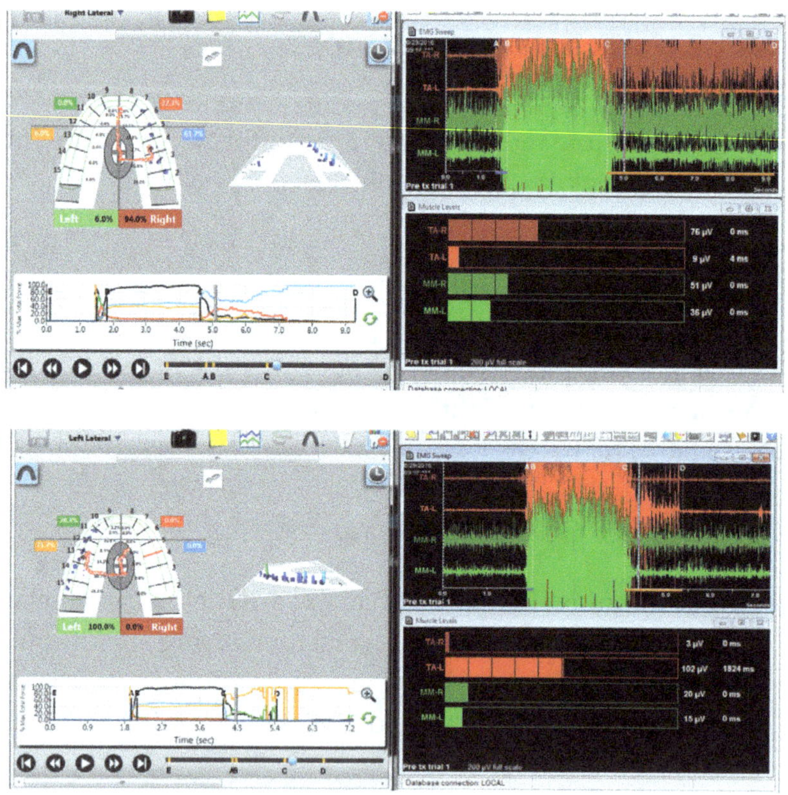

Figure 12. (a) The preoperative right excursive T-Scan/BioEMG data showed (in the T-Scan left pane) prolonged disclusion time with mostly working and minimal balancing excursive frictional occlusal contacts present in the 2D and 3D ForceViews. Between C and D (in the EMG data right pane), there was very high muscle contractions visible in the two masseter MM-R MM-L and right temporalis muscles TA-R, as the patient moved laterally across their teeth toward the right canine. The nonworking (left temporalis TA-L) does not fire in the right excursion. The right disclusion time pretreatment was 3.58 s long, causing this high muscle firing and the MPDS symptoms the patient has been forced to live with since her bite changed after the upper premolar fillings were done. (b) The preoperative left excursive T-Scan/ BioEMG data showed (in the T-Scan left pane) prolonged disclusion time with only working side excursive frictional occlusal contacts present in the 2D and 3D ForceViews the total force (black) line "step downs," indicating sharp force drops as the patient's posterior teeth frequently stopped the mandible from moving freely laterally. Between C and D (in the EMG data right pane), there was very high muscle contractions left temporalis TA-L muscle with right temporalis TA-R spasm visible for the same duration the left temporalis hyperfunctions. The right and left masseters MM-R and MM-L both fired excursively well above rest. The left disclusion time pretreatment was 1.37 s long causing the visible high muscle firing and the MPDS symptoms the patient has been forced to live with since her bite changed after the upper premolar fillings were done.

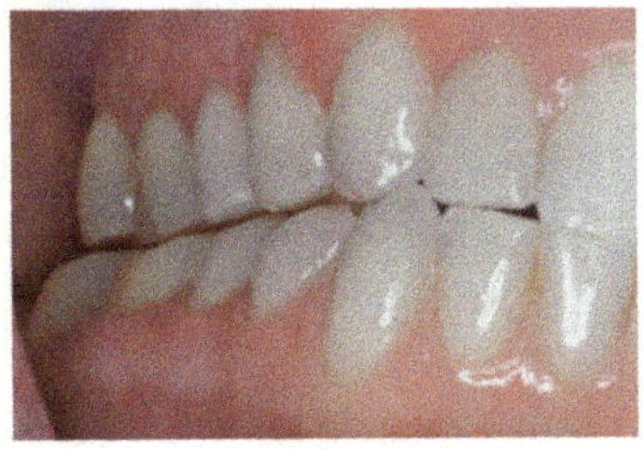

(a)

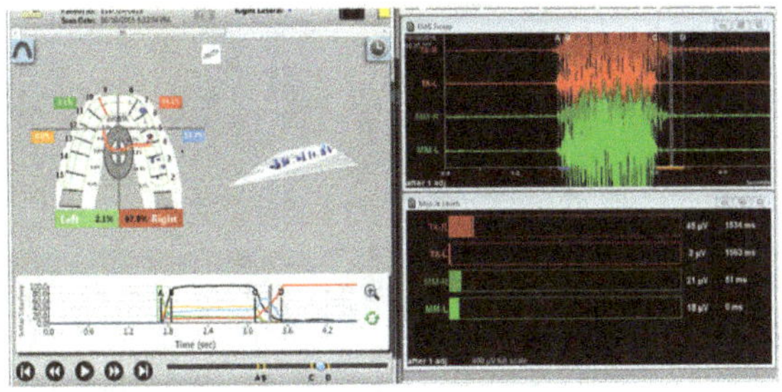

(b)

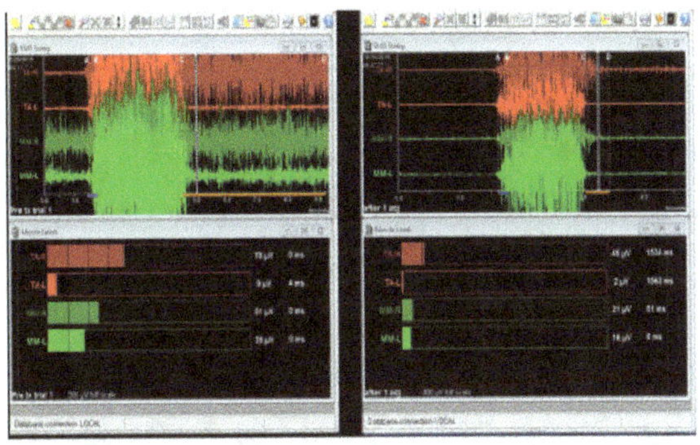

(c)

Figure 13. (a) The post-ICAGD right excursion showing slight space between the group function teeth that was not there before performing of the ICAGD coronoplasty. (b) The right excursion after ICAGD. The disclusion time equaled 0.45 s duration, which reduced the right temporalis and right and left masseter excursive hyperactivity dramatically compared to pretreatment. (c) Right excursive EMG improvements from pretreatment (left pane) to after ICAGD (right pane), where there is markedly lowered muscle activity levels post treatment at rest (before A), and in the excursion (to the right of C). With lessened excursive muscular hyperactivity, the muscle physiology can heal and MPDS symptoms can then abate.

component present, as well. Her symptoms came on after having two fillings placed in her two upper premolar teeth #s 14 and 15. Muscular pain ensued shortly after the fillings were done as they changed her occlusal contact comfort. Since then, further occlusal adjusting to the teeth involved did not resolve her MPDS symptoms.

8.3. Previous unsuccessful treatments

The patient reported wearing an appliance for 10 months nightly, but also reported symptom worsening with his attempted regular appliance use. She felt it made her clench more than if it was not worn. As such, she stopped wearing the appliance some months before consultation. Anti-inflammatory and pain medication gave her some marginal relief that would last only for a few hours.

The following figures (**Figures 12–15**) detail the patients in preoperative occlusal and muscle physiology status, as well as her post-ICAGD disclusion time reduction changes. For brevity, only the right and left excursions were illustrated, and protrusive excursions were not described.

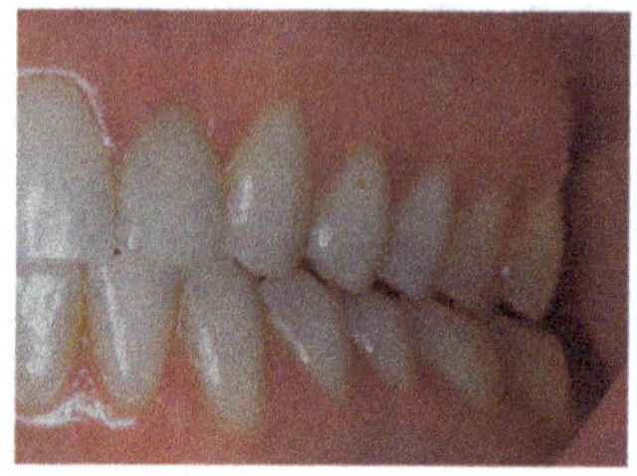

(a)

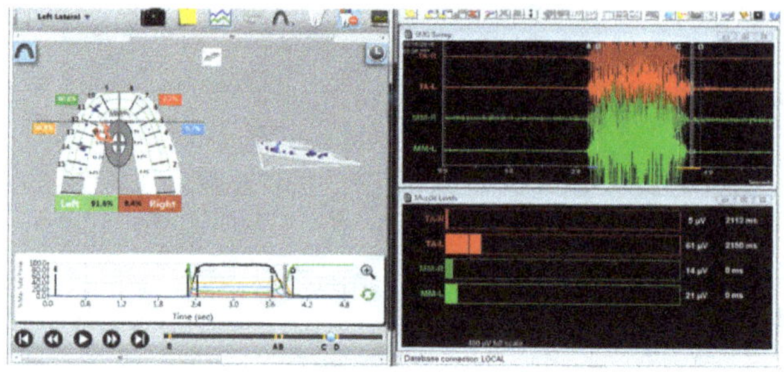

(b)

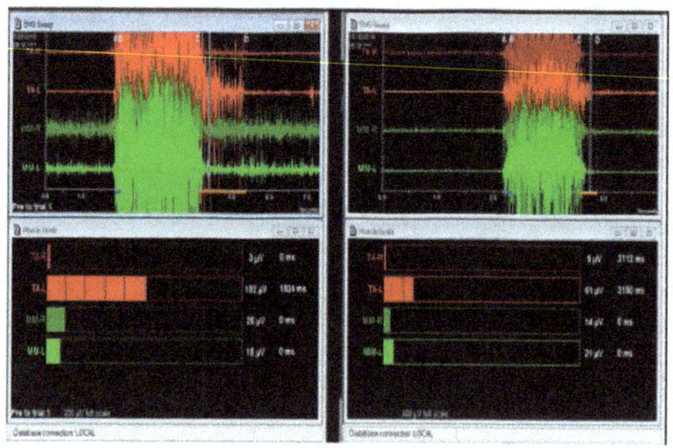

(c)

Figure 14. (a) The post ICAGD left excursion showing slight space between the group function teeth that was not there before performing of the ICAGD coronoplasty. (b) The left excursion after ICAGD when the disclusion time equaled to 0.34 s. The excursive EMG improvements show markedly lowered muscle activity levels post-treatment at rest (before A), and in the excursion (to the right of C). (c) The left excursive EMG improvements from pretreatment (left pane) to after ICAGD (right pane), where there is markedly lowered muscle activity levels present at rest (before A), and in the excursion post-treatment (to the right of C). With lessened excursive muscular hyperactivity, the muscle physiology can heal and MPDS symptoms can then abate.

With the pretreatment T-Scan/BioEMG data showing prolonged disclusion times and very high levels of excursive muscular hyperactivity, the patient was a good candidate to undergo the ICAGD coronoplasty. She was a Class I MPDS patient with adequate bilateral canine contact present to be safely treated with ICAGD.

It is through the measurement of the occlusion and muscles together using the T-Scan 9/BioEMG III synchronized occlusal measurement technologies so that these diagnostic and treatment improvements demonstrated within this case can become clinically predictable in managing MPDS patient. By quantifying occlusal function and muscle function together, the therapeutic effectiveness the ICAGD measured occlusal adjustment procedure has a dramatic effect on the central nervous system (CNS) that greatly reduces muscle activity levels and quickly lessens many common MPDS symptoms.

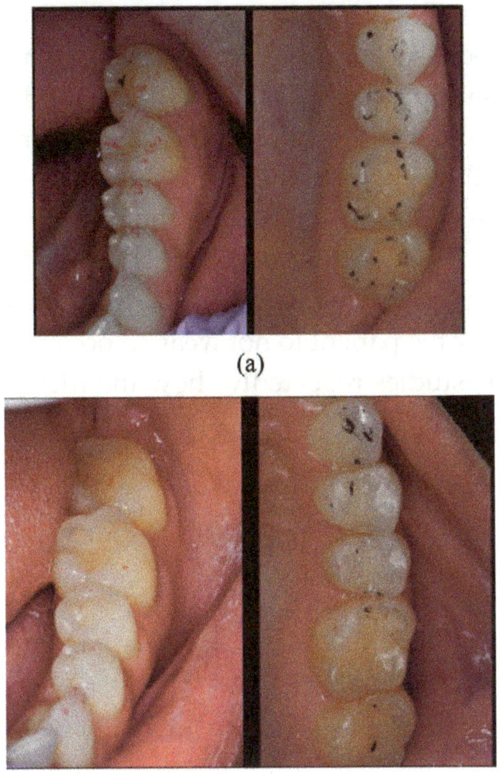

(a)

(b)

Figure 15. (a) Opposing occlusal surfaces with many pre-ICAGD articulating paper ink lines that describe that long disclusion time friction is present on all upper and lower posterior opposing occlusal surfaces (teeth #s 28–24 and #s 38–34). Note the very long red ink line visible on #37 distolingual occlusal incline. Its counterpart frictionally prolonged contact is the #27 distopalatol black ink line. (b) Post-ICAGD articulating paper markings showing 1–2 short disclusion time red and black pinpoint closure contacts per tooth, present on the opposing posterior occlusal surfaces (teeth #s 28–24 and #38–34). There are anterior guidance ink tracks visible across the occluding canine surfaces (#s 23 and 33). The small posterior closure contacts allow for the minimum posterior excursive contact, which are indicative of a disclusion time of <0.4 s. This small overall volume of tooth contact posteriorly is how the ICAGD coronoplasty controls the repetitive PDL mechanoreceptor neuronal action potential from heading into the CNS. Without the neural input, muscle contractions are dramatically lessened (**Figures 13c** and **14c**).

9. Final thoughts

This chapter describes in detail how the peripheral neural receptors that are located in and around the posterior teeth periodontal ligaments and in the dental pulp create ongoing masticatory muscle hyperactivity that can lead to the clinical appearance of myofascial pain dysfunction syndrome symptoms. MPDS commonly afflicts the masticatory musculature with chronic muscular pain, frequent temporal headaches, chewing pain and weakness, opening limitations, and frequent clenching and bruxing of teeth. Because unmeasured, published Occlusal Equilibration studies did not predictably treat the MPDS condition, conventional MPDS treatments have focused on lessening MPDS symptoms without treating the occlusion directly. The use of occlusal splints, physical therapy, and trigger point injections has been predominant. However, since the development of the T-Scan system in the 1980s, and the discovery of prolonged posterior disclusion time, a computer-guided alternative coronoplasty to occlusal equilibration, has evolved to treat MPDS (known as disclusion time reduction (DTR) with the ICAGD coronoplasty).

DTR is an etiologically based treatment aimed at reducing prolonged occlusal surface friction, which drastically limits the tooth socket compressions and pulpal occlusal contact impacts that the posterior teeth sustain multiple times on a daily basis (and nightly, if there is parafunction). By cutting down the volume of socket compressions and impacts, the molar and premolar peripheral action potential response to the occlusal contacts is drastically lessened, which remove the stimulus that the occlusion inputs into the central nervous system (CNS) to fire muscles and create ischemia. This limiting neurophysiologic change allows the masticatory muscles to calm down and relax physiologically, because the ischemia reverses intramuscularly from within the CNS, requiring the patient to not wear an occlusal splint. In short order following the ICAGD coronoplasty, studies repeatedly show the MPDS symptoms, then abate, and lessen in severity and frequency.

Author details

Serdar Gözler

Address all correspondence to: serdargozler@aydin.edu.tr

TMD Clinic, Dentistry Faculty of Istanbul Aydin University, Istanbul, Turkey

References

[1] Lipton JA, Dionne RA. National institutes of health technology assessment conference statement: Management of temporomandibular disorders, April 29-May 1, 1996. Oral Surgery, Oral Medicine, Oral Pathology, Oral Radiology [Internet]. 1996;**83**(1):177-183 Available from: http://cat.inist.fr/?aModele=afficheN&cpsidt=2551680

[2] Kerstein RB. Disclusion time measurement studies: A comparison of disclusion time between chronic myofascial pain dyfunction patients and nonpatients: A population analysis. The Journal of Prosthetic Dentistry. 1994;**72**:473-480

[3] Kerstein RB. Treatment of myofascial pain dysfunction syndrome with occlusal therapy to reduce lengthy disclusion time—A recall evaluation. CRANIO® [Internet]. 1995 Apr 1; **13, 105**(2):15. DOI: 10.1080/08869634.1995.11678053

[4] Baldini A, Nota A, Cozza P. The association between occlusion time and temporomandibular disorders. Journal of Electromyography & Kinesiology [Internet]. 2015;**25**(1):151-154. DOI: 10.1016/j.jelekin.2014.08.007

[5] Bennett R. Myofascial pain syndromes and their evaluation. Best Practice & Research: Clinical Rheumatology. 2007;**21**(3):427-445. Available from: http://www.ncbi.nlm.nih.gov/pubmed/17602992

[6] Palla S. Trigger points as a cause of Orofacial pain. J Musculoskelet Pain. 2004;**12**(3-4):29-36

[7] Ge HY, Monterde S, Graven-Nielsen T, Arendt-Nielsen L. Latent myofascial trigger points are associated with an increased intramuscular electromyographic activity during synergistic muscle activation. Journal of Pain. 2014;**15**(2):181-187. DOI: 10.1016/j.jpain.2013.10.009

[8] Svensson P. Pain mechanisms in myogenous temporomandibular disorders. Pain Forum. 1997;**6**(3):158-165. Available from: http://www.sciencedirect.com/science/article/pii/S1082317497700102

[9] Kerstein RB. Disclusion time-reduction therapy with immediate complete anterior guidance development to treat chronic myofascial pain-dysfunction syndrome. Quintessence International. 1992;**23**(11):735-747

[10] Fricton J. Myofascial pain: Mechanisms to management. Oral and Maxillofacial Surgery Clinics of North America. 2016;**28**(3):289-311. DOI: 10.1016/j.coms.2016.03.010

[11] Farella M, Michelotti A, Bocchino T, Cimino R, Laino A, Steenks MH. Effects of orthognathic surgery for class III malocclusion on signs and symptoms of temporomandibular disorders and on pressure pain thresholds of the jaw muscles. International Journal of Oral and Maxillofacial Surgery. 2007;**36**(7):583-587

[12] De Rossi SS, Stern I, Sollecito TP. Disorders of the masticatory muscles. Dental Clinics of North America. 2013;**57**(3):449-464. DOI: 10.1016/j.cden.2013.04.007

[13] Schindler H, Eckehard S, Spiess WEL. Standardization of the registration and analysis of mastication: Proposal for clinical application. Turker K, editor. Journal of Prosthetic Dentistry. 2016;**9**(3):1-7. DOI: 10.1016/j.prosdent.2014.04.032

[14] Gözler S. Aggregating stimulus increases the activity in motoneurons causing spasm a case from our study. In: 10th Biennial International Motoneuron Meeting, Istanbul-Motoneuron Congress. 2017

[15] Kerstein RB, Wright NR. Electromyographic and computer analysis of patients suffering from chronic myofascial pain-dysfunction syndrome: Before and after treatment with immediate complete anterior guidance development. The Journal of Prosthetic Dentistry. 1991;**66**:677-686

[16] Kerstein RB, Radke J. Average chewing pattern improvements following disclusion time reduction. Cranio: The Journal of Craniomandibular Practice. 2016;**9634**(February):1-17. DOI: 10.1080/08869634.2016.1190526

[17] Olesen J. The international classification of headache disorders, 3rd edition. Cephalagia. 2013;**33**(9):629-808. Available from: http://www.ncbi.nlm.nih.gov/pubmed/18808500%5Cnhttp://www.ncbi.nlm.nih.gov/pubmed/24409431%5Cnhttp://www.ncbi.nlm.nih.gov/pubmed/22325197%5Cnhttp://www.ncbi.nlm.nih.gov/pubmed/16805756%5Cnhttp://www.ncbi.nlm.nih.gov/pubmed/24238370%5Cnhttp://www.ncbi.nlm

[18] Dawson PE. A classification system for occlusions that relates maximal intercuspation to the position and condition of the temporomandibular joints. The Journal of Prosthetic Dentistry. 1996;**75**(1):60-66

[19] De Rossi SS, Stern I, Sollecito TP, Fushima K, Gallo LM, Krebs M, et al. The relationship between skull morphology, masticatory muscle force and cranial skeletal deformation during biting. Journal of Prosthodontic Research. 2016;**25**(3):51-59. DOI: 10.1016/j.jfoodeng.2016.06.008

[20] Learreta JA, Beas J, Bono AE, Durst A. Muscular activity disorders in relation to intentional occlusal interferences. Cranio: The Journal of Craniomandibular Practice. 2007;**25**(3):193-199

[21] van der Bilt A. Assessment of mastication with implications for oral rehabilitation: A review. Journal of Oral Rehabilitation. 2011;**38**(10):754-780

[22] Meyer RA. Chapter 163 The Temporomandibular Joint Examination. 2017. pp. 2-4

[23] Fricton JR. Etiology and management of masticatory miofascial pain. Musculoskeletal Pain. 1999;**7**(1/2):143-160

[24] Fuentes AD, Sforza C, Miralles R, Ferreira CL, Mapelli A, Lodetti G, et al. Assessment of electromyographic activity in patients with temporomandibular disorders and natural mediotrusive occlusal contact during chewing and tooth grinding. Cranio: The Journal of Craniomandibular Practice. 2016;**9634**(February 2017):1-10. DOI: 10.1080/08869634.2016.1173312

[25] Wickwire NA, Gibbs CH, Jacobson AP, Lundeen HC. Chewing patterns in normal children. The Angle Orthodontist. 1981;**51**(1):48-60

[26] Kuwahara T, Besette R, Maruyama T. Characteristic chewing parameters for specific types of TMJ internal derangements, Kuwahara et al.pdf. Cranio: The Journal of Craniomandibular Practice. 1996;**14**(1):9086871

[27] National Institutes of Health Tecnology Assesment Conference Statment. Management of Temporomandibular disorders. Journal of the American Dental Association (1939). 1996;**127**(11):1595-1606

[28] De Abreu M, Domingues M, Furtado F, Pereira G, Prado R, Mestriner W, et al. ScienceDirect masticatory efficiency and bite force in individuals with normal occlusion. Archives of Oral Biology. 2014;**59**(10):1065-1074

[29] Gözler S. Stomatognatik Sistemin Nöromüsküler Fizyolojisi. In: Çalıkkocaoğlu PDS, editor. Tam Protezler. 5th ed. Istanbul: Gnatoloji Derneği; 1989. pp. 89-105

[30] Gözler S, Tüzer E, Çalıkkocaoğlu S. Nöromüsküler mekanizmanın protetik diş hekimliğindeki yeri. İstanbul Üniversitesi Diş Hekimliği Fakültesi Dergisi. 1982;**16**(1):83-114

[31] Huguenin LK. Myofascial trigger points: The current evidence. Physical Therapy in Sport. 2004;**5**(1):2-12

[32] Cummings M, Baldry P. Regional myofascial pain: Diagnosis and management. Best Practice & Research. Clinical Rheumatology. 2007;**21**(2):367-387

[33] Türker KS, Brinkworth RSA, Abolfathi P, Linke IR, Nazeran HA. Device for investigating neuromuscular control in the human masticatory system. Journal of Neuroscience Methods. 2004;**136**:141-149

[34] Trulsson M, Gunne HS. Food-holding and -biting behavior in human subjects lacking periodontal receptors. Journal of Dental Research. 1998;**77**(4):574-582

[35] Trulsson M. Sensory-motor function of human periodontal mechanoreceptors. Journal of Oral Rehabilitation. 2006;**33**(4):262-273

[36] Bessette RW, Mohl ND, Bishop B. Contribution of periodontal receptors to the masseteric silent period. Journal of Dental Research. 1974;**53**(5):1196-1204

[37] Dessem D, Iyadurai OD, Taylor A. The role of periodontal receptors in the jaw-opening reflex in the cat. The Journal of Physiology. 1988;**406**:315-330

[38] Schindler HJ, Stengel E, Spiess WEL. Feedback control during mastication of solid food textures—A clinical-experimental study. The Journal of Prosthetic Dentistry. 1998;**80**(3):330-336

[39] McCulloch CA, Lekic P, McKee MD. Role of physical forces in regulating the form and function of the periodontal ligament. Periodontology 2000. 2000;**24**:56-72

[40] Barczyk M, Bolstad AI, Gullberg D. Role of integrins in the periodontal ligament: Organizers and facilitators. Periodontology 2000. 2013;**63**(1):29-47

[41] Zent R, Pozzi A. Cell-extracellular matrix interactions in cancer. Cell-extracellular Matrix Interact Cancer. 2010:1-314

[42] Windhorst U. Muscle proprioceptive feedback and spinal networks. Brain Research Bulletin. 2007;**73**(4-6):155-202

[43] Ji RR, Kohno T, Moore KA, Woolf CJ. Central sensitization and LTP: Do pain and memory share similar mechanisms? Trends in Neurosciences. 2003;**26**(12):696-705

[44] Harden RN, Bruehl SP, Gass S, Niemiec C, Barbick B. Signs and symptoms of the myofascial pain syndrome: A national survey of pain management providers. Clinical Journal of Pain. 2000;**16**(1):64-72. Available from: http://www.scopus.com/inward/record.url?eid=2-s2.0-0034015338&partnerID=tZOtx3y1

[45] Rhudy JL, Meagher MW. Fear and anxiety: Divergent effects on human pain thresholds. Pain. 2000;**84**(1):65-75

[46] Rahn EJ, Guzman-Karlsson MC, David Sweatt J. Cellular, molecular, and epigenetic mechanisms in non-associative conditioning: Implications for pain and memory. Neurobiology of Learning and Memory. 2013;**105**:133-150. DOI: 10.1016/j.nlm.2013.06.008

[47] Greene SA. Chronic pain: Pathophysiology and treatment implications. Topics in Companion Animal Medicine. 2010;**25**(1):5-9. DOI: 10.1053/j.tcam.2009.10.009

[48] Greene CS, Laskin DM. Splint therapy for the myofascial pain-dysfunction (MPD) syndrome: A comparative study. Journal of the American Dental Association. 1972;**84**(3): 624-628. DOI: 10.14219/jada.archive.1972.0090

[49] Donovan TE, Anderson M, Becker W, Cagna DR, Hilton TJ, JR MK. Annual review of selected scientific literature: report of the committee on scientific investigation of the American Academy of Restorative Dentistry. Journal of Prosthetic Dentistry. 2012; **108**(1):15-50. DOI: 10.1016/S0022-3913(10)60087-X

[50] Conti PCR, De Alencar EN, Da Mota Corrêa AS, Lauris JRP, Porporatti AL, Costa YM. Behavioural changes and occlusal splints are effective in the management of masticatory myofascial pain: A short-term evaluation. Journal of Oral Rehabilitation. 2012; **39**(10):754-760

[51] Gozler S, Vanlioglu B, Evren B, Gozneli R, Yildiz C, Ozkan YK. The effect of temporary hydrostatic splint on occlusion with computerized occlusal analysis system. Indian Journal of Dental Research: Official Publication of Indian Society for Dental Research. 2012;**23**:617-622

[52] Aldemir K, Üstüner E, Erdem E, Demiralp AS, Oztuna D. Ultrasound evaluation of masseter muscle changes in stabilization splint treatment of myofascial type painful

temporomandibular diseases. Oral Surgery, Oral Medicine, Oral Pathology, Oral Radiology. 2013;**116**(3):377-383. DOI: 10.1016/j.oooo.2013.06.011

[53] Wang C, Yin X. Occlusal risk factors associated with temporomandibular disorders in young adults with normal occlusions. Oral Surgery, Oral Medicine, Oral Pathology, Oral Radiology. 2012;**114**(4):419-423. DOI: 10.1016/j.oooo.2011.10.039

[54] Lauritzen AG, Bodner GH. Variations in location of arbitrary and true hinge axis points. Journal of Prosthetic Dentistry. 1961;**11**(2):224-229. Available from: http://linkinghub.elsevier.com/retrieve/pii/0022391361901962

[55] Helms RB, Katona TR, Eckert GJ. Do occlusal contact detection products alter the occlusion? Journal of Oral Rehabilitation. 2012;**39**(5):357-363

[56] Mongini F. Condylar remodeling after occlusal therapy. The Journal of Prosthetic Dentistry. 1980;**43**(5):568-577

[57] Mongini F. Anatomic and clinical evaluation of the relationship between the temporomandibular joint and occlusion. The Journal of Prosthetic Dentistry. 1977;**38**(5):539-551

[58] Condylator C. Gerber-Condylator Gerber-Condylator [Internet]. Available from: www.condylator.com/en/articles/advantages_of_the_condylator.pdf

[59] Garrido García VC, García Cartagena A, González Sequeros O. Evaluation of occlusal contacts in maximum intercuspation using the T-Scan system. Journal of Oral Rehabilitation. 1997;**24**(12):899-903

[60] Da Silva Martins MJ, Caramelo FJ, Ramalho da Fonseca JA, Gomes Nicolau PM. In vitro study on the sensibility and reproducibility of the new T-Scan®III HD system. Revista Portuguesa de Estomatologia, Medicina Dentária e Cirurgia Maxilofacial. 2014;**55**(1):14-22. DOI: 10.1016/j.rpemd.2014.01.001

[61] Kerstein RB, Lowe M, Harty M, Radke J. A force reproduction analysis of two recording sensors of a computerized occlusal analysis system. Cranio. 2006;**24**(1):15-24

[62] Kerstein RB, Chapman R, Klein M. A comparison of ICAGD (immediate complete anterior guidance development) to mock ICAGD for symptom reductions in chronic myofascial pain dysfonction patients. Cranio: The Journal of Craniomandibular Practice. 1997;**15**(January 1997):21-37

[63] Koos B, Höller J, Schille C, Time AG. Dependent analysis and representation of force distribution and occlusion contact in the masticatory. Cycle. 2012;**73**(3):3-4

[64] Svetlana K. Case report T-scan III computed guided occlusal adjustment in orthodontic relapse patient. The procedure description. EC Dental Science. 2016;**2**:1297-1308

[65] Qadeer S, Yang L, Sarinnaphakorn L, Kerstein RB. Comparison of closure occlusal force parameters in post-orthodontic and non-orthodontic subjects using T-Scan(R) III DMD occlusal analysis. Cranio. 2016;**9634**(April):1-7. DOI: 10.1080/08869634.2015.1122277

[66] Makofsky HW, Sexton TR, Diamond DZ, Sexton MT. The effect of head posture on muscle contact position using the T-Scan system of occlusal analysis. Cranio: The Journal of Craniomandibular Practice. 1991;**9**:316-321

[67] Qadeer S, Abbas AA, Sarinnaphakorn L, Robert B. Comparison of excursive occlusal force parameters in post-orthodontic and non-orthodontic subjects using T-Scan® III. Cranio®. 2016;(**9634**, January):1-8. DOI: 10.1080/08869634.2016.1259785

[68] Lund JP. Mastication and its control by the brain stem. Critical Reviews in Oral Biology & Medicine. 1991;**2**(1):33-64. Available from: http://cro.sagepub.com/content/2/1/33.short

[69] Kerstein RB, Radke J, Dmd RBK, Mba JR. Average chewing pattern improvements following Disclusion Time reduction. Cranio®. 2017;**9634**(January):1-17. DOI: 10.1080/08869634.2016.1190526

[70] Yiannios N, Kerstein RB, Radke J. Treatment of frictional dental hypersensitivity (FDH) with computer-guided occlusal adjustments. Cranio®. 2016;**9634**(November):1-11 Available from: https://www.tandfonline.com/doi/full/10.1080/08869634.2016.1251692

[71] Thumati P, Kerstein R, Thumati R. Disclusion time reduction therapy in treating occluso-muscular pains. Journal of Indian Prosthodontic Society. 2016. Available from: http://www.j-ips.org/preprintarticle.asp?id=194948

[72] Kerstein RB, Chapman R, Klein MA. Comparison of ICAGD (immediate complete anterior guidance development) to mock ICAGD for symptom reductions in chronic myofascial pain dysfunction patients. Cranio. 1997;**15**:21-37

[73] Kerstein RB, Radke J. Masseter and temporalis excursive hyperactivity decreased by measured anterior guidance development. Cranio: The Journal of Craniomandibular Practice. 2012;**30**(4):243-254

[74] Thumati P, Manwani R, Mahantshetty M. The effect of reduced disclusion time in the treatment of myofascial pain dysfunction syndrome using immediate complete anterior guidance development protocol monitored by digital analysis of occlusion. Cranio: The Journal of Craniomandibular Practice. 2014;**32**(4):289-299

[75] Goodman P, Greene CS, Laskin DM. Response of patients with myofascial pain-dysfunction syndrome to mock equilibration. Journal of the American Dental Association. 1976;**92**(4):755-758. Available from http://www.ncbi.nlm.nih.gov/pubmed/1068180

[76] Forssell H, Kirveskari P, Kangasniemi P. Effect of occlusal adjustment on mandibular dysfunction. A double-blind study. Acta Odontologica Scandinavica. 1986;**44**(2):63-69. Available from http://www.ncbi.nlm.nih.gov/pubmed/3524093

[77] Wenneberg B, Nystrom T, Carlsson GE. Occlusal equilibration and other stomatognathic treatment in patients with mandibular dysfunction and headache. The Journal of Prosthetic Dentistry. 1988;**59**(4):478-483

[78] Tsolka P, Morris RW, Preiskel HW. Occlusal adjustment therapy for craniomandibular disorders: A clinical assessment by a double-blind method. The Journal of Prosthetic Dentistry. 1992;**68**(6):957-964

[79] Kerstein RB, Neff PA. A comparison of traditional occlusal equilibration and immediate complete anterior guidance development. Cranio®. 1993;**11**(2):126-140. DOI: 10.1080/08869634.1993.11677954

6

Internal Derangements of the Temporomandibular Joint: Diagnosis and Management

Ufuk Tatli and Vladimir Machon

Abstract

Millions of individuals worldwide suffer from temporomandibular joint (TMJ) disorders and are characterized by pain and joint dysfunction. TMJ internal derangement (ID) is the most frequent type of temporomandibular disorders (TMDs). The ID of TMJ is defined as a joint dysfunction associated with an abnormal disc position. Identification and elimination of the causes of tissue breakdown of the TMJ that lead to ID are the key factors for successful treatment. The common causes for TMJ ID are trauma and parafunctional habits which lead to joint overload and degenerative changes in the articular structures, increased friction, and gradual disc displacement. Local and systemic inflammatory/degenerative arthropathies may also affect TMJ and cause ID. The aim of this chapter is to give comprehensive knowledge about the contemporary perspective of TMJ ID including diagnostic and therapeutic developments and innovations. Clinicians should establish the correct diagnosis and cause of the disease for appropriate management so that patients do not suffer from ineffective treatments. As an innovative development, TMJ replacements with alloplastic joint prosthesis and tissue-engineered structures hold promise for the future of management of TMJ ID.

Keywords: internal derangement, temporomandibular joint, TMJ, conservative treatment, TMJ surgery

1. Introduction

Millions of individuals worldwide suffer from temporomandibular joint (TMJ) disorders and are characterized by pain and joint dysfunction. TMJ internal derangement (ID) is the most frequent type of temporomandibular disorders (TMDs), including 41.1% of patients with TMD [1]. The ID of TMJ is defined as a joint dysfunction associated with an abnormal disc position [2]. Identification and elimination of the causes of tissue breakdown of the TMJ that lead to ID are the key factors for successful treatment. The common causes for TMJ ID are trauma and parafunctional habits which lead to degenerative changes in the articular structures, increased friction, and gradual disc displacement [2]. Systemic degenerative arthropathies may also affect TMJ and cause ID. Moreover, some kind of infections and tumors can cause the nonspecific symptoms and may mimic TMJ ID.

The natural course of TMJ ID without treatment was shown that some patients heal spontaneously and the length of time for symptoms to resolve is variable, but generally 1 year. This is thought to be associated with the adaptation capacity of the joint and the healing capacity of the individuals. However, it is not possible to predict the patients who are likely to have a return to asymptomatic condition. The older patients, the patients with longer time of disease onset, and those with magnetic resonance imaging (MRI) evidence of advanced TMD are at a higher risk for not improving spontaneously [3].

This chapter gives comprehensive knowledge about the contemporary perspective of TMJ ID including diagnostic and therapeutic developments and innovations with an emphasis on tissue engineering strategy for joint reconstruction.

2. Definition of the internal derangement of the temporomandibular joint

The most popular definition of ID of TMJ can be explained as the joint dysfunction associated with an abnormal disc position and damage to the internal structures of the joint [2]. The signs and symptoms of ID are nonspecific and can be caused by multiple etiologic factors.

For the diagnosis and management of TMJ ID, updated guidelines and classification systems such as Wilkes staging [4] and Diagnostic Criteria for TMDs (DC/TMD) [5] are available. The Wilkes staging system for ID of TMJ is frequently used by oral and maxillofacial surgeons to provide a guide for treatment based on the severity of the joint damage (**Table 1**). The DC/TMD classification system underwent extensive testing (in terms of sensitivity and specificity) and validated for different languages (the validated translations of DC/TMD into different

Stage	Clinical findings	Radiological findings
I (Early)	Painless clicking, no limitation of motion	Slight disc displacement with early reduction, normal disc morphology
II (Early/intermediate)	Occasional painful clicking, intermittent locking, related headache	Moderate disc displacement with late reduction, mild disc deformity
III (Intermediate)	Frequent pain, joint tenderness, restriction of motion, closed locks	Disc displacement without reduction, deformity of disc, no hard tissue changes
IV (Intermediate/late)	Chronic pain, restriction of motion	Severe disc displacement (without reduction), Severe deformity of disc, degenerative changes
V (Late)	Variable and episodic joint pain, chronic restriction of motion, crepitus	Gross deformity and/or perforation of disc, degenerative arthritic changes, osteophyte deformity subcortical cyst formation

Table 1. Wilkes classification for internal derangement of temporomandibular joint [4].

languages are available at http://www.rdc-tmdinternational.org). The current update of DC/TMD was released in 2014 [5]. This diagnostic system has AXIS 1 for classification of the physical categories of the TMDs, and AXIS 2 for classification of psychosocial behavioral aspects of patients with TMDs. According to the last update of DC/TMD Axis 1, TMJ ID is defined in four stages: disc displacement with reduction (DDwR), disc displacement with reduction with intermittent locking, disc displacement without reduction (DDwoR) with limited mouth opening, and disc displacement without reduction without limited mouth opening. The weakness of these classification systems is that there is no causative information associated with the corresponding stages. However, understanding the true cause of damage to the joint structures is essential for proper treatment. Without useful categorization of cause and pathogenesis, treatments often fail because causative factors persist.

In a physiologically normal joint, the disc is positioned between mandibular condyle and the posterior slope of articular eminence when the jaw is closed. When the jaw is opened, the disc slides into a position between condyle and top of the eminence. The attachments of the disc prevent its displacement during opening. The ID of TMJ can be divided into two subgroups basically: disc displacement with reduction and disc displacement without reduction (**Figure 1**). In the DDwR case, disc has slight deformation and forward displacement when the jaw is closed. The displaced disc reduces to normal position at maximal mouth opening (first click noise appears). When the jaw is intended to close, the disc displaces forward again (second click noise—reciprocal click—appears). The patient with DDwR has symptoms of TMJ pain with clicking, intermittent locking, and orofacial pain without limitation on mouth opening. The disc displacement and reduction can be observed in open- and closed-mouth MRI examination (**Figure 2**). In the DDwoR case, disc has moderate to severe deformation and forward displacement when the jaw is closed. During mouth opening, the disc cannot return to its normal position and is compressed between condyle and eminence so as the disorder progresses (**Figure 3**). The patient with DDwoR

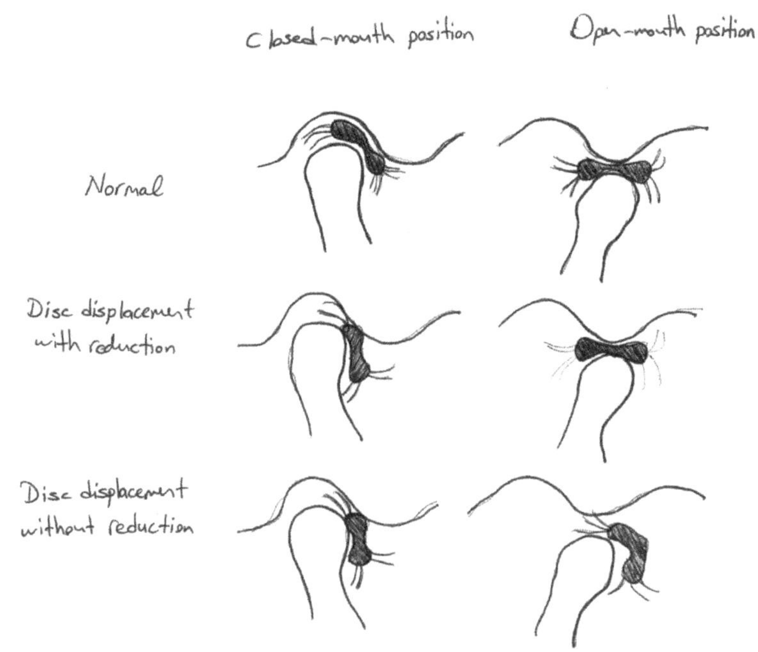

Figure 1. The hand-sketch TMJ figure showing normal condyle-disc relationship, disc displacement with reduction, and without reduction in closed- and open-mouth positions.

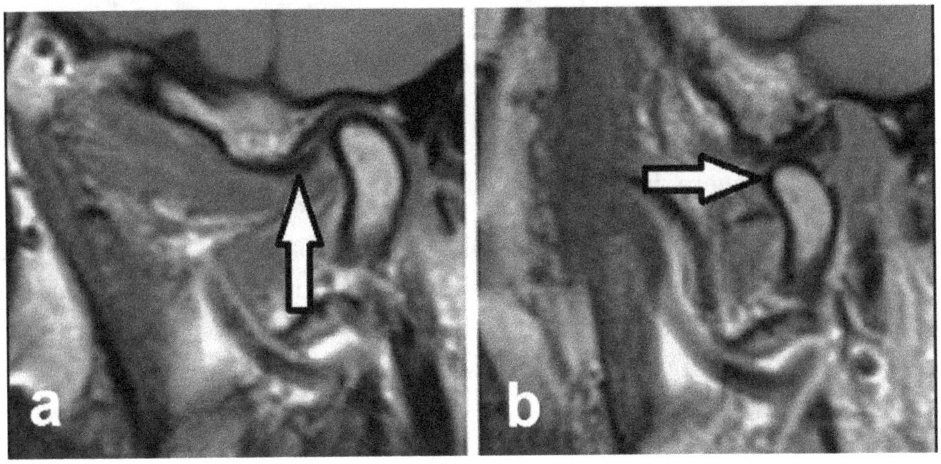

Figure 2. T1-weighted MRI of a TMJ showing anterior disc displacement with reduction; (a) closed-mouth position (anterior displacement of the disc) and (b) open-mouth position (reduction of the disc). White arrow shows articular disc.

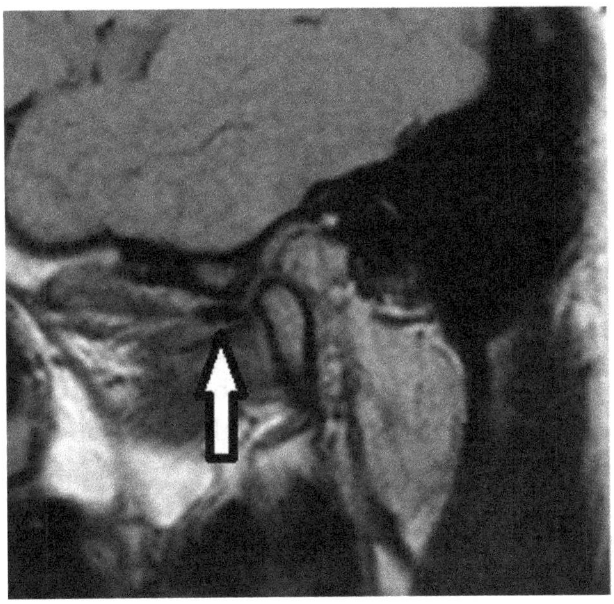

Figure 3. T1-weighted MRI of a TMJ showing anterior disc displacement without reduction in an open-mouth position. Note that the disc is still in a displaced position. White arrow shows articular disc.

has symptoms of increased TMJ and orofacial pain with restricted mandibular motion. The click noise disappears, however; in advanced cases, crepitation noise appears as a result of degenerative changes. In unilateral case, the patient shows restricted controlateral jaw movement while ipsilateral movement is normal. In advanced stages of DDwoR, increased degenerative changes including disc perforation and abrasion of the underlying bone occur.

3. Pathogenesis of internal derangement of temporomandibular joint

The displaced disc can degenerate, become misshaped, perforated, or even torn. If the patient cannot achieve proper treatment, ID gets progressively worse with time, inflammation accompanied, and osteoarthritic changes (abrasion of articular cartilage and underlying bone, flattening of articular surfaces, less pronounced articular eminence, osteophyte formation, subchondral cyst, and resorption of the condyle) occur [5, 6]. Several inflammatory mediators (such as tumor necrosis factor-α, interleukin 1-β, prostaglandin E2, etc.) play crucial roles in the pathogenesis of ID [7, 8]. The more detailed explanations about the inflammatory mediator background of the ID were discussed in another chapter of this book.

The challenge for clinicians is to diagnose the accurate condition that causes the ID. Once identified, the basis for the treatment is to relieve the patient's symptoms and to improve healing while simultaneously removing the causal factors. The following causal factors or diseases may lead to ID and should be addressed carefully: the excessive loading of the joint, and systemic and localized arthropathies may cause ID of TMJ [2].

3.1. Excessive loading

Joint overload is the most common cause of ID. The joint overload (often caused by stress-mediated parafunction, acute or chronic trauma, unstable occlusion, and increased joint friction) deteriorates cartilage metabolism. This pathologic process causes the fibrillation of cartilage and ultimately leads to biomechanical failure impairing the sliding of the articular surfaces. Clinically, joint noise (clicking) is detected in this stage. The individuals who have persistent parafunction continue to overload articular structures beyond their adaptive capacity leading to pain, synovitis, intra-articular adhesions, osteoarthritis, and disc perforation [2]. Thus, the key principles in the management of ID caused by joint overloading are the reduction of joint loading and inflammation, maximizing joint mobility, and relieving pain. If the patients with ID have the signs of joint overload and if all other causal factors are ruled out, these patients should be managed by an intense 2–3 week regimen of conservative therapies as described below. If the symptoms begin to resolve, then conservative treatment should be continued. However, if the symptoms persist, minimally invasive surgical interventions should be considered. The advanced stages of ID leading to fibrosis, disc deformation or perforation, and TMJ ankylosis require arthrotomy.

3.2. Systemic arthropathy

A number of systemic and rheumatoid disorders play a role of causal factor and can contribute to inflammatory/degenerative arthropathy and ID. Since systemic disorders affect the structure and function of articular tissues, TMJ of the patients with systemic arthropathy may fail under normal joint loads. Thus, clinicians should be aware of this issue when considering patient management. The examples of systemic disorders, which can cause ID, include rheumatoid arthritis, psoriatic arthritis, juvenile idiopathic arthritis, pseudogout, ankylosing spondylitis, polymyalgia rheumatica, chondrocalcinosis, Ehler-Danlos syndrome, Lyme disease, lupus erythematosus, and other connective tissue disorders [2, 9, 10]. For these patients, management of systemic disorders is essential for the treatment of TMJ ID and requires coordination between a maxillofacial surgeon and a rheumatologist. Conservative therapies and arthrocentesis or arthroscopy can relieve symptoms. Moreover, arthroscopic biopsy led to the diagnosis.

3.3. Localized arthropathy

This term describes an articular disorder that is atypical and not caused by joint overloading or systemic disease. A localized atypical arthropathy usually affects one joint only. The clinical signs and symptoms are nonspecific and include joint pain, noise, limited function, and changes in the occlusion. The imaging techniques and arthroscopic biopsy show unusual findings (multiple loose calcifications or synovial effusions) and confirm the diagnosis. The localized arthropathy of TMJ can be summarized as follows: osteochondroma, synovial chondromatosis, crystal deposition disease, and synovial cyst. The localized arthropathies may cause or mimic TMJ ID. The secondary inflammatory component from neighboring regions (otitis, tonsillitis, and maxillary sinusitis) can affect TMJ and cause ID [2, 11]. The correct diagnosis is crucial in these kinds of disorders and treatment usually includes arthroscopy or arthrotomy.

4. Diagnosis of internal derangement of temporomandibular joint

4.1. History and physical examination

Complete medical history, clinical, and radiological examinations are essential for correct diagnosis. The most frequent signs and symptoms related to ID are pain on TMJ region, decrease in mouth opening (the normal values of maximum inter-incisal mouth opening are between 35 and 50 mm) and laterotrusive movements (the normal values of the ipsi- and contra-lateral movements of the joint are between 5 and 10 mm), TMJ noise (clicking and crepitation), intermittent lock of the joint, deflexion or deviation of the mandible during mouth opening [5]. The tenderness of the masticatory muscles may accompany.

4.2. Imaging methods

Imaging of TMJ is necessary to establish the proper diagnosis, to select the appropriate treatment, and to assess the treatment results. For imaging purposes, the following contemporary techniques are frequently used.

4.2.1. Panoramic radiography or arthrography

Orthopantomography (OPG) and/or arthrography are used to assess hard tissues of TMJ including condyle, glenoid fossa, and articular eminence. For detailed examination, computed tomography (CT)/cone-beam computed tomography (CBCT) is preferred.

4.2.2. Computed tomography or cone-beam computed tomography

CT or CBCT is useful to assess bone abnormalities such as ankylosis, degenerative changes, osteoarthritis, growth abnormalities, fractures, and tumors. A stereolithographic model of a patient's TMJ skeleton can be prefabricated using three-dimensional (3D) technology for reconstructive purposes.

4.2.3. Magnetic resonance imaging

MRI is the standard imaging technique for visualization of TMJ. It is used to assess retrodiscal tissue, disc position and morphology, displacement and reduction of the disc, bone marrow changes, degenerative involvements, and joint effusion [12]. Recently, the potential use of MRI-CBCT image fusion technique was introduced in order to improve the reliability and accuracy of assessment of disc positions [13]. Contemporarily, real-time MRI imaging of TMJ allows comprehensive data about the dynamics of all articular structures during jaw movement and offers more reliable diagnosis for ID of TMJ [14]. MRI is contraindicated in claustrophobic patients and those with pacemakers.

4.2.4. *Single photon emission computed tomography*

This technique is used to detect metabolic activity and inflammation on the joint structures. The single photon emission computed tomography (SPECT) can be used for conventional evaluation of osteoarthritis of TMJ (which is the further stage of ID) [15].

4.2.5. *Electromyography*

This method is used to assess masticatory and cervical muscles' activities when bruxism or muscle-mediated joint overload is suspected as a causal factor for TMD [16].

4.2.6. *Ultrasonography*

The ultrasonography (USG) is used as an alternative imaging technique for the diagnosis of TMD. On USG images, condyle and glenoid fossa are hyperechoic (high reflection of sound waves) and appear white, bone marrow is hypoechoic (low reflection of sound waves) and appears black, connective tissues (joint capsule and retrodiscal tissue) and muscles (lateral pterygoid and masseter muscles) are isoechoic (intermediate reflection) and appear heterogeneously gray, and the disc appears as a thin area of hyperechogenity surrounded by a hypoechoic halo [17]. Diagnostic accuracy of USG was reported to be 54–100% for disc displacement, 72–95% for joint effusion, and 56–93% for osteoarthrosis [17]. The USG can be used to assess the thickness of the masticatory muscles in order to evaluate their causal effects for TMD [18]. Moreover, USG can also be used as an image guide for injection into the superior and lower joint space [19, 20].

4.2.7. *Other methods*

If the clinician suspects systemic involvement (such as rheumatoid arthritis or juvenile idiopathic arthritis), appropriate tests including human leukocyte antigen-B27, anti-nuclear factors, and rheumatoid factors should be ordered [10].

4.3. Differential diagnosis

Some kinds of extra-articular disorders may mimic clinical signs and symptoms of TMJ ID and should be considered as differential diagnosis. These pathologic entities can be summarized as headache, neuralgia, migraine, atypical orofacial pain, ear disorders, coronoid process hyperplasia, trismus following inferior alveolar nerve anesthesia or muscle trauma, deep-space infections of maxillofacial region, radiation fibrosis, myositis ossificans, and metastasis of other regions' cancer [2, 5].

5. The treatment methods of internal derangements of temporomandibular joint

The most frequently used diagnostic classification system in order to decide proper management for ID of TMJ is Wilkes classification (**Table 1**) [4]. Wilkes defined five stages with clinical and radiographic features of ID and offered different treatment methods according to the stages of the disorder [4]. The treatment methods of TMJ ID can be basically divided into two subgroups: conservative and surgical. According to Wilkes classification [4], early stages of ID can be managed with conservative or minimally invasive methods; however, advanced stages (IV or V) might require open joint surgery. The principle of treatment consists of removal of the factors which can cause ID, reduction of symptoms, and also promote the healing of the articular structures. The disc displacement does not always cause mechanical obstruction. In the literature, MRI studies [21, 22] showed a high percentage of disc displacement in asymptomatic patients (about 32–38%) and thus it is controversial whether repositioning the disc into normal position should be a treatment goal or not.

The conservative and surgical treatments should never be considered separately. The two therapeutic options should always be taken into account. The lack of control of causal factors such as joint overload usually causes failure of the treatment.

5.1. Conservative methods

The conservative treatment is a fundamental therapeutic element. Mostly, it is also the first-line therapeutic step (except for the ankylosis, tumor diseases and cysts. For the corresponding diseases, the primary treatment method is the open surgery). The basis of the conservative therapy is the reduction of the joint loading and pain and also improvement of healing. If the causal factor of ID is diagnosed as excessive joint loading, most of these patients can be successfully managed with conservative methods. The conservative therapy includes a number of different treatment methods:

5.1.1. Patient education

The most important aspect of conservative treatment is to inform and educate the patients about the natural course, etiology, and pathogenesis of the ID. The diet modification, improved sleeping, and awareness of mandibular parafunction should be established by patient education. Patient education is the first and essential part of the management and makes the patients important partners for their care. The education of patients is crucial for control of all causal factors (especially excessive loading) leading to ID.

5.1.2. Drug treatment

This therapy includes several groups of drugs:

a. **Analgesic drugs:** They are used to reduce pain (most often non-steroidal anti-inflammatory—NSAI—drugs). NSAI drugs are also used to reduce inflammation.

b. **Anti-spasmodic and muscle relaxants:** They are used to reduce muscle spasm accompanying a number of painful conditions (in addition to reducing the skeletal muscle tone, it is also effective to reduce emotional stress).

c. **Chondroprotective drugs:** These drugs are capable of restoration of the metabolic balance in articular cartilage cells; their anti-inflammatory and analgesic effects are also described [8]. In our previous study [8], we concluded that glucosamine-chondroitin combination, which are structural molecules of joint cartilage and necessary for proteoglycan and glycosaminoglycan synthesis, significantly increases the mouth opening and decreases the inflammatory cytokine levels of synovial fluid in ID of TMJ. Moreover, this chondroprotective combination provides efficient pain relief as well as narcotic analgesics.

d. **Antidepressant drugs:** High prevalence of stress, depression, and anxiety is associated with TMD. Antidepressant medications are used to solve stress-related causal factors of TMD. These drugs have adjunct effects in improving sleep quality and reducing stress-related parafunctional habits including bruxism and clenching [23]. Low doses of antidepressant drugs have also analgesic effects.

e. **Antibiotics:** These drugs are only indicated in the event of accompanying infectious diseases of the joint (septic arthritis).

5.1.3. Physiotherapy

This is one of the basic therapeutic methods. The indications include discopathy and the hypermobility of the joint. The position of the dislocated disc can be improved by physiotherapy in discopathy cases. In hypermobility cases, the physiotherapy supports the strengthening of the ligaments of the articular capsule, thus reducing the excessive movement in the joint. Physiotherapy techniques are also used to improve the mobility in the masticatory and cervical spine muscles [6]. During physiotherapy, following cautions should be applied: the exercises should be performed at short time intervals (three to five times in a row) and multiple times in a day, which is better than exercising once a day for a longer time period (which can lead to the overload of the joint and occurrence and/or progression of the pain). Moreover, the exercise should always be done to the pain limit—avoid trying to overcome the pain by the movement. Aside from the reduction of joint loading, it is crucial to perform passive-motion exercises for a minimum of 2 months after surgical interventions [2]. The basis of the physiotherapy consists in

a. **Isometric exercises:** Exercises against palm resistance during which the active muscle groups are strengthened, strengthening the muscles and ligaments of the articular capsule.

b. **Post-isometric relaxation exercises:** Relaxation of muscle groups for the treatment of the increased muscle tone due to the emotional stress.

c. **Repositioning exercises:** These exercises are indicated for the alignment of the dislocated disc and mobilization of the joint (restoration of the jaw motion, indicated for the luxation of the jaw—the *Hippocrates maneuver* as well as for the acute dislocation of the disc).

d. **Massages of the chewing muscles:** These exercises are used to improve muscle blood flow, thus enhancing functions of the muscles and reducing their pain; they contribute to the movement coordination and to the stretching of spastic muscle fibers. These exercises are also used for rehabilitation of the opening, the most often used method in the post-operative care. It is divided into the passive one (when patients open their mouths using some aids or fingers) and the active ones (when the mouth opening is accompanied with the actual activities of the muscles).

5.1.4. Thermotherapy

Thermal stimuli—cold or heat—can be used in the treatment of ID. Cold causes reduction in passing of nerve impulses on nerve endings, thus reducing perception of pain. Furthermore, it causes local vasoconstriction and it acts as an anti-inflammatory agent. Cold is indicated mainly for bacterial inflammations. The use of cold may include compresses or the application of cooling sprays. The application of heat effects pain receptors in muscles and synovium, thus reducing the pain accompanying aseptic inflammations (such as arthritis and osteoarthritis). Heat is most often used in the form of hot compresses.

5.1.5. Bio-stimulating laser therapy

Low-level laser therapy (LLLT) supports reparation processes; it acts as the analgesic and anti-inflammatory agent (it stimulates mitochondria, supporting the production of aminisine triphosphate, increasing the blood flow in tissues, and increasing the lymphatic drainage). Moreover, the laser application stimulates blood microcirculation and reduces muscle contraction [24]. The bio-stimulation laser is indicated especially for aseptic arthritis and degenerative changes. The advantages of LLLT for the management of ID are that it provides aseptic, noninvasive, painless, non-pharmaceutical therapy without postoperative discomfort [24]. However, long-term effectiveness of LLLT for the management of TMD is limited [25].

5.1.6. Occlusal splint

This is a removable appliance of plastic material (most often resin) with a thickness of 1.5–3 mm. The splint can be made on the superior or inferior dental arch, while the splint on the inferior dental arch is preferred as it is better hidden and patients consider it better (**Figure 4**). The splints can be partial (covering only a part of the dental arch) or total (covering the dental arch completely). The treatment effect consists in the reduction in intra-articular pressure (thus reducing overload and pain), balancing of the occlusion, relaxation of the muscle spasm, and creation of the environment for easier alignment of the dislocated disc. It should be kept in mind that continuous and/or long-term use of an appliance may develop a malocclusion and must be avoided. An occlusal splint must meet several conditions:

- It must ensure a symmetrical, bilateral articulating contact of dental arches.
- It must be strong enough, with smooth edges and good retention.
- It should cover only the teeth; it must not irritate the periodontium.
- It must not be a functional obstacle, restrict the movement of the tongue, phonation, and swallowing.

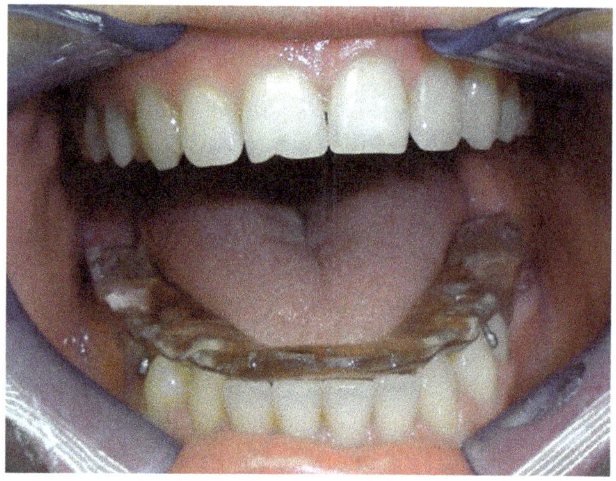

Figure 4. Clinical view of occlusal splint therapy used for conservative treatment of ID of TMJ.

The indications for the occlusal splint include the discopathy as well as inflammatory and degenerative changes. The splint is also used for patients with para-functional activities (night guard). In our previous clinical study [26], we observed that stabilization splint therapy provided significant improvements in pain relief, joint mobility (mouth opening and laterotrusive movements), disability, and psychological status of the patients with DDwoR after 6 months of treatment. However, the success rate of splint therapy was shown to be 60% for DDwoR. Splint therapy can be used alone or in combination with arthrocentesis. Our recent study showed that simultaneous splint application following arthrocentesis (success rate was 95%) has no significant additional effect on arthrocentesis alone (success rate was 92.5) for the treatment of DDwoR [26].

5.1.7. Inter-maxillary fixation

It is used to restrict the jaw motion, thus soothing inflammatory affections of the joint, leading to the reduction of pain. The inter-maxillary fixation (IMF) is most often used in the form of inter-maxillary screws and elastic bands. The indications for the IMF include, in particular, septic arthritis. Another application consists in a conservative treatment of articular eminence fractures, and it is further used for non-cooperating patients with recurrent luxations of the TMJ.

5.2. Surgical methods

The surgical treatment is provided in the event when the conservative treatment does not have any effects (the painful symptoms as well as joint dysfunctions still persist) for a period of 3–6 months. The risk of surgical intervention is the injury to the surrounding anatomic structures (in particular the facial nerve). The surgical treatments for ID consist in the following:

5.2.1. Arthrocentesis

This is the mini-invasive surgical method in order to perform the lavage of the superior joint space [27]. The intervention is performed directly into the joint structures; however, the operation input is limited to the injection needle only (**Figure 5**). It can be performed under local

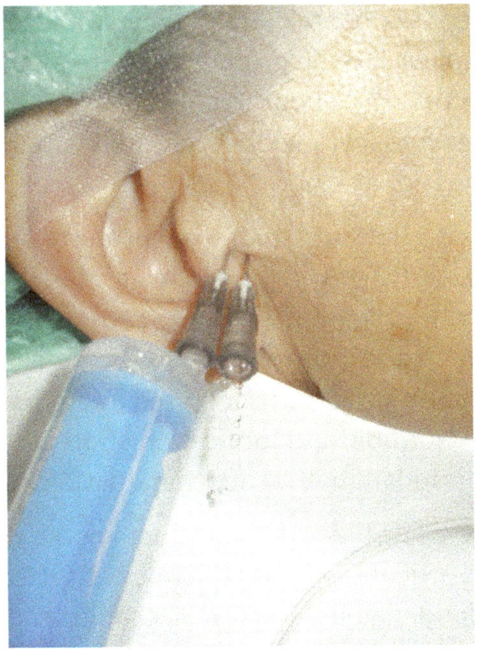

Figure 5. Clinical view of TMJ arthrocentesis used as a minimally invasive surgical treatment method of ID.

anesthesia alone or in combination with conscious sedation. The procedure can be performed in two different ways:

a. **Single-needle technique:** This is also called pumping arthrocentesis. The irrigation fluid is introduced into the joint with a single needle and subsequently removed through it.

b. **Two-needle technique:** One needle is used to introduce the fluid into the joint, whereas through the other needle the fluid escapes from the joint cavity.

The aim of the lavage is to flush out inflammatory mediators and loose particles from the joint space (to reduce pain), lysis of the adhesions in the joint, expand the joint cavity (to facilitate the alignment of the dislocated disc), change negative intra-articular pressure to positive pressure (to release the adhering disc), and irrigate micro-particles of the degenerative-changed cartilage (which otherwise irritate the joint synovium and lead to the development of inflammatory changes). Ringer's solution is used as the irrigation fluid (100–400 ml). Arthrocentesis requires less surgical skill and is an economic treatment method, but does not permit direct visualization and removal of pathologic intra-articular tissues and is less effective for lavage and removal of adhesions compared to arthroscopy. At the end of arthrocentesis, intra-articular application of the therapeutic drugs (corticosteroids, sodium hyaluronate, platelet-rich plasma (PRP), etc.) is also possible. It was reported that arthrocentesis was reliable for treating Wilkes II and III stages of ID, and the treatment results were better in patients with advanced stage [28].

5.2.2. Intra-articular application of drugs

The application of a number of medications directly into the superior synovial joint cavity (the space between the disc and glenoid fossa) is a treatment method. The following medications may be used for intra-articular application:

a. **Glucocorticoids:** These medications are used for their anti-inflammatory effects. They reduce the synthesis of prostaglandins and the production of antibodies, thus decreasing joint effusion and pain. After arthrocentesis, about 1 ml betamethasone can be used for anti-inflammatory purpose. The indications include osteoarthritic symptoms, rheumatoid arthritis, and inflammatory degenerative joint disease.

b. **Sodium hyaluronate:** This is a buffered solution of hyaluronate acid sodium salt, which is an essential component of the cartilage and the synovial fluid. It acts against the disintegration of the extracellular matrix. It activates reparation processes of the cartilage, improves the condition of chondrocytes, and the viscosity of the synovial fluid (it reduces friction), and it features an anti-inflammatory effect (through the inhibition of inflammatory cytokines). The hyaluronate has chondrotropic and lubrication effects. It is indicated for the treatment of osteoarthritic symptoms, inflammatory degenerative joint disease, and discopathy.

c. **Platelet-rich plasma (PRP):** The blood platelets obtained by centrifugation of the venous blood can be applied intra-articularly. The principle of the treatment consists in the growth factors contained in the blood platelets that cause changes in the cell proliferation, regulate the cellular metabolism, and affect chondrogenous activities. The indications of PRP in the TMJ include inflammatory degenerative diseases [29].

5.2.3. Arthroscopy

This is a method, in which the endoscope is introduced into the joint cavity; the endoscope allows examination of the intra-articular cavity through the transmission of the intra-articular image to the display (**Figure 6**). The endoscopes intended for the TMJ arthroscopy usually have a diameter of 1.9–2.7 mm. Typically, only the arthroscopy of the superior synovial cavity (the cavity between the disc and glenoid fossa) is performed; the arthroscopy of the inferior joint space (the cavity between the disc and condyle) is carried out less often due to the difficult access. The arthroscopy technique yields superior efficacy compared to arthrocentesis in removing articular adhesions, increasing joint function, and decreasing pain for the management of ID [30]. According to the performed intervention, the following is carried out:

a. **Diagnostic arthroscopy:** It consists in the visualization of each part of the joint space, while lysis of the adhesions and joint lavage are also carried out during the arthroscopy. In addition

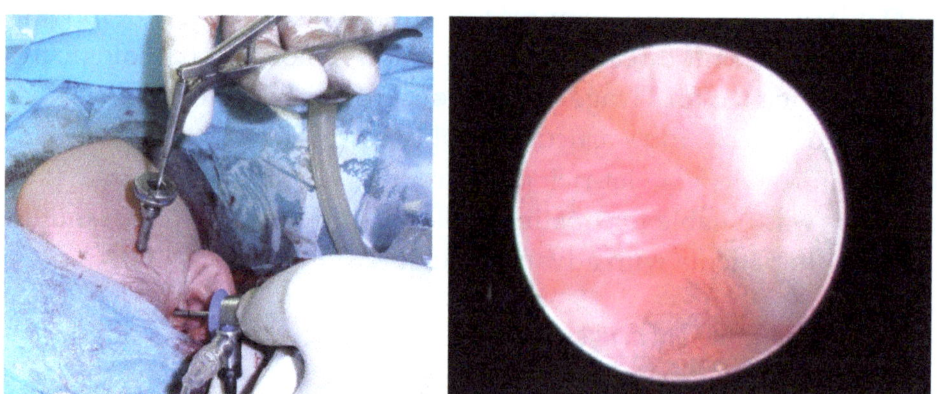

(a) (b)

Figure 6. TMJ arthroscopy: (a) clinical view and (b) endoscopic view of the joint.

to the endoscope, the needle used to release the irrigation fluid is introduced into the joint during the diagnostic arthroscopy. Through arthroscopic joint visualization, diagnosis of ID stage and identification of osteoarthritic changes can be established. The needle can also be used for the direct injection of medications into the inflammatory-changed synovial tissue and the retrodiscal tissue. In our previous clinical study [31], we observed that patients with a longer duration of symptoms of DDwoR had more advanced levels of fibrous adhesion and inflammatory and degenerative changes of the articular structures under arthroscopic view. The patients with a shorter duration of ID benefit more from arthroscopic lysis and lavage than those with longer duration of disease onset [31].

b. **Surgical arthroscopy:** It consists in the surgical intervention in the joint under arthroscopic view. In addition to the endoscope and the needle for releasing, the working (surgical) input for surgical tools (hook, probe, scissors, forceps, laser fiber, and shaver) is also introduced into the joint. The surgical arthroscopy is used to remove adhesions and to align and fix the disc, for synovectomy, discectomy (surgical removal of herniated disc material), or eminectomy (removal of the articular tubercle) procedures [32]. As shown in our recent technical note, hand-made alternative mini-instruments, which are made from stainless steel wire of 0.5 mm in diameter, can be used for the removal of adhesions during arthroscopic surgery [33]. It is also possible to obtain specimens for histopathologic examinations.

5.2.4. *Open joint surgery*

Open surgery is indicated only in the event that the conservative therapy, arthrocentesis, or arthroscopy does not have effects repeatedly (approximately 5% of the TMD patients) [34]. Generally, it can be concluded that the open surgery is indicated if all possibilities have been exhausted and the patient's condition has not improved or has even deteriorated. The exceptions include ankylosis, dislocated fractures of the articular eminence, tumors, and developmental anomalies (in which the surgical treatment is the first therapeutic step). The open joint surgery operations for TMJ ID can be performed on the soft and/or hard tissues of the joint. The most common for ID, open joint surgery may include discectomy, reshaping of the articular surface, and implementation of autologous or alloplastic materials [35]. Briefly, the following surgical interventions can be performed:

a. **Discopexy:** The open repositioning of the dislocated disc and its fixation in a suitable position related to the condyle (with a suture, pin, screw, and anchor).

b. **Discoplicacy:** This is another method to solve the dislocation of the disc. It is based on the assumption that the dislocation of the disc causes stretching of the retrodiscal tissue. During the discoplicacy, the rear part of the retrodiscal tissue is excised and then the remaining parts are approximated to each other with a suture. Thus, the disc is aligned and fixed back in its physiologic position.

c. **Discoplasty:** The reparation of the disc perforation accompanying degenerative changes consists in closing of small perforations (with a suture or its overlap). It is indicated only for young patients.

d. **Discectomy:** The removal of the disc is indicated for extensive degenerative changes (disc perforation) or if the patients have persistent symptoms after discoplasty treatment

(**Figure 7**). In ID patients showing no improvement with previous mini-invasive modalities, discectomy offers regaining jaw motion and reducing orofacial pain and may be followed with disc replacement.

e. **Condyloplasty:** The removal of unevenness from the condyle, grinding, and smoothing. It is indicated for accompanying degenerative changes.

f. **Condylar shaving:** The removal of 3–5-mm bone tissue from the top of the condyle is indicated for condylar hyperplasia at the active stage of the growth (**Figure 8**).

g. **Condylectomy:** The removal of the condyle in the event of extensive degenerative changes (**Figure 9**).

h. **Eminoplasty or Eminectomy:** These methods are basically introduced for the treatment of joint hypermobility. However, the osteoplasty or the removal of the articular tubercle can also be performed for the treatment of TMJ ID, for repositioning of the dislocated disc. In the TMJ ID cases, the disc is caught between the condyle and articular eminence; thus, eminectomy procedure expands the space between the bony structures so the disc can be aligned back to its original position.

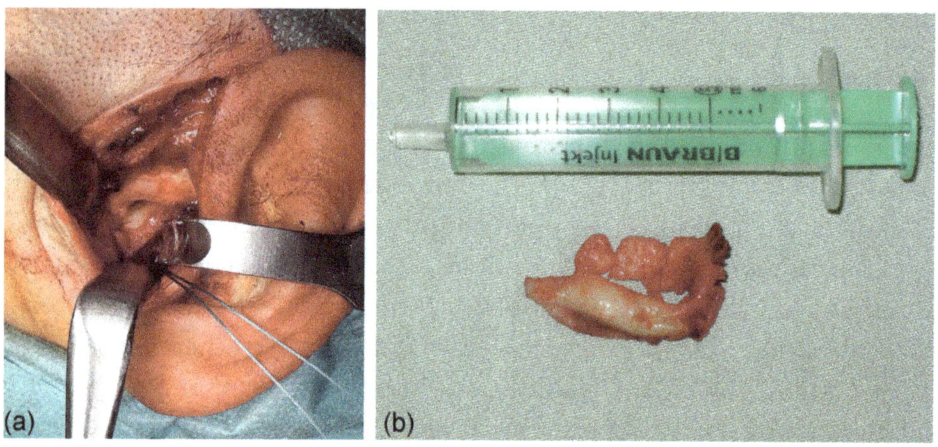

Figure 7. TMJ discectomy as a surgical treatment method of ID; (a) surgical (preauricular) approach, (b) removed articular disc tissue.

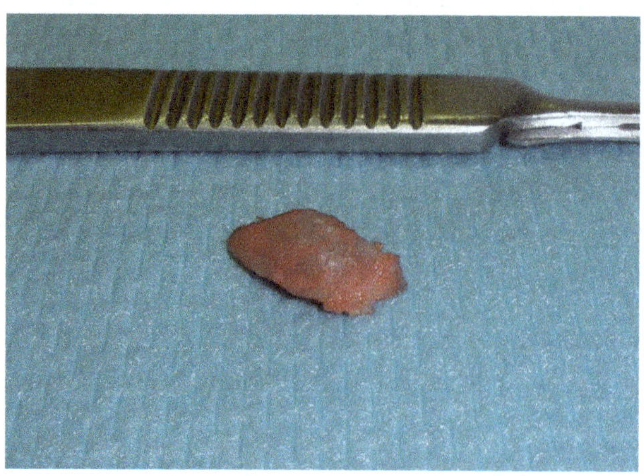

Figure 8. Condylar shaving is the removal of 3–5-mm bone tissue from the top of the condyle.

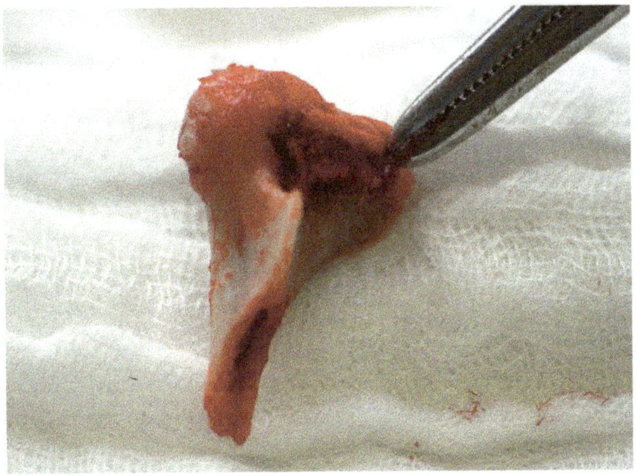

Figure 9. Condylectomy is the removal of the condyle. This technique can be used in the event of extensive degenerative changes caused by advanced stages of ID of TMJ.

i. **Reconstruction of the joint:** It can be divided into the reconstructions of the disc, condyle, and articular fossa:

- **Disc reconstruction:** The reconstruction of articular disc is performed after the discectomy. The subsequent direct contact of the condyle with the fossa can lead to the progression of the degenerative changes and the occurrence of the ankylosis. This is prevented by the interposition material, which is inserted into the joint cavity. For disc replacement, a variety of tissues and materials are used including abdominal fat graft, auricular cartilage, temporalis muscle or fascia, silastic, and proplast-teflon disc implants [6].

- **Fossa reconstruction:** The reconstruction of the glenoid fossa is performed using fossa prosthesis. The fossa prosthesis is made of metal alloys; the fossa is fixed with mini-screws to the zygomatic arch. It is described for degenerative changes.

- **Condyle reconstruction:** The reconstruction of the condyle is performed after resection of the condyle. The reconstructive materials are fixed to the branch of the inferior jaw. The autologous (costochondral, sternoclavicular, metatarsophalangeal bone grafts, especially indicated for young patients due to the growth activity of graft materials) and alloplastic (made of metal alloys) materials are used for the reconstruction.

- **Total joint reconstruction:** The total joint prosthesis combines the replacement of the fossa and the condyle at the same time. The condyles are made of chromium-cobalt alloy (and they are fixed to the branch of the inferior jaw with mini-screws). The fossa is made of the high-polymerized polyethylene (and it is fixed with mini-screws to the zygomatic arch). The articular prostheses are available in the form of stock prosthesis (where there is a number of fossa and condyle sizes available) and custom prosthesis (which are made individually according to the patient's CT-based stereolithographic model) (**Figure 10**). It is clearly evident that the individual prostheses are more convenient. However, their use is limited by a higher price compared to stock prostheses [36].

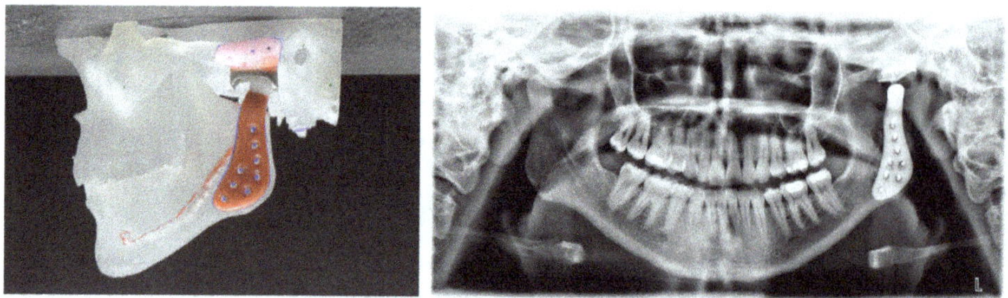

(a) (b)

Figure 10. The total joint reconstruction combines the replacement of the fossa and the condyle at the same time; (a) production stage of custom-made TMJ prosthesis which is made individually according to the patient's CT-based stereolithographic model, (b) postoperative OPG of a patient with custom-made TMJ prosthesis.

6. Tissue engineering in temporomandibular joint reconstruction

In the current century, the main topic of new studies searching the contemporary treatment methods of TMJ ID is the repair and replacement of joint structures by using tissue engineering methods. The main objective is to produce joint components (such as mandibular condyle or articular disc) that have the ability to perform functional articulation. The main research areas are cell sourcing, biomaterials for scaffolding, and bioactive stimuli [6]. Using tissue engineering techniques, it is intended to produce joint components capable of adaptation to functional articulation and possessing the biochemical, biomechanical, and geometric properties of healthy TMJ tissues [6].

The possible indications for bioengineered articular structures can be summarized as untreatable condylar trauma, condylar hyperplasia, TMJ pathology in skeletally immature patients, and history of metal hypersensitivity (a contraindication for TMJ alloplastic replacement), and TMJ ID [37]. Bioengineered replacements have the potential to be able to grow with the patients, so tissue engineering technology may particularly offer significant benefits for skeletally immature patients requiring TMJ reconstruction. On the other hand, growth potential of bioengineered tissues should be considered cautiously. In terms of TMJ ID, surgical implantation of bioengineered articular disc may be a promising management for patients with unsalvageable disc (Wilkes stages III–V).

The possible contraindications for bioengineered TMJ reconstruction can be summarized as unresolved causal factors such as parafunctional habits, ankylosis (recurrence of ankylosis may occur in bioengineered articular structures as in autografts), history of multiple-failed TMJ arthroplasty (scar tissue can impede vascularization of bioengineered tissue), and autoimmune diseases (the underlying disease such as rheumatoid arthritis might destroy bioengineered tissue).

7. Conclusion

The TMJ disorders are widespread in population and ID is the most frequent type of TMD. The etiologic factors of ID are joint overload and localized and systemic arthropathies.

The real causal factors and correct diagnosis should be established in order to provide appropriate management. In early stages of TMJ ID, conservative methods are considered. If the derangement becomes more severe or refractory to conservative therapies, and in some special situations, proper surgical techniques should be considered. In these situations, the timing of surgical treatment and performing proper technique is crucial for long-term success. Otherwise, patients require repeat treatments indicating low promise for successful management. In terms of open joint surgery, it should be kept in mind that arthroplasty may be resulted in degenerative changes in the future and the patient may need further surgical treatments including total joint replacement. Currently, contemporary researches focus on replacing the disc or condyle in terms of tissue engineering therapy. However, it seems that there are many steps to solve in order to insert this technology into clinical practice.

Author details

Ufuk Tatli[1]* and Vladimir Machon[2]

*Address all correspondence to: dr.ufuktatli@gmail.com

1 Department of Oral and Maxillofacial Surgery, Çukurova University Faculty of Dentistry, Adana, Turkey

2 Department of Oral and Maxillofacial Surgery, Charles University and General University Hospital, Prague, Czech Republic

References

[1] Manfredini D, Guarda-Nardini L, Winocur E, Piccotti F, Ahlberg J, Lobbezoo F. Reasearch diagnostic criteria for temporomandibular disorders: A systematic review of axis I epidemiologic findings. Oral Surgery, Oral Medicine, Oral Pathology, Oral Radiology and Endodontics. 2011;**112**:453-462. DOI: 10.1016/j.tripleo.2011.04.021

[2] Israel HA. Internal derangement of the temporomandibular joint: New perspectives on an old problem. Oral and Maxillofacial Surgery Clinics of North America. 2016;**28**:313-333. DOI: 10.1016/j.coms.2016.03.009

[3] Kurita K, Westesson PL, Yuasa H, Toyama M, Machida J, Ogi N. Natural course of untreated symptomatic temporomandibular joint disc displacement without reduction. Journal of Dental Research. 1998;**77**:361-365. DOI: 10.1177/00220345980770020401

[4] Wilkes CH. Internal derangements of the temporomandibular joint. Pathological variations. Archives of Otolaryngology – Head & Neck Surgery. 1989;**115**:469-477. DOI: 10.1001/archotol.1989.01860280067019

[5] Schiffman E, Ohrbach R, Truelove E, Look J, Anderson G, Goulet JP, List T, Svensson P, Gonzalez Y, Lobbezoo F, Michelotti A, Brooks SL, Ceusters W, Drangsholt M, Ettlin D, Gaul C,

Goldberg LJ, Haythornthwaite JA, Hollender L, Jensen R, John MT, De Laat A, de Leeuw R, Maixner W, van der Meulen M, Murray GM, Nixdorf DR, Palla S, Petersson A, Pionchon P, Smith B, Visscher CM, Zakrzewska J, Dworkin SF, International RDC/TMD Consortium Network, International association for Dental Research; Orofacial Pain Special Interest Group, International Association for the Study of Pain. Diagnostic criteria for temporomandibular disorders (DC/TMD) for clinical and research applications: Recommendations of the International RDC/TMD Consortium Network and Orofacial Pain Special Interest Group. Journal of Oral & Facial Pain and Headache. 2014;**28**:6-27. DOI: 10.11607/jop.1151

[6] Murphy MK, MacBarb RF, Wong ME, Athanasiou KA. Temporomandibular disorders: A review of etiology, clinical management, and tissue engineering strategies. The International Journal of Oral & Maxillofacial Implants. 2013;**28**:e393-e414. DOI: 10.11607/jomi.te20

[7] Ernberg M. The role of molecular pain biomarkers in temporomandibular joint internal derangement. Journal of Oral Rehabilitation. 2017;**44**:481-491. DOI: 10.1111/joor.12480

[8] Damlar I, Esen E, Tatli U. Effects of glucosamine-chondroitin combination on synovial fluid IL-1β, IL-6, TNF-α and PGE2 levels in internal derangements of temporomandibular joint. Medicina Oral, Patologia Oral y Cirugia Bucal. 2015;**20**:e278-e283. DOI: 10.4317/medoral.20242

[9] Sidebottom AJ, Salha R. Management of the temporomandibular joint in rheumatoid disorders. British Journal of Oral and Maxillofacial Surgery. 2013;**51**:191-198. DOI: 10.1016/j.bjoms.2012.04.271

[10] Kalaykova SI, Klitsie AT, Visscher CM, Naeije M, Lobbezoo F. A retrospective study on possible predictive factors for long-term temporomandibular joint degeneration and impaired mobility in juvenile arthritis patients. Journal of Oral & Facial Pain and Headache. 2017;**31**:165-171. DOI: 10.11607/ofph.1656

[11] Araz Server E, Onerci Celebi O, Hamit B, Yigit O. A rare complication of tonsillitis: Septic arthritis of the temporomandibular joint. International Journal of Oral and Maxillofacial Surgery. 2017;**46**:1118-1120. DOI: 10.1016/j.ijom.2017.04.007

[12] Bertram S, Rudisch A, Innerhofer K, Pümpel E, Grubwieser G, Emshoff R. Diagnosing TMJ internal derangement and osteoarthritis with magnetic resonance imaging. Journal of the American Dental Association. 2001;**132**:753-761. DOI: 10.14219/jada.archive.2001.0272

[13] Al-Saleh MA, Alsufyani NA, Lagravere M, Nebbe B, Lai H, Jaremko JL, Major PW. MRI alone versus MRI-CBCT registered images to evaluate temporomandibular joint internal derangement. Oral Surgery, Oral Medicine, Oral Pathology and Oral Radiology. 2016;**122**:638-645. DOI: 10.1016/j.oooo.2016.07.024

[14] Krohn S, Frahm J, Merboldt KD, Wassmann T, Joseph AA, Bürgers R. Diagnosis of disk displacement using real-time MRI: Clinical report of two patients. Journal of Prosthetic Dentistry. DOI: 10.1016/j.prosdent.2017.03.022 [Epub ahead of print]

[15] Park KS, Song HC, Cho SG, Kang SR, Kim J, Jun HM, Song M, Jeong GC, Park HJ, Kwon SY, Min JJ, Bom HH. Open-mouth bone scintigraphy is better than closed-mouth bone

scintigraphy in the diagnosis of temporomandibular osteoarthritis. Nuclear Medicine and Molecular Imaging. 2016;**50**:213-218. DOI: 10.1007/s13139-016-0407-z

[16] Choi KH, Kwon OS, Jerng UM, Lee SM, Kim LH, Jung J. Development of electromyographic indicators for the diagnosis of temporomandibular disorders: A protocol for an assessor-blinded cross-sectional study. Integrative Medicine Research. 2017;**6**:97-104. DOI: 10.1016/j.imr.2017.01.003

[17] Manfredini D, Guarda-Nardini L. Ultrasonography of the temporomandibular joint: A literature review. International Journal of Oral and Maxillofacial Surgery. 2009;**38**:1229-1236. DOI: 10.1016/j.ijom.2009.07.014

[18] Strini PJ, Strini PJ, Barbosa Tde S, Gavião MB. Assessment of thickness and function of masticatory and cervical muscles in adults with and without temporomandibular disorders. Archives of Oral Biology. 2013;**58**:1100-1108. DOI: 10.1016/j.archoralbio.2013.04.006

[19] Dayisoylu EH, Cifci E, Uckan S. Ultrasound-guided arthrocentesis of the temporomandibular joint. British Journal of Oral and Maxillofacial Surgery. 2013;**51**:667-668. DOI: 10.1016/j.bjoms.2013.05.144

[20] Levorova J, Machon V, Hirjak D, Foltan R. Ultrasound-guided injection into the lower joint space of the temporomandibular joint. International Journal of Oral and Maxillofacial Surgery. 2015;**44**:491-492. DOI: 10.1016/j.ijom.2014.12.013

[21] Larheim TA, Westesson P, Sano T. Temporomandibular joint disk displacement: Comparison in asymptomatic volunteers and patients. Radiology. 2001;**218**:428-432. DOI: 10.1148/radiology.218.2.r01fe11428

[22] Katzberg RW, Westesson PL, Tallents RH, Drake CM. Anatomic disorders of the temporomandibular joint disc in asymptomatic subjects. Journal of Oral and Maxillofacial Surgery. 1996;**54**:147-153. DOI: 10.1016/S0278-2391(96)90435-8

[23] Rajan R, Sun YM. Reevaluating antidepressant selection in patients with bruxism and temporomandibular joint disorder. Journal of Psychiatric Practice. 2017;**23**:173-179. DOI: 10.1097/PRA.0000000000000227

[24] Marini I, Gatto MR, Bonetti GA. Effects of superpulsed low-level laser therapy on temporomandibular joint pain. The Clinical Journal of Pain. 2010;**26**:611-616. DOI: 10.1097/AJP.0b013e3181e0190d

[25] Douglas De Oliveira DW, Lages FS, Guimarães RC, Pereira TS, Botelho AM, Glória JC, Tavano KT, Gonçalves PF, Flecha OD. Do TMJ symptoms improve and last across time after treatment with red (660 nm) and infrared (790 nm) low level laser treatment (LLLT)? A survival analysis. Cranio. DOI: 10.1080/08869634.2017.1292176 [Epub ahead of print]

[26] Tatli U, Benlidayi ME, Ekren O, Salimov F. Comparison of the effectiveness of three different treatment methods for temporomandibular joint disc displacement without reduction. International Journal of Oral and Maxillofacial Surgery. 2017;**46**:603-609. DOI: 10.1016/j.ijom.2017.01.018

[27] Nitzan DW, Dolwick MF, Martinez GA. Temporomandibular joint arthrocentesis: A simplified treatment for severe, limited mouth opening. Journal of Oral and Maxillofacial Surgery. 1991;**49**:1163-1167. DOI: 10.1016/0278-2391(91)90409-F

[28] Ungor C, Atasoy KT, Taskesen F, Pirpir C, Yilmaz O. Long-term outcome of arthrocentesis plus hyaluronic acid injection in patients with Wilkes stage II and III temporomandibular joint internal derangement. Journal of Craniofacial Surgery. 2015;**26**:2104-2108. DOI: 10.1097/SCS.0000000000002078

[29] Hegab AF, Ali HE, Elmasry M, Khallaf MG. Platelet-rich plasma injection as an effective treatment for temporomandibular joint osteoarthritis. Journal of Oral and Maxillofacial Surgery. 2015;**73**:1706-1713. DOI: 10.1016/j.joms.2015.03.045

[30] Al-Moraissi EA. Arthroscopy versus arthrocentesis in the management of internal derangement of the temporomandibular joint: A systematic review and meta-analysis. International Journal of Oral and Maxillofacial Surgery. 2015;**44**:104-112. DOI: 10.1016/j.ijom.2014.07.008

[31] Machoň V, Sedý J, Klíma K, Hirjak D, Foltán R. Arthroscopic lysis and lavage in patients with temporomandibular anterior disc displacement without reduction. International Journal of Oral and Maxillofacial Surgery. 2012;**41**:109-113. DOI: 10.1016/j.ijom.2011.07.907

[32] McCain JP, Hossameldin RH, Srouji S, Maher A. Arthroscopic discopexy is effective in managing temporomandibular joint internal derangement in patients with Wilkes stage II and III. Journal of Oral and Maxillofacial Surgery. 2015;**73**:391-401. DOI: 10.1016/j.joms.2014.09.004

[33] Machon V, Levorova J, Foltan R, Hirjak D, Sidebottom A. Mini-instruments for minimally invasive arthroscopy of the temporomandibular joint: A technical note. British Journal of Oral and Maxillofacial Surgery. 2015;**53**:662-663. DOI: 10.1016/j.bjoms.2015.04.015

[34] Dolwick MF, Dimitroulis G. Is there a role for temporomandibular joint surgery? British Journal of Oral and Maxillofacial Surgery. 1994;**32**:307-313. DOI: 10.1016/0266-4356(94)90052-3

[35] Dolwick MF. The role of temporomandibular joint surgery in the treatment of patients with internal derangement. Oral Surgery, Oral Medicine, Oral Pathology, Oral Radiology and Endodontics. 1997;**83**:150-155. DOI: 10.1016/S1079-2104(97)90106-2

[36] Mercuri LG. Custom TMJ TJR devices. In: Mercuri LG, editor. Temporomandibular Joint Total Joint Replacement – TMJ TJR. A Comprehensive Reference for Researchers, Materials Scientists, and Surgeons. Switzerland: Springer; 2016. pp. 91-130. DOI: 10.1007/978-3-319-21389-7

[37] Salash JR, Hossameldin RH, Almarza AJ, Chou JC, McCain JP, Mercuri LG, Wolford LM, Detamore MS. Potential indications for tissue engineering in temporomandibular joint surgery. Journal of Oral and Maxillofacial Surgery. 2016;**74**:705-711. DOI: 10.1016/j.joms.2015.11.008

7

Optimizing the Management Outcomes in Patients with Temporomandibular Disorder

Buket Aybar, Yusuf Emes and Guhan Dergin

1. Introduction

Being one of the most controversial topics in dentistry, treatment of temporomandibular disorders (TMDs) requires the clinician to determine the patients' needs and try to help the patient based on the most recent scientific evidence. TMDs are today commonly considered as a collection of various conditions of the temporomandibular joint (TMJ) or the masticatory muscles, which have different etiologies and mechanisms but presenting with similar symptoms [1]. Temporomandibular joint (TMJ) is affected by musculoskeletal disorders of the neck and masticatory system [2], and it is important for the clinical practitioner to tell the difference between the complaint originating from a musculoskeletal disorder and a complaint caused by an intra-articular disorder. By making this discernment, the patient can receive the optimal management and is protected from going under unnecessary surgical interventions.

There are several classification systems for the TMDs. The most recent and the most commonly used classification is the research diagnostic criteria for temporomandibular disorders (RDC-TMD) [3]. The most common intra-articular disorders are known to be reducing and nonreducing anterior disc displacements.

Anterior disc displacement is a condition in which the disc is positioned anteriorly to the mandibular condyle. If the disc reduces on opening, this is called anterior disc displacement with reduction. If the disc does not reduce on opening, then this is called anterior disc displacement without reduction (irreductible disc displacement) which is closely related to acute closed lock [1, 4].

Anteriorly displaced discs are common findings in the asymptomatic patients too. Studies by Larheim et al. [5] and Davant et al. [6] reported that magnetic resonance imaging (MRI) shows that about one third of the asymptomatic patients have displaced discs. It is also known that anteriorly displaced discs are most of the time displaced medially too [7], and it is important to evaluate the patient's complaints and try to resolve the symptoms which are joint sounds, pain, and limited mouth opening. Chronic disc displacement can lead to the adhesion of the disc to the articular fossa. Pain in the TMJ is present in the 10% of the adult population and found more often in women [8]. However, it must be kept in mind that prior to initiating the treatment of a TMD patient, any possibilities of benign and malign tumors, developmental disorders, and fractures should be out-ruled.

If the overloading of the TMJ continues (parafunctional habits, bruxism) remodeling, mechanism is triggered. When overloading exceeds the limits of remodeling, degenerative process of the articular surfaces may begin leading to the osteoarthritis of the TMJ [9].

General consensus in treatment is that the most conservative and the most reversible method should be the initial treatment of choice. This is because temporomandibular disorders have a tendency of improving over time, and clinical experience shows that sometimes conservative treatments are as effective as invasive methods in relieving the patient's symptoms [10].

When a patient is referred to a dentist for a complaint of temporomandibular disorder, oral history must be taken, and the patient should initially be examined for medical pathologies of the head and neck, including intraoral examination to search for a pain of dentoalveolar origin, type of occlusion, and any indicator of parafunctional habits such as bruxism. Imaging studies should be performed if necessary. The patients should also be evaluated for neurological and psychological conditions and should be referred to a specialist if necessary [11].

Management of the TMD patient may require a multidisciplinary approach. Physical therapy, cognitive behavioral intervention, educating the patients on self-care, and sometimes referring the patient to a psychologist or psychiatrist are all parts of the management. However, in most of the cases, a dental practitioner can begin the initial management. Using a step-by-step approach, a wide range of treatment modalities may be applied alone or in combination with each other. When conservative methods are ineffective in treating the patient, more invasive methods are applied, and open surgery may be indicated in patients not responding to other treatments. The practitioner should know that duration of symptoms is an important factor in the treatment success even in open surgery; earlier interventions have a higher chance for success [12].

Being an important aspect of the management of the patients with TMD, patient education requires full compliance of the patient because the treatment may fail due to the non-cooperative behavior of the patient.

The patient should be informed not to contact the teeth during rest (preventing clenching at daytime), being aware of parafunctional habits such as nail biting, lip-cheek chewing, and jaw protrusion [1].

The patient must be informed that he/she should have a soft diet and should limit the range of mouth opening. Slow chewing, decreasing the amount of daily tea, and coffee consumption are all parts of the treatment [1, 13]. Biting the food using incisors should be avoided, and biting on the effected side is recommended in case of joint pain [1].

Self-management is another important part of the management process. Self-massage is the initial self-management therapy, which is found to be very helpful in pain management especially in patients with masticatory muscle-originated pain [14, 15]. In myofascial pain massaging, the trigger points especially lead to improvement in pain even though it is temporary, and the massage must be continued to keep the benefits obtained from it [13].

Another self-management method is the application of moist heat or application of ice especially in cases of local myalgia and myofascial pain [1]. As a simple method, 20 minutes of hot bath is found to be effective in decreasing muscle pain.

Another method that can be used is the application of a hot pack to the tender site for 20 minutes three times a day. Heat relaxes the muscles and provides increased blood flow to the muscles. Also when cold is applied, as a reaction in order to increase the heat in the cold-applied muscle, the brain increases the blood flow to the muscle by vasodilatation providing an improvement in pain. Most of the studies on cold application are about acute pain, so there is little data on the application of cold for the management of chronic pain [16].

Pharmacological therapy is a part of TMD management. Nonsteroidal anti-inflammatory drugs (NSAIDs), analgesics, muscle relaxants, anxiolytic drugs, local anesthetics, antidepressants, and corticosteroids are indicated in TMD treatment.

2. Nonsteroidal anti-inflammatory drugs

Analgesics and NSAIDs form an important part of the pharmacological treatment of the osteoarthritic TMJ. The American College of Rheumatology guidelines recommend the use of paracetamol as the first medication of choice for the osteoarthritic hip and knee [17–19]. The use of paracetamol is also recommended for the management of osteoarthritis by some authors; however, they conclude that paracetamol is effective in osteoarthritis only at very high, near toxicity level doses. Ibuprofen and naproxen are recommended agents in osteoarthritis of the TMJ, but in the management of chronic pain, cox-2 inhibitors such as celecoxib or meloxicam should be preferred, not only for their effectiveness in chronic pain but also for less gastrointestinal effects, for they may require a prolonged use in chronic pain [20].

NSAIDs provide anti-inflammatory effects and analgesia for the TMD patients with osteoarthritis, capsulitis, synovitis, myositis, and pain related to reducing and nonreducing disc displacements [21].

Naproxen, ibuprofen, and diclofenac are the most often used NSAIDs [22]. Mejersjo and Wenneberg [23] have studied the effects of diclofenac 50 mg, given orally 3 ×1 in patients with TMJ arthritis. Their findings at the end of 3 months produced results similar to efficacy of occlusal appliances.

Anti-inflammatory properties of corticosteroids are greater than that of NSAIDs. Because the long term systemic use of corticosteroids may lead to complications such as Cushing's syndrome, diabetes, and osteoporosis, they must be used only for a short time [24]. Anxiolytics is also recommended for a limited period of use because of their potential for dependency. Their sedative and muscle relaxant properties help reduce the effects of masticatory parafunctional habits such as bruxism. They help patients cope with stress, which is an important etiologic factor of TMD, stress-induced muscular hyperactivity, and dysfunction [22, 25]. A recent animal study has shown that the benzodiazepines also have effects on the biochemical content of the TMJ [26].

Usually used in combination with NSAIDs, centrally acting muscle relaxants help relax the masticatory muscles, and the patients may also benefit from their sedative properties [22]. The aim of using the muscle relaxants in the TMD patient is not only to manage acute muscle pain but also to decrease muscle activity for a limited period [27, 28].

The mechanism via which the muscle relaxants help the TMD patients is not totally clear. The prescribed doses are not high enough when taken orally to relax masticatory muscles locally. So, it is believed that their sedative and stress-reducing effects are more effective in helping the TMD patient [27].

Chlorzoxazone, cyclobenzaprine, methocarbamol, and diazepam are the most commonly used centrally acting muscle relaxants. All of these drugs have sedating effects, so the patients should preferably take them at bedtime [29].

Tizanidine is a spasmolytic agent, and there is so far only one clinical trial studying its effectiveness in the TMDs. Alencar et al. [30] have reported that tizanidine and cyclobenzaprine have effects similar to placebo on myofascial pain patients.

Even though there is little scientific evidence to support the efficacy of opioid analgesics in TMDs, they are usually prescribed together with non-opioid analgesics, in the management of TMJ pain. However, they must be used with caution for their tendency to create dependence in the patients. Opioid analgesics should be used only for short periods such as 2–3 weeks [22].

Hydrocodone is an opioid analgesic used in combination with a non-opioid analgesic or a NSAID in order to manage moderate to severe pain [31]. However, hydrocodone is not very effective in chronic pain cases. Codeine, morphine, oxycodone, hydromorphone, and fentanyl are also among the opioid analgesics preferred in the management of pain. The use of opioid analgesics is considered safe in some forms of noncancer pain as long as patients are selected carefully, well monitored for adverse effects, and onset of dependence [32].

However, it is still a subject of debate, which kind of opioids to use in the management of TMJ pain. Opioids are classified as short-acting and long-acting opioids. Short-acting opioids have the advantage of rapid onset of pain relief; however, they have a higher risk of drug-related adverse effects [33]. Long-acting opioids also help improve pain, and there is less reported drug-related adverse effects in patients [34]. However, Argoff and Silvershein [35] have not found any differences between the two types of drugs for efficacy.

Currently, due to lack of enough randomized controlled clinical trials on the clinical efficiency of pharmacological agents on TMD-related pain, it must be kept in mind that the pharmacological treatment in TMD patients is mostly empirical [36, 37].

Occlusal splints are the most commonly used treatment modality in the management of TMDs. Occlusal splints help in relieving the muscle hyperactivity originating from bruxism. Occlusal appliances also provide relief from occlusal overload to the TMJ and inhibit strain [38].

Casares et al. have [39] measured the effects of occlusal splints on intra-articular pressure using a pressure transducer, and they have concluded that stabilization splints significantly reduced the intra-articular pressure in the upper joint compartment. They have also reported better joint function as an outcome of splint treatment.

Conti et al. [40] have reported that even though behavioral treatment improves symptoms in patients with myofascial pain in short term, occlusal splints may accelerate the process, helping the patients to get positive results earlier. Another study even has hinted that occlusal splints may be helping improve the psychological status of the TMD patients [41].

First described for the temporomandibular joint by Nitzan et al. [42], arthrocentesis is simply the irrigation of the superior TMJ compartment using two needles and is considered to be an efficient process with low morbidity rate [43]. When applied for the treatment of TMJ osteoarthritis, this process removes degradation products and inflammatory mediators from the joint [44, 45]. However, Laskin [44] has stated that intra-articular lavage may also remove the favorable agents such as hyaluronic acid from the intra-articular space too. TMJ arthrocentesis may inhibit pain and increase the range of mandibular motion [42, 46, 47].

Two needles are used for irrigation and outflow of the irrigation solution, which is in most cases ringers lactate solution [9]. The amount of ringer's solution is a subject of debate and varies between 60 ml [48] and 200 ml [49] in the literature.

The current understanding in the management of TMDs positions arthrocentesis after the initial conservative treatment modalities. When the conservative treatment fails, then arthrocentesis is indicated. However, some studies have evaluated the outcomes of arthrocentesis as an initial treatment. Vos et al. [50] have studied 80 patients in which 40 patients had arthrocentesis as an initial treatment, and the other 40 received conservative treatment as control. They have reported a more rapid improvement in symptoms following arthrocentesis, whereas the conservative treatment group showed a more gradual improvement. Their study has also shown that both methods produced similar results at the end of 26 weeks. However, they have discussed that this might be partially due to conservative treatment being dependent on patient compliance, whereas arthrocentesis is not, which may affect the outcome of the study. Machon et al. [45] have reported arthrocentesis to be more effective when combined with splint therapy.

Arthrocentesis may be performed in combination with the injection of various agents such as sodium hyaluronate [51] and corticosteroids (It has been previously reported that corticosteroids have positive effects on pain and function when injected intra-articularly) [52, 53]. For this reason, corticosteroid injection alone or in combination with arthrocentesis is used for treatment of the internal derangements of the TMJ. However, the injection of corticosteroids into the TMJ is still controversial due to reported complications such as bone necrosis, destruction of the cartilage, and progression of the degenerative disease [54–56]. These complications are reported to be mostly due to multiple injections or high-dose injections, and single injections are considered to be safe [57].

Sodium chlorate injections are also commonly used in the TMDs [58–61]. They are either used in single injections or multiple injections, and multiple arthrocenteses followed by multiple injections of sodium hyaluronate have been found to be beneficial in patients with internal derangement [62, 63].

However, Manfredini et al. [51] have stated that a single dose of sodium hyaluronate injection following single arthrocentesis produced benefits similar to multiple interventions.

Emes et al. [64] have compared the effects of arthrocentesis to tenoxicam injection alone and reported no differences between the groups. However, their groups consisted of patients who did not respond to a previous arthrocentesis.

Sipahi et al. [48] have injected morphine and tramadol following arthrocentesis into the TMJs of patients with TMJ pain and have concluded that injection of morphine has significantly increased pain relief for 6 months. They have had similar pain relief with tramadol too, but this relief period was shorter in tramadol when compared to morphine.

Arthroscopy of the TMJ is an invasive surgical technique, which is used for the diagnosis and treatment of internal derangements of the TMJ [9]. It also has a low risk of degenerative articular change in the long term, which makes it a safe procedure (has lower complications than open surgery and less invasive than open surgery) [65]. However, it is not beneficial in examining the lower joint compartment. When there is a degenerative process affecting the lower joint compartment, usually an open surgery is indicated. Arthroscopy and arthrocentesis have similar benefits in TMDs, but arthroscopy is the technique of choice in the diagnosis and management of rheumatoid disorders affecting the TMJ [66]. It can also be used for techniques other than simple lysis and lavage; for example, Murakami et al. [67] have reported that arthroscopic lateral release of the capsule and anterior discal release were more effective than arthrocentesis in increasing the range of mouth opening.

Several studies show that the majority of TMDs can be managed by nonsurgical methods. When these methods fail to help the patient with his/her symptoms, then invasive techniques, such as arthrocentesis and arthroscopy, or open joint surgery are indicated [68]. Open procedures are used in order to reposition the anteriorly displaced disc, remove the anteriorly displaced disc, or remove and replace it (by temporalis flap, auricular cartilage, or an alloplastic material) [69, 70]. Several studies conclude that, in the treatment of the internal derangement of TMJ, open surgery is more effective in decreasing pain when compared to arthroscopic surgery [69, 70–73].

3. Conclusion

The treatment of the TMD patient is challenging for the clinician because of the complex pathophysiology of the disorder, and deciding the optimal method for these patients is a difficult task. Our current treatment modalities all have some degree of placebo properties, and due to lack of randomized controlled clinical trials with placebo, our treatment protocols may fall within the boundaries of empirical treatment. In most cases, optimal treatment is the treatment targeting the patient's individual needs, a step-by-step approach, avoiding aggressive, radical surgical protocols as much as possible, will be beneficial for the patient and increase the successful outcomes of our treatment.

Author details

Buket Aybar[1], Yusuf Emes[1]* and Guhan Dergin[2]

*Address all correspondence to: yusufemes@yahoo.com

1 Faculty of Dentistry, Department of Oral and Maxillofacial Surgery, Istanbul University, Turkey

2 Faculty of Dentistry, Department of Oral and Maxillofacial Surgery, Marmara University, Turkey

References

[1] McNeill C, Rudd PA. Diagnosis and non-surgical management of orofacial pain. In: Andersson L, Kahnberg K, Pogrel MA, editors. Oral and Maxillofacial Surgery. West Sussex: Blackwell; 2010. pp. 1175-1197

[2] Lipton JA, Ship JA, Larach-Robinson D. Estimated prevalence and distribution of reported orofacial pain in the United States. Journal of the American Dental Association (1939). 1993;**124**(10):115-121

[3] Schiffman E, Ohrbach R, Truelove E, Look J, Anderson G, Goulet JP, et al. Diagnostic criteria for Temporomandibular disorders (DC/TMD) for clinical and research applications: Recommendations of the international RDC/TMD consortium network* and orofacial pain special interest group. Journal of Oral & Facial Pain and Headache. 2014 Winter;**28**(1):6-27

[4] Sidebottom AJ. How do I manage restricted mouth opening secondary to problems with the temporomandibular joint? The British Journal of Oral & Maxillofacial Surgery. 2013 Sep;**51**(6):469-472

[5] Larheim TA, Westesson PL, Sano T. Temporomandibular joint disk displacement: Comparison in asymptomatic volunteers and patients. Radiology. 2001;**218**(2):428-432

[6] Davant TSI, Greene CS, Perry HT, Lautenschlager EP. A quantitative computer-assisted analysis of the disc displacement in patients with internal derangement using sagittal view and magnetic resonance imaging. Journal of Oral and Maxillofacial Surgery. 1993;**51**(9):974-979

[7] Kurita K, Westesson PL, Tasaki MM, Liedberg J. Temporomandibular joint: Diagnosis of medial and lateral disc displacement with anterioposterior arthrography. Correlations with cryosections. Oral Surgery, Oral Medicine, Oral Pathology, Oral Radiology, and Endodontics. 1992;**73**(3):364-368

[8] LeResche L. Epidemiology of temporomandibular disorders: Implications for the investigation of etiologic factors. Critical Reviews in Oral Biology and Medicine. 1997; **8**(3):291-305

[9] Holmlund A. Arthroscopy and arthroscopic surgery. In: Andersson L, Kahnberg K, Pogrel MA, editors. Oral and Maxillofacial Surgery. West Sussex: Blackwell; 2010. pp. 1197-1208

[10] Greene CS. Management of patients with TMDs: A new standard of care. The International Journal of Prosthodontics. 2010;**23**(3):190-191

[11] De Boever JA, Nilner M, Orthlieb JD, et al. Recommendations by the EACD for examination, diagnosis, and management of patients with temporomandibular disorders and orofacial pain by the general dental practitioner. Journal of Orofacial Pain. 2008; **22**(3):268-278

[12] Al-Moraissi EA. Open versus arthroscopic surgery for the management of internal derangement of the temporomandibular joint: A meta-analysis of the literature. International Journal of Oral and Maxillofacial Surgery. 2015 Jun;**44**(6):763-770

[13] Wright EF. Self-management Therapy. In: Manual of Temporomandibular Disorders. Iowa: Wiley-Blackwell; 2010. pp. 209-225

[14] Riley JL 3rd, Myers CD, Currie TP, Mayoral O, Harris RG, Fisher JA, Gremillion HA, Robinson ME. Self -care behaviors associated with myofascial temporomandibular disorder pain. Journal of Orofacial Pain. 2007;**21**(3):194-202

[15] DeBar LL, Vuckovic N, Schneider J, Ritenbaugh C. Use of complementary and alternative medicine for temporomandibular disorders. Journal of Orofacial Pain. 2003;**17**(3):224-236

[16] Clark GT. Differential diagnosis and management of masticatory myogenous pain and dysfunction. In: Clark GT, Dione RA, editors. Orofacial Pain: A Guide to Medications and Management. West Sussex: Blackwell; 2012. pp. 271-294

[17] Hochberg MC, Altman RD, Brandt KD, Clark BM, Dieppe PA, Griffin MR, et al. Guidelines for the medical management of osteoarthritis. Part I. Osteoarthritis of the hip. Arthritis and Rheumatism. 1995;**38**(11):1535-1540

[18] Hochberg MC, Altman RD, Brandt KD, Clark BM, Dieppe PA, Griffin MR, et al.; American College of Rheumatology. Guidelines for the medical management of osteoarthritis. Part II. Osteoarthritis of the knee. Arthritis and Rheumatism. 1995;**38**(11):1541-1546

[19] Lane NE, Thompson JM. Management of osteoarthritis in the primary-care setting: An evidence-based approach to treatment. The American Journal of Medicine. 1997; **103**(6A):25S-30S

[20] Teruel A, Broussard JS, Clark GT. Temporomandibular joint arthritis: Implications, diagnosis, and management. In: Clark GT, Dione RA, editors. Orofacial Pain: A Guide to Medications and Management. West Sussex: Blackwell; 2012. pp. 271-294

[21] Syrop S. Pharmacologic management of myofascial pain and dysfunction. Oral and Maxillofacial Surgery Clinics of North America. 1995;**7**:87-97

[22] Karlis V, Glickman R. Nonsurgical management of temporomandibular disorders. In: Miloro M, Ghali GE, Larsen PE, Waite PD, editors. Peterson's Principles of Oral and Maxillofacial Surgery. Second ed. Vol. 2. Ontario, Canada: BC Decker; 2004. pp. 949-961

[23] Mejersjo C, Wenneberg B. Diclofenac sodium and occlusal splint therapy in TMJ osteoarthritis: A randomized controlled trial. Journal of Oral Rehabilitation. 2008;**35**(10):729-738

[24] Streeten DHP. Corticosteroid therapy, complication and therapeutic indication. JAMA. 1975;**232**(10):1046-1059

[25] Scrivani SJ, Keith DA, Kaban LB. Temporomandibular disorders. The New England Journal of Medicine. 2008;**359**(25):2693-2705

[26] Figueroba SR, Desjardins MP, Nani BD, et al. Effect of diazepam on temporomandibular joints in rats with increased occlusal vertical dimension. The British Journal of Oral & Maxillofacial Surgery. 2014;**52**(5):438-444

[27] Dionne RA. Pharmacologic approaches. In: Laskin DM, Greene CS, Hylander WL, editors. Temporomandibular Disorders: An Evidence-Based Approach to Diagnosis and Treatment. Hanover Park, IL: Quintessence; 2006. pp. 347-357

[28] Winocur E, Gavish A, Voikovitch M, Emodi -Perlman A, Eli I. Drugs and bruxism: A critical review. Journal of Orofacial Pain. 2003;**17**(2):99-111

[29] Wright EF. Pharmacological management. In: Manual of Temporomandibular Disorders. Iowa: Wiley-Blackwell; 2010. pp. 251-264

[30] Alencar FG Jr, Viana PG, Zamperini C, Becker A. Patient education and self-care for the management of jaw pain upon awakening: A randomized controlled clinical trial comparing the effectiveness of adding pharmacologic treatment with cyclobenzaprine or tizanidine. Journal of Oral & Facial Pain and Headache. 2014 Spring;**28**(2):119-127

[31] Clark GT, Richeimer SH Opioids for chronic orofacial pain with a focus on nonmalignant chronic pain. In: Clark GT and Dione RA editors. Orofacial Pain: A Guide to Medications and Management. West Sussex: Blackwell; 66-83

[32] Bouloux GF. Use of opioids in long-term management of temporomandibular joint dysfunction. Journal of Oral and Maxillofacial Surgery. 2011;**69**(7):1885-1891

[33] Simon S. Opioids and treatment of chronic pain: Understanding pain patterns and the role for rapid-onset opioids. Med. Genetics in Medicine. 2005;**7**(4):54

[34] McCarberg B, Barkin R. Long-acting opioids for chronic pain: Pharmacotherapeutic opportunities to enhance compliance, quality of life, and analgesia. American Journal of Therapeutics. 2001;**8**(3):181

[35] Argoff C, Silvershein D. A comparison of long-and short-acting opioids for the treatment of chronic noncancer pain: Tailoring therapy to meet patient needs. Mayo Clinic Proceedings. 2009;**84**(7):602-612

[36] Cascos-Romero J, Va'zquez-Delgado E, Va'zquez-Rodrı'guez E, Gay-Escoda C. The use of tricyclic antidepressants in the treatment of temporomandibular joint disorders: systematic review of the literature of the last 20 years. Medicina Oral, Patología Oral y Cirugía Bucal. 2009;**14**(1):E3-E7

[37] List T, Axelsson S, Leijon G. Pharmacologic interventions in the treatment of temporomandibular disorders, atypical facial pain, and burning mouth syndrome. A qualitative systematic review. Journal of Orofacial Pain. 2003;**17**(4):301-310

[38] Kuttila M, Le Bell Y, Savolainen-Niemi E, Kuttila S, Alanen P. Efficiency of occlusal appliance therapy in secondary otalgia and temporomandibular disorders. Acta Odontologica Scandinavica. 2002;**60**(4):248-254

[39] Casares G, Thomas A, Carmona J, Acero J, Vila CN. Influence of oral stabilization appliances in intra-articular pressure of the temporomandibular joint. Cranio. 2014; **32**(3):219-223

[40] Conti PC, de Alencar EN, da Mota Corrêa AS, et al. Behavioural changes and occlusal splints are effective in the management of masticatory myofascial pain: A short-term evaluation. Journal of Oral Rehabilitation. 2012;**39**(10):754-760

[41] Costa YM, Porporatti AL, Stuginski-Barbosa J, Bonjardim LR, Conti PC. Additional effect of occlusal splints on the improvement of psychological aspects in temporomandibular disorder subjects: A randomized controlled trial. Archives of Oral Biology. 2015;**60**(5):738-744

[42] Nitzan DW, Dolwick MF, Martinez GA. Temporomandibular joint arthrocentesis: A simplified treatment for severe, limited mouth opening. Journal of Oral and Maxillofacial Surgery. 1991;**49**(11):1163-1167

[43] Al-Belasy FA, Dolwick MF. Arthrocentesis for the treatment of temporomandibular joint closed lock: A review article. International Journal of Oral and Maxillofacial Surgery. 2007;**36**(9):773-782

[44] Laskin DM. Arthrocentesis for the treatment of internal derangements of the temporomandibular joint. The Alpha Omegan. 2009;**102**(2):46-50

[45] Machon V, Hirjak D, Lukas J: Therapy of the osteoarthritis of the temporomandibular joint. Journal of Cranio-Maxillo-Facial Surgery. 2011;**39**(2):127-130

[46] Currie R. Temporomandibular joint arthrocentesis and lavage. Evidence-Based Dentistry. 2009;**10**(4):110

[47] Monje-Gil F, Nitzan D, Gonzalez-Garcia R: Temporomandibular joint arthrocentesis. Review of the literature. Medicina Oral Patologia Oral y Cirugia Bucal. 2012;**17**(4): 575-581

[48] Sipahi A, Satilmis T, Basa S. Comparative study in patients with symptomatic internal derangements of the temporomandibular joint: Analgesic outcomes of arthrocentesis with or without intra-articular morphine and tramadol. The British Journal of Oral & Maxillofacial Surgery. 2015;**53**(4):316-320

[49] Sidebottom AJ. How do I manage restricted mouth opening secondary to problems with the temporomandibular joint? The British Journal of Oral & Maxillofacial Surgery. 2013;**51**(6):469-472

[50] Vos LM, Huddleston Slater JJ, Stegenga B. Arthrocentesis as initial treatment for temporomandibular joint arthropathy: A randomized controlled trial. Journal of Cranio-Maxillo-Facial Surgery. 2014;**42**(5):134-139

[51] Manfredini D, Rancitelli D, Ferronato G, et al. Arthrocentesis with or without additional drugs in temporomandibular joint inflammatory-degenerative disease: Comparison of six treatment protocols. Journal of Oral Rehabilitation. 2012;**39**(4):245-251

[52] Hersh EV, Balasubramaniam R, Pinto A. Pharmacologic management of temporomandibular disorders. Oral and Maxillofacial Surgery Clinics of North America. 2008;**20**(2): 197-210

[53] Dimitroulis G, Dolwick MF. Temporomandibular disorders. Part3. Surgical treatment. Australian Dental Journal. 1996;**41**(3):16-20

[54] Haddad IK. Temporomandibular joint osteoarthrosis. Histopathological study of the effects of intra-articular injection of triamcinolone acetonide. Saudi Medical Journal. 2000;**21**(7):675-679

[55] Lida K, Kurita K, Tange K, Yoshida K. Necrosis of the articular tubercle after repeated injections of sodium hyaluronate in the temporomandibular joint. A case report. International Journal of Oral and Maxillofacial Surgery. 1998;**27**(4):278-279

[56] Aggarwal S, Kumar A. A cortisone-wrecked and bony ankylosed temporomandibular joint. Plastic and Reconstructive Surgery. 1989;**83**(6):1084-1085

[57] Toller PA. Use and misuse of intra-articular corticosteroids in treatment of temporomandibular joint pain. Proceedings of the Royal Society of Medicine. 1977;**70**(7):461-463

[58] Mountziaris PM, Kramer PR, Mikos AG. Emerging intra-articular drug delivery systems for the temporomandibular joint. Methods. 2009;**47**(2):134-140

[59] Bertolami CN, Gay T, Clark GT, Rendell SV, Liu C, et al. Use of sodium hyaluronate in treating temporomandibular joint disorders: A randomized, double-blind, placebo-controlled clinical trial. Journal of Oral and Maxillofacial Surgery. 1993;**51**(3):232-242

[60] Hepguler S, Akkoc YS, Pehlivan M, Ozturk C, Celebi G, Saracoglu A, et al. The efficacy of intra-articular sodium hyaluronate in patients with reducing displaced disc of the temporomandibular joint. Journal of Oral Rehabilitation. 2002;**29**(1):80-86

[61] Yeung RW, Chow RL, Samman N, Chiu K. Short-term therapeutic outcome of intraarticular high molecular weight hyaluronic acid injection for nonreducing disc displacement of the temporomandibular joint. Oral Surgery, Oral Medicine, Oral Pathology, Oral Radiology, and Endodontics. 2006;**102**(4):453-461

[62] Guarda-Nardini L, Cadorin C, Frizziero A, Ferronato G, Manfredini D: Comparison of 2 hyaluronic acid drugs for the treatment of temporomandibular joint osteoarthritis. Journal of Oral and Maxillofacial Surgery. 2012;**70**(11):2522-2530

[63] Tuncel U. Repeated sodium hyaluronate injections following multiple arthrocenteses in the treatment of early stage reducing disc displacement of the temporomandibular joint: A preliminary report. Journal of Cranio-Maxillo-Facial Surgery. 2012;**40**(8):685-689

[64] Emes Y, Arpınar IŞ, Oncü B, et al. The next step in the treatment of persistent temporomandibular joint pain following arthrocentesis: A retrospective study of 18 cases. Journal of Cranio-Maxillo-Facial Surgery 2014;**42**(5):65-69

[65] Israel HA. The use of arthroscopic surgery for treatment of temporomandibular joint disorders. Journal of Oral and Maxillofacial Surgery. 1999;**57**(5):579-582

[66] Sidebottom AJ, Salha R. Management of the temporomandibular joint in rheumatoid disorders. The British Journal of Oral & Maxillofacial Surgery. 2013;**51**(3):191-198

[67] Murakami K, Hosaka H, Moriya Y, Segami N, Iizuka T. Short-term treatment outcome study for the management of temporomandibular joint closed lock. A comparison of arthrocentesis to nonsurgical therapy and arthroscopic lysis and lavage. Oral Surgery, Oral Medicine, Oral Pathology, Oral Radiology, and Endodontics. 1995;**80**(3):253-257

[68] Schiffman EL, Look JO, Hodges JS, Swift JQ, Decker KL, Hathaway KM, et al. Randomized effectiveness study of four therapeutic strategies for TMJ closed lock. Journal of Dental Research. 2007;**86**(1):58-63

[69] Dolwick MF, Sanders B. TMJ Internal Derangement and Arthrosis: Surgical Atlas. St. Louis: Mosby; 1985

[70] Witsenburg B, Freihofer HP. Replacement of the pathologic temporomandibular articular disc using autogenous cartilage of the external ear. International Journal of Oral Surgery. 1984;**13**(5):401-405

[71] Politi M, Sembronio S, Robiony M, Costa F, Toro C, Undt G. High condylectomy and disc repositioning compared to arthroscopic lysis, lavage, and capsular stretch for the treatment of chronic closed lock of the temporomandibular joint. Oral Surgery, Oral Medicine, Oral Pathology, Oral Radiology, and Endodontics. 2007;**103**(1):27-33

[72] Undt G, Murakami K, Rasse M, Ewers R. Open versus arthroscopic surgery for internal derangement of the temporomandibular joint: A retrospective study comparing two centres' results using the jaw pain and function questionnaire. Journal of Cranio-Maxillo-Facial Surgery. 2006;**34**(4):234-241

[73] Marciani RD, Ziegler RC. Temporomandibular joint surgery: A review of fifty-one operations. Oral Surgery, Oral Medicine, Oral Pathology, Oral Radiology, and Endodontics. 1983;**56**(5):472-476

8

Temporomandibular Joint Pathology and its Indication in Clinical Orthodontics

Bakr M. Rabie, Jeremy Ho and Qianfeng Li

Abstract

Temporomandibular joint (TMJ) pathology has been an area of study in dentistry specifically a research interest in clinical orthodontics in which treatment option has been a dilemma for practitioners. Discussion between 'dos' and 'don'ts' in growth modification has drawn spread however opposite opinions from different schools of thoughts in whether growth modification itself is working. To provide a better illustration of biological process within TMJ, this chapter discussed aspects including overall condylar growth; the histological structure of endochondral bone of condyle; extracellular factors that regulate proliferation, differentiation, hypertrophy, terminal maturation and apoptosis of chondrocytes; and molecular regulation of the entire process. An understanding of the pathology, histology, cellular and molecular events related to the morphology and growth of TMJ forms through reading over this chapter; the emphasis of the mechanotransduction mediators and the influence of mechanical strain on the level of expression of genes were presented in details. Novel studies using virus vector stimulating condylar growth through enhancing angiogenesis within a time limit were discussed; also clinical implications in treatment options in relation to mandibular advancement were briefly compared.

Keywords: temporomandibular joint pathology, condylar growth, orthodontics, gene therapy, growth modification

1. Introduction

More than 700 of 6000 known hereditary syndromes involve dental or craniofacial disorders; temporomandibular disorders (TMDs) are one subgroup [1]. TMDs are a class of musculoskeletal disorders related to mouth opening and closing, chewing and other mandibular processes necessitating the involvement of the temporomandibular joint (TMJ) and any of its associated structures [2]. Currently, one of the most widely used diagnostic criteria remains to be the RDC/TMJ criteria, axis 1 diagnoses by Manfredini et al. which classifies TMJ cases into one of three categories: musculoskeletal issues [3], TMJ disc displacements and joint pain (arthralgia). There are also other classifications of TMDs which focus on inflammation, injury and systemic conditions (**Table 1**) [3–5].

As TMDs have implications on the quality of life and well-being of affected individuals and their families, it is of major interest to clarify the etiology of TMDs. Several issues have arisen with the understanding of the etiology, treatment options and preventative measures of TMDs. There is a great variability in symptoms of TMDs (ranging from pain and inflammation to limitations of jaw movements) which can even vary in prevalence between genders—as

I. Musculoskeletal issues
A. Myofascial pain: pain or ache in the jaw, temples, face, preauricular area or inside the ear at rest or during function and pain in response to palpation of three muscle sites of the mandible with at least one of the painful sites on the same side as the complaint of pain [3, 4]
B. Myofascial pain with limited opening: myofascial pain with pain-free unassisted mandibular opening 40 mm and maximum assisted opening (passive stretch) 5 mm greater than pain-free unassisted opening [3, 4]
C. Ankylosis: joint stiffness potentially from disease and injury or a consequence of surgery [4, 5] and can be divided into fibrous, fibro-osseous and osseous conditions [4, 5]
II. TMJ disc displacements
A. Disc displacement with reduction: reciprocal clicking in TMJ or clicking in TMJ on both vertical ranges of motion in two of three consecutive trials [3, 4]
B. Disc displacement without reduction with limited opening: history of significant limitation in opening, maximum unassisted opening 35 mm, passive stretch increases opening by 4 mm over maximum unassisted opening, contralateral excursion 7 mm or uncorrected deviation to ipsilateral side on opening and the absence of joint sound or joint sounds not meeting criteria for disc displacement with reduction [3, 4]
C. Disc displacement without reduction, without limited opening: history of limitation of mandibular opening, maximum unassisted opening 35 mm, passive stretch increases opening by 5 mm over maximum unassisted opening, contralateral excursion 7 mm, the presence of joint sounds not meeting criteria for disc displacement with reduction, imaging conducted by either arthrography or magnetic resonance reveals disc displacement without reduction [3, 4]
III. Arthralgia, osteoarthritis and osteoarthrosis
A. Arthralgia: pain in one or both joint sites during palpation; one or more self-reports of pain; for simple cases, coarse crepitus must be absent [3, 4]
B. Osteoarthritis of the TMJ: arthralgia, coarse crepitus in the joint or radiologic signs of arthrosis, classified as a degenerative joint disorder [3–5]
C. Osteoarthrosis of the TMJ: the absence of all signs of arthralgia; coarse crepitus in the joint or radiologic signs of arthrosis; classified as a degenerative joint disorder [3–5]
III. External causes
A. Inflammation: can be acute, chronic or, a third option, infectious, which can be nonspecific or specific to a type of disease [3, 4]
B. Tumors: can be benign or malignant [4, 5]
C. Systemic conditions: include rheumatoid, juvenile and psoriatic arthritis, scleroderma and mixed connective tissue disease [4, 5]

Table 1. General classification of temporomandibular disorders (TMDs).

Etiological factors of TMDs
A. Predisposing factors: factors of structure (decrease in calibration, disc erosion or improper alignment, patterns of occlusion and bruxism); tissue quality; systemic diseases such as rheumatoid arthritis (RA), gout and fibromyalgia; facial typology; as well as age [5, 7]
B. Triggering factors: trauma at the macro and micro levels (e.g. injury to the jaw joint, osteoarthritis), bruxism as well as excess ability of articular tolerance [5, 7]
C. Perpetuating factors: underlying behavioral, social and emotional stresses [7]

Table 2. Classification of etiological factors of TMJ [5, 7].

females have been found to be more susceptible to TMDs compared to males [6]. This has resulted in treatment options being too broad or general, such as cognitive behavior therapy, nonsteroidal anti-inflammatory drugs (NSAIDs) and physiotherapy [6]. While there have been efforts for classification of the etiological factors including a widely known classification by de Boever et al. (**Table 2**) [7], current literature has shifted its focus to anatomical and histological examination of the structures within the TMJ, to identify contributing factors for TMDs, which will be the focus of this chapter.

2. Anatomy of the TMJ

The temporomandibular joint (TMJ) is an articular disc between the cranium and mandible and, more specifically, centered within the orofacial system, a functional group of structures which includes the masticatory and stomatognathic systems as well as the maxilla-mandibular apparatus (**Figure 1**) [5, 8]. The TMJ contains the glenoid fossa, TMJ disc (center, anterior and

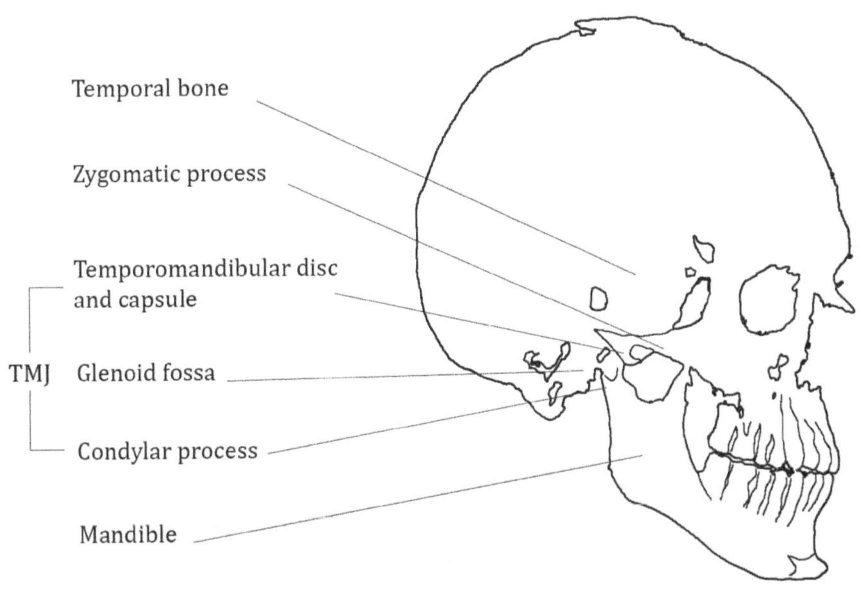

Figure 1. Schematic representation of the TMJ and associated structures in the human skull. The temporomandibular disc and capsule, glenoid fossa, neck of the condylar process and articular eminence (not labeled) are adjacent to each other and comprise the TMJ.

posterior), porous bone and mandibular condyle. It is a synovial joint and is unique in that it is one bone that is composed of two bilateral joints which cannot move independently of each other [6, 9]. Between the two joints is synovial fluid which promotes the hinge and sliding movements of the mandibular condyles required for mouth opening and closing and occlusion of the teeth [6].

The major function of the TMJ includes the coordination of individual tooth positions and other features of the orofacial system [8]. This is accomplished by lateral ligaments which are attached inside of joint capsules, being the structures which stabilize the intra-articular discs [10, 11]. The capsule is surrounded by fibrocartilage (rather than hyaline cartilage) and contrasts in thickness—the anteromedial and medial aspects are thin (0.7 mm), while the lateral and posterior aspects are thick (1.8 mm) [5, 9]. The capsule extends from the glenoid fossa to the neck of the mandible, preventing excessive displacement of the TMJ [5]. The majority of blood supply originates from the trail of superficial temporal, superior articular, anterior tympanic, and pterygoid arteries [5].

2.1. Glenoid fossa

The glenoid fossa is a concave portion of the temporal bone [8]. It borders the articular eminence anteriorly and the tympanic plate posteriorly [5, 9]. The glenoid fossa, similar to the disc and condyle, is a site of angiogenesis when subjected to mechanical stimuli [5, 9]. However, its histological composition has striking differences. Histological examination of the glenoid fossa has recorded fewer posterior layers of chondrocytes than the condyle. As chondrocytes are involved in chondrogenesis in the formation of cartilage to support the growth of the bone by means of endochondral ossification, the glenoid fossa may undergo a reduced level of endochondral ossification and a greater level of intramembranous ossification [5].

2.2. TMJ disc

The disc is fibrocartilaginous and biconcave and takes on a bow-tie morphology [5]. The two ridges of the disc are referred to as bands which attach to different structures. The smaller and shorter anterior band connects with the joint capsule, condylar head and articular eminence [5]. On the other hand, the larger and longer posterior band attaches to the condyle and the temporal bone [9]. The disc attaches to the capsule and neck of the condyle medially. The disc facilitates jaw opening in which the disc moves between the head of the mandible and the articular eminence [5].

2.3. Mandibular condyles

The articular surface of the mandible borders the anterior surface of the mandibular condyles [12]. The mandibular condyles are structures of the human mandible, covered with fibrous tissue composed of predominantly type I collagen, which present a surface for interaction with the articular disc of the temporomandibular joint, composed of avascular fibrous tissue including collagen and fibroblasts [12]. Below this resting, the fibrous layer of the condyles is four layers of cartilage: the proliferative, chondroblast, hypertrophic and erosive layers [12].

Extending further posteriorly than anteriorly, the condyles are convex laterally with a long axis situated medially and partially backwards [13]. The convex lateral extremities of the condyles are connected to small tubercles for attachment to the ligament of the TMJ [13].

Human condyles grow to 15–20 mm laterally and 8–10 mm anteroposteriorly in adulthood [5]. The growth of condyles is attributed to the condylar cartilage which acts as a template for bone growth [12]. The mandibular condyles are unique in that the cartilage (predominantly type II collagen) is known as secondary, compared to main and primary cartilage [12]. Another categorization of the condylar cartilage is articular [14]. However, unlike other types of the articular cartilage such as the synovial or epiphyseal cartilage, it has a striking difference of undergoing adaptive changes in response to external stimuli including mechanical or positional changes (e.g. repositioning of the condyles and/or the mandible, the functioning of the articular discs and the mechanical loading of the condyles) [15–17]. Some of the adaptive changes are related to growth and remodeling such as endochondral ossification and altering or regenerating chondrogenesis [14]. While these changes can occur during or after the natural growth period, there has been study that in adult rats, the remnant condylar cartilage serves more 'articular' function than 'growth' function as the adult rat condyle stops growth or becomes inactive of endochondral ossification [14]. Additionally, Luder studied adult human condyle structures and found that the cellular layers of organization did not resemble that of growing condyles and attributed the discrepancy to articular remodeling from mechanical loading [18]. As it was determined that articular tissue differed considerably between areas of loading and non-loading, Luder proposed that adult condyles should be divided differently and into three zones of organization—superficial, intermediate and deep [18]. Luder completed a follow-up study and found that features of the articular tissue in the condyles were subject to changes based on age [19]. Most tissue features were altered between 15 and 30 years of age and generally remained stable beyond this age range [19]. During this time, there was a progressive cartilaginification of the newly formed superficial zone, disappearance of the hypertrophic growth plate, appearance of the grid-fibrous fibrocartilage accompanied by a decline in endochondral ossification as well as formation of the subchondral bone plate [19]. From middle age to older age, there was a decrease in cellularity and some senescence and a progressive fibrosis of the intermediate zone. It was determined that the extent of maturation and remodeling and changes experienced in later age were related to articular load bearing [19].

Recently, there has been a spotlight on the mandibular condyles as major contributing factors to TMDs. As active growth sites of the mandible, impaired growth of the condyles has been associated with the development of TMDs [14]. Impairment of condylar development can result in mandibular asymmetry (e.g. hemifacial macrosomia and retrognathia) and problems in mastication, breathing and facial harmony which can lead to the onset of TMDs [14]. As it is evident that the etiological causes of TMDs are multifactorial, an evaluation of the influences and treatment options in the context of condylar growth is of great importance for affected individuals and their respective practitioners. Of major interest in condylar growth is the condylar cartilage for its influence in the growth of the mandible and its adaptive remodeling of the condyles in orthodontic intervention [14]. An understanding of the process of condylar growth and the involvement of cartilage in growth is therefore essential.

3. Steps in mandibular condylar growth

Given the fact that the anatomy of the condyles is clinically relevant in addressing TMDs, it is of importance to distil the major steps and cell types involved in the condylar growth process. There are two major processes involved in the growth of the mandibular condyles: chondrogenesis (cartilage formation) and osteogenesis (bone formation).

Mesenchymal cells eventually undergo one of two processes of osteogenesis by means of endochondral or intramembranous ossification, the latter of which is completed in the absence of the cartilage (**Figure 2**). In the former process, the mesenchymal cells will first differentiate into prechondrocytes which will mature into terminally hypertrophic chondroblasts [20–22]. This sequence of steps is collectively known as chondrogenesis. The chondroblasts eventually calcify and die, resulting in the bone replacing the cartilage by the bone through the invasion of osteoprogenitors which differentiate into osteoblasts [20]. This final step is known as endochondral ossification [23, 24]. Conversely, in intramembranous ossification, mesenchymal cells recruited from neovascularization migrate to the subperiosteal connective tissue and directly differentiate into osteoblasts to give rise to new bone (**Table 3**) [25].

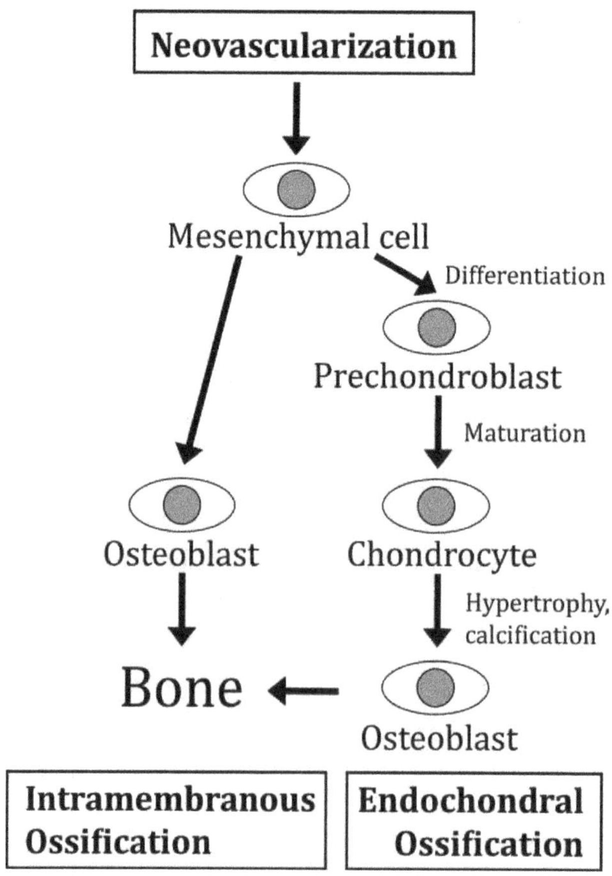

Figure 2. Schematic of the effects of VEGF during chondrogenesis, neovascularization and osteogenesis.

I. Chondrogenesis: mesenchymal cells

A. Fibrous layer [20]: differentiation into prechondroblasts [20]; can replicate up to 38 ± 4 times, and its quantity (dictated by various cellular and molecular factors) influences the growth potential [21, 26]; affected by mechanical forces [27]

B: Proliferative layer [21]: differentiates into chondroblasts and chondrocytes to maintain cartilage [21, 22]; affected by mechanical forces [27]

C: Erosive layer [21]: recruited with neovascularization and migrates to the subperiosteal connective tissue to directly give rise to osteoblasts through intramembranous ossification for the remodeling and repair of the bone [12, 21, 25, 28]

II. Chondrogenesis: prechondroblasts

Proliferative layer [12]: expresses type II collagen [12]; multipotential—can switch to differentiation of osteoblasts if articulate functioning is limited which can increase growth as articulate functioning retards growth versus condylar unloading which stimulates growth [23]

III. Chondrogenesis: hypertrophic chondrocytes

Hypertrophic layer, erosive layer [29–32]: maturation facilitates the transition from chondrogenesis to osteogenesis to serve as a regulatory point for growth [33], impacts cartilage formation and influences the growth of the condyle [34]; intercellular matrix calcification inhibits diffusion of nutrients, ultimately causing the death of the hypertrophic chondrocytes [20]

IV. Neovascularization

Refer to 3.1.

Va. Osteogenesis: endochondral ossification

Beneath erosive layer [20]: facilitates postnatal condylar growth and replaces degrading cartilage with the bone [20]

Vb. Osteogenesis: intramembranous ossification

Subperiosteal connective tissue [25]: unlike endochondral ossification, the cartilage is not present with this process of ossification which also serves the purpose for forming new bone [25]

Table 3. Analysis of the major processes involved in condylar growth and the corresponding stages within each process.

3.1. Neovascularization

Neovascularization is an essential step in endochondral or intramembranous ossification which occurs in the hypertrophic and erosive layers of the condylar cartilage as well as the glenoid fossa and the TMJ disc [28]. It is quantitatively correlated with endochondral ossification and is an indicator of osteogenesis in the replacement of dying cartilage with new bone [20]. Neovascularization functions by replenishing the population of mesenchymal cells for osteogenesis as blood vessels are the regions where progenitor cells are able to diffuse out and into the surrounding tissues [28].

While neovascularization has been determined to play a major role in condylar bone formation, it is of future interest to investigate the glenoid fossa and the TMJ disc, regions also characterized by mesenchymal cells and chondrocytes [5], as additional potential regions of neovascularization and subsequent bone growth. However, irrespective of anatomical location, an understanding of the factors influencing each of the steps in bone growth in the condyles and its associated regions is of major relevance for improving the management of TMDs.

4. Factors influencing condylar growth

Factors influencing the growth of condylar cartilage can be categorized into cellular (**Table 4**) and molecular factors (**Table 5**).

4.1. Factors at the cellular level

Cellular factors can be defined as factors that exert their activity at the extracellular level, including growth factors, cytokines, extracellular matrix (ECM) and other types of proteins. Growth factors and cytokines serve as local mediators in response to mechanical and inflammatory stimuli, while ECM serve as intercellular structural support [14].

I. Growth factors

A. Insulin-like growth factor (IGF): found in chondrocytes [35, 36], mediates growth and development of the cartilage and bone [14, 37]

B. Fibroblast growth factor (FGF): found in proliferating and chondroblast layers [14, 36]; regulates skeletal development and postnatal osteogenesis (e.g. FGF-2 promotes angiogenesis, inhibits the terminal differentiation of chondrocytes and reduces the formation of the bone) [14]

C. Vascular endothelial growth factor (VEGF): refers to 4.1.1

D. Connective tissue growth factor (CTGF): found in hypertrophic layer [38], regulates cartilage ECM and VEGF-A expression [38]; CTGF null or deficiency impairs endochondral ossification [39]

II. Cytokines

A. TGF-β: found in site of endochondral ossification, articular cartilage and growth plate [40, 41]; stimulatory and inhibitory roles dependent on concentration, culture period and state of cellular differentiation [42–44]; generally inhibits chondrocyte maturation and hypertrophy and alkaline phosphatase activity [45–47]

B. Bone morphogenetic protein (BMP): BMP-2 and BMP-4 are involved with cellular proliferation by regulating endochondral ossification [48]; activity of BMP-2 can be inhibited by Wnt signaling [14]

III. Extracellular matrix

A. Type II collagen: supports cartilage formation [12]

B. Type III collagen: regulates bone repair and development [49]; cross links are weaker than type I collagen and therefore can support replacement by type I collagen in remodeling [28]

C. Type X collagen: short-chain collagen [20]; correlated to the hypertrophic phenotype and marks the transition to osteogenesis [20]

IV. Other proteins

A. Parathyroid hormone-related protein (PTHrP): refers to 4.1.2

B. Indian hedgehog (Ihh): refers to 4.1.3

C. Matrix metalloproteinases (MMP-1, MMP-9): found in hypertrophic layer [50]; mediates the transition to osteogenesis, angiogenesis and further proliferation of the hypertrophic chondrocytes [20, 50]; facilitates remodeling of the bone by degrading matrix [51]

Table 4. Analysis of the cellular factors involved in condylar growth and, if applicable, the localizations of its respective activities.

I. Transcription factors
A. Core binding factor A1 (CBFA1): found in erosive layer [21]; essential for chondrocyte differentiation as the earliest regulator of transcription [21, 68, 69] can induce premature hypertrophy of chondrocytes [68]; mediates VEGF-A in endochondral ossification as its overexpression increases VEGF expression [38, 70]
B: SOX-9: refers to 4.2.1
II. Novel genes specific for condylar growth
A. Mustang, alpha B-crystallin (CryAB): associated with increased mesenchymal cell and osteoblast differentiation in response to mechanical strain [64]
B: Noggin: prevents apoptosis of chondrocytes [71]
C: Chondroadherin (CHAD): increases type II collagen expression in response to mechanical strain [64]
D: Nephroblastoma overexpressed (NOV): improves cartilage formation and integrity by positive modulation of type X collagen [64]
III. Other proteins
A: Wnt family: found in proliferative and hypertrophic layers [72]; controls mesenchymal cell differentiation into chondrocytes (e.g. Wnt1 and Wnt7a block chondrocyte differentiation, while Wnt4 blocks chondrogenesis but accelerates chondrocyte differentiation) [72–74]
B: Proliferating cell nuclear antigen (PCNA): found in hypertrophic layer [14]; increases the DNA replication of mesenchymal cells and is the marker for cell proliferation [14]
C: D-type cyclins: 'gatekeeper' of the G1 phase of the cell cycle which regulates the DNA replication of mesenchymal cells [72]

Table 5. Analysis of the molecular factors involved in condylar growth and, if applicable, the locations of its respective activities.

4.1.1. Vascular endothelial growth factor (VEGF)

VEGF is one of the most prominent regulators of mandibular condylar growth. It is found mainly in the hypertrophic layer of the condylar cartilage [24, 28, 52, 53], but traces have been discovered in the proliferative layer [54]. VEGF serves multiple functions in supporting the growth of the condyles including the coordination of the death of chondrocytes, function of chondroblasts, remodeling of ECM, secretion of growth factors and cytokines, angiogenesis as well as formation of the bone [12, 25, 26, 55].

Observing each of the functions of VEGF in greater detail, the coordination of chondrocyte death is accomplished by guiding of mesenchymal cell differentiation towards osteogenesis by bringing the cells to the mineralization front for calcification [24, 56, 57]. Additionally, VEGF-A has been the main isoform which facilitates the progression of angiogenesis [12]. VEGF in general supports rapid vascularization essential to healing and induction of bone associated with bone matrix that has been demineralized [58]. With respect to supporting bone formation, VEGF has been noted to increase mandibular length, and its expression has been correlated with the quantity of newly formed bone in the posterior of the condyle [12]. It is therefore evident that VEGF is a major therapeutic target of interest in research towards regulation of condylar growth.

4.1.2. Parathyroid hormone-related protein (PTHrP)

Another major regulator of condylar growth, PTHrP, is found in the transition zone between the proliferative and hypertrophic layers [59, 60]. It controls the condylar bone formation by facilitating and mediating the biomolecular pathway through which chondrogenic phenotype is shifted to osteogenesis [20]. This is accomplished by slowing down the hypertrophy of mature chondrocytes to promote further maturation and to provide more time to develop the cartilage in preparation for osteogenesis [33, 61]. By promoting further maturation and delaying the transition from chondrogenesis to osteogenesis, the population of chondrocytes continues to rise, leading to an increase in cartilage volume and subsequently bone formation.

Additionally, PTHrP induces the differentiation of mesenchymal cells through SOX-9, a transcription factor which serves to positively regulate the growth of the condyles [33].

4.1.3. Indian hedgehog (Ihh)

Compared to other factors at the cellular level, Ihh functions as a highly dynamic mechanotransduction factor which increases in expression in response to mechanical stimuli [12]. It is expressed by prechondroblasts and early hypertrophic chondrocytes in the proliferative layer [12, 62]. Ihh has a variety of effects on the TMJ and condyles including supporting early development [63] by regulating mesenchymal cell and chondrocyte proliferation and cartilage development (most notably type II collagen) in chondrogenesis as well as the transition to osteogenesis under mechanical strain [34, 64–66]. Interestingly, Ihh can also function as a molecular factor by shortening the turnover and enhancing the renewal of condylar cells [34] by upregulating cyclin D1, the 'gatekeeper' of the transition from the G1 to the S phases of the cell cycle [65, 67].

4.1.4. PTHr/Ihh negative feedback loop

Rabie et al. postulated that PTHrP and Ihh activities are linked through a negative feedback loop which regulates the development of the growth plate [5]. In the feedback loop, when PTHrP production is fleeting and not sufficiently stimulating chondrocytes, chondrocytes stop proliferating and maturing [66]. The chondrocytes begin to synthesize Ihh in the hypertrophic layer which acts on the chondrocytes by means of receptor-mediated signaling [66]. Ihh increases the proliferative rate of the chondrocytes and stimulates the production of PTHrP at the terminus of the bone. PTHrP then maintains the chondrocytes in a proliferative state and delays further maturation and differentiation which delays Ihh production [34]. As a result, the PTHrP/Ihh negative feedback loop modulates the pace of proliferation and differentiation of the chondrocytes to regulate cartilage and eventual bone formation [12].

4.2. Factors at the molecular level

Molecular factors can be defined as factors that operate within the cell by means of genetic and other intracellular factors. Such factors can be categorized into transcription factors, novel genes specific for condylar growth and other intracellular proteins. Transcription factors control genetic expression, while intracellular proteins control signal transduction and cell cycling pathways.

4.2.1. SOX-9

Targeted in PTHrP signaling, SOX-9 is a transcription factor that regulates the differentiation process from mesenchymal cells to hypertrophic chondrocytes [12]. Additionally, SOX-9 prevents premature differentiation and regulates type II collagen synthesis and cartilage formation through activation of the enhancer region of Col1a2 and Col2a1 [20, 75–77]. It is able to accomplish its activities by recognizing the DNA sequence of CCTTGAG and other members of the high mobility group (HMG) box class of DNA-binding proteins [71].

To understand how SOX-9 facilitates differentiation, it is vital to recognize that SOX-9 is expressed in mesenchymal cells, prechondroblasts and early differentiated chondrocytes but not in hypertrophic chondrocytes [78]. In mesenchymal cells, SOX-9 is required for differentiation into prechondroblasts. Later in the prechondroblast stage, SOX-9 supports the proliferation and further differentiation into early and proliferating chondrocytes. At the same time, SOX-9 regulates the expression of Noggin, an anti-apoptotic gene to support the proliferation of the chondrocytes [71]. After this stage, SOX-9 inhibits the transition from proliferative to hypertrophic chondrocytes to control subsequent endochondral ossification. Overall, SOX-9 is involved in cell proliferation of successive cell types in the earlier stages of chondrogenesis, but it also serves to prevent the hypertrophy of chondrocytes (**Figure 3**).

5. Interventions to address condylar growth

Given the working understanding of the stages and factors involved in condylar growth, researchers have found the condyles to be clinically relevant to the development and morphology of the orofacial complex [14, 20]. The condyles have been studied as a therapeutic target in addressing TMD and craniofacial issues in general. Two leading interventions to reactivate and control condylar growth have been the use of the recombinant adeno-associated virus (rAAV) vector and the application of mandibular advancement orthodontic appliances.

5.1. Intervention by the rAAV vector

The rAAV vector has become of interest in in vivo TMD therapy as it has been shown to overcome many limitations involved in the gene therapy of the cartilage and bone [79, 80]. Some advantages of the vector include reduced pathogenicity and immunogenicity, which supports long-term expression of transgenes which can be restricted to defined anatomical locations including specific oral tissues and success in transfecting many types of dividing and nondividing cells due to its size of 22–25 nm [55, 79, 81]. At this small size, rAAV-VEGF has been demonstrated as a suitable in vivo vector to significantly induce condylar growth by diffusing through the layers of the cell surface and infect with regular and hypertrophic chondrocytes to promote VEGF-mediated growth [79]. The systemic safety of the rAAV-VEGF vector has also been studied as exogenous VEGF was not identified in reverse-transcribed RNA samples of remote organs (e.g. heart, spleen and kidney) of transfected subjects [79].

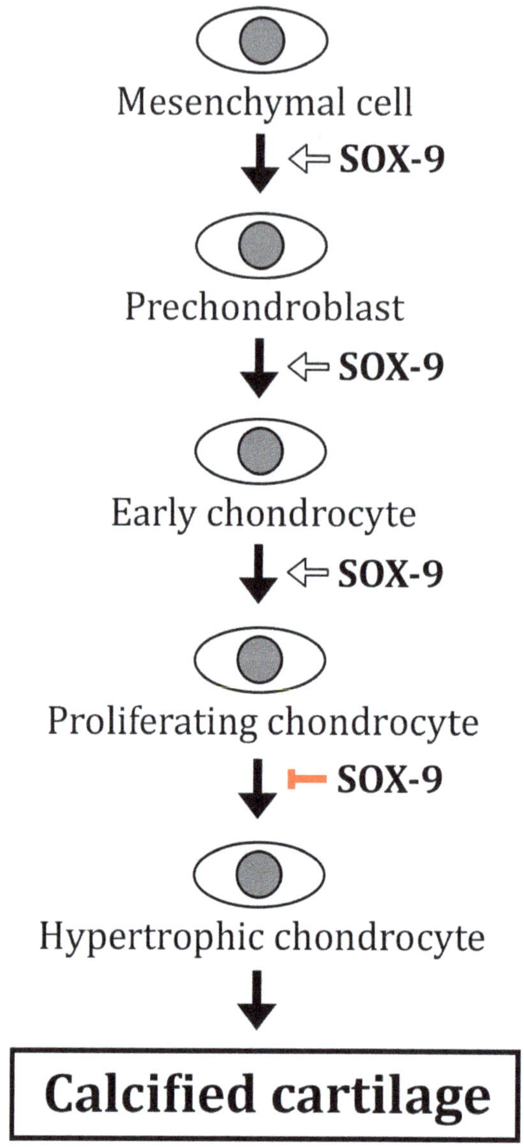

Figure 3. The roles of SOX-9 in each successive step of chondrogenesis towards endochondral ossification in the condyles. SOX-9 functions to commit mesenchymal cells to differentiate into prechondroblasts and supports the transition of prechondroblasts to early and proliferating chondrocytes but inhibits hypertrophy of the chondrocytes prior to the calcification of the cartilage.

Rabie et al. investigated the effect of in vivo rAAV-mediated VEGF administration on female Sprague–Dawley rats and found increases of the length of the condylar process axis (B-F) and the mandibular length from day 30 post-surgery and beyond [55]. The condylar width and length also increased during the same time period [55]. The growth of the condyle was upwards and backwards such that the greatest cellular response was found in the posterior condyle compared to the anterior surface [55]. This supported the adaptability of the condyle in directional changes in the growth of the mandible [24]. In addition, other studies have found a gain of function of VEGF, or VEGF gene has been associated with increases in neovascularization and regeneration of the bone in defective condyles [82, 83]. This has also reinforced the significance of rAAV-mediated VEGF as an appropriate option in contributing to neovascularization and endochondral ossification [28].

Most notably, it was determined that there was a delay in morphological effects of rAAV vector such that VEGF levels were increased on day 14 while chondrogenesis and osteogenesis occurred on days 21 and 30, respectively [55]. This finding had clinical implications in terms of understanding that gene therapy required a careful balance of inhibition or reinjection of the viral vector to address the potential consequences of overgrowth or relapse [55].

5.2. Intervention by mandibular advancement orthodontic devices

Recently, it has been proposed that condylar growth can be induced by forward mandibular advancement which has been noted to mirror natural growth [21]. Animal studies of mandibular advancement treatment on rats have reported the enhancement of chondrocyte maturation and endochondral ossification which give rise to new bone and condylar growth [84].

Three major factors of consideration include the age of the patient, the length of the treatment and stepwise versus single-step mandibular advancement. First, there have been recommendations of using functional appliances during or after the peak pubertal period to observe the greatest stability of treatment results [85–87]. Second, recommendations have been made to extend the commonly studied period of mandibular advancement of 6 months to 1 year in order to support the maturity of type I collagen [88–90]. Two other separate studies also noted that the treatment length was correlated to the maintenance of the effects of the orthodontic intervention [91, 92]. However, there have been mixed conclusions on the effect of lengthening the treatment period. Hagg et al. and Phan et al. found opposing trends of the length of treatment on the maxilla and the mandible, increasing the effect for the former and decreasing the effect for the latter [93, 94].

5.2.1. Stepwise versus single-step mandibular advancement

There has been extensive literature for the comparison of two approaches of mandibular advancement: stepwise versus single-step advancement. Currently, stepwise advancement has been determined as being the preferable therapy.

One of the reasons supporting stepwise advancement is the improvement in skeletal effect, most notably the sagittal jaw relationship with the maxilla, assuming a more forward positioned mandible due to more growth than single-step advancement [21, 95]. This improvement may be attributed to work completed by Petrovic et al. who found that the forward repositioning of the mandible periodically increases the rate and amount of growth in the condylar cartilage [96]. Van Lam and Rabie also found that stepwise treatment was correlated with significantly greater new bone formation [21].

From a cellular and molecular perspective, stepwise advancement that exceeded a minimum threshold of mechanical strain resulted in increases in Ihh, type II collagen, PTHrP and VEGF [34, 57, 97–100]. Thus, stepwise treatment involves repeated cycles of mechanical strain and increases neovascularization which results in increases in eventual new condylar bone formation [57]. Studies have shown that manipulating the amplitude of mechanical strain by stepwise advancement can significantly impact VEGF production by chondrocytes [55]. Moreover, the later stages of stepwise treatment are responsible for more VEGF production and subsequent condylar bone formation [57]. The extent of condylar growth modification from mandibular advancement has been determined through changes in measurements of the condyle and documented effects at the cellular and molecular levels (**Table 6**).

One modality of stepwise advancement in orthodontic treatment is the Herbst appliance; due to the advantages of stepwise treatment, it has been recommended to be included in an

---

I. Chondrogenesis

A. Mesenchymal cells: increase in quantity and rate of replication which is correlated to increased bone formation [12, 101]; cells deformed and oriented in the direction of the strain in the proliferative layers [84]

B: Prechondroblasts: reactivation of cells and chondrogenesis to promote growth of the condyle [12], which leads to an increase of osteogenesis [102, 103]

C: Hypertrophic chondrocytes: enhances but does not accelerate (a point that has not been clarified) [104] the hypertrophy of the cells towards osteogenesis [23]

D: Neovascularization: increased by means of VEGF expression which preceded the peaks of chondrogenesis and osteogenesis [55]; angiogenesis in the erosive layer during the enhanced, not accelerated (a point that has not been clarified) [104], transition towards osteogenesis [23]

II. Osteogenesis

Endochondral ossification: reactivation in the posterior aspect of the condyle leading to formation of new bone [12]

III. Cellular factors

A. IGF: increases expression of IGF-I and IGF-II [105]

B. VEGF: refers to 'neovascularization' in I (chondrogenesis)

C. Type II collagen: increases in expression [104]

D. Type X collagen: 540% increase in the posterior condyle which is correlated with 319% increase in bone formation [102, 106] by means of a similar temporal pattern when compared to natural growth [23]; maximal expression coinciding with that of Cbfa [88]

E. PTHrP: increases in expression which is associated with an increase in new chondrocyte population level [33]

F. Indian hedgehog (Ihh): immediate increase in expression due to deformation of the ECM and subsequent cellular cytoskeleton [62, 84, 107]; mechanical strain can reactivate dormant condylar growth [12], but the extent of reactivation of the condyle and glenoid fossa reduced with increasing age [108–110]; promotes chondrocyte proliferation, increased expression of cyclin D [72]

IV. Molecular factors

A. Cbfa1: upregulation of expression despite similar pattern of expression, coinciding with the maximal expression of type X collagen [21]

B. SOX-9: increases in expression which increased mesenchymal cell commitment to endochondral ossification [12, 33]

C. Novel condylar genes: increase in expression of Mustang, CryAB, NOV, Noggin and CHAD [64]

V. Morphology

Mandibular condyles: bending of the bone elongates [111, 112] the length and width of the condylar process and length of the mandible [55] with most change in direction posteriorly [24, 55]; there is potential to target the superior condylar layer to regulate upward condylar growth [55]

Table 6. Analysis of the factors affected by means of orthodontic mandibular advancement.

orthodontist's armamentarium [72]. The Herbst appliance has been evaluated with young adult patients and has yielded promising results in the treatment of Class II malocclusion [12]. It has been identified to operate by reactivating prechondroblast activity [12]. However, Pancherz has found several limitations of the Herbst appliance. The appliance has been met with concerns of relapse in cephalometric angle measurements after treatment [88, 90]. Additionally, it is most effective with Class II cases and thus cannot be used by individuals who have fully completed growth [90]. Thus, Pancherz has recommended the use of removable functional appliances post-treatment to maintain the effects from the Herbst appliance [90].

6. Conclusion

There have been considerable efforts to elucidate the etiological factors of TMDs and understand the factors regulating the growth of the TMJ and mandibular condyles at both the cellular and molecular levels. Current approaches to stimulating and controlling the growth of the condyles to address craniofacial abnormalities and/or TMDs have proven to be promising. Further research will be required to develop orthodontic treatment modalities that can be applied in a clinical setting on a case-to-case basis.

Author details

Bakr M. Rabie[1], Jeremy Ho[2] and Qianfeng Li[2*]

*Address all correspondence to: qianfengjennifer@gmail.com

1 Faculty of Dentistry, The University of Hong Kong, Hong Kong

2 The University of Hong Kong, Hong Kong

References

[1] Thyagarajan T, Totey S, Danton MJ, Kulkarni AB. Genetically altered mouse models: The good, the bad, and the ugly. Critical Reviews in Oral Biology and Medicine. 2003;**14**:154-174. DOI: 10.1177/154411130301400302

[2] Tanaka E, Detamore MS, Mercuri LG. Degenerative disorders of the temporomandibular joint: Etiology, diagnosis, and treatment. Journal of Dental Research. 2008;**87**:296-307. DOI: 10.1177/154405910808700406

[3] Manfredini D, Guarda-Nardini L, Winocur E, Piccotti F, Ahlberg J, Lobbezoo F. Research diagnostic criteria for temporomandibular disorders: A systematic review of axis I epidemiologic findings. Oral Surgery, Oral Medicine, Oral Pathology, Oral Radiology, and Endodontics. 2011;**112**:453-462. DOI: 10.1016/j.tripleo.2011.04.021

[4] Edvitar L, Oksana J, Ülle V-O. Temporomandibular joint arthroscopy versus arthrotomy. In: Bagaria V, editor. Regional Arthroscopy. Estonia: Tartu University, Tartu University Hospital; 2013. pp. 61-95. DOI: 10.5772/55011

[5] Schiffman E, Ohrbach R, Truelove E, et al. Diagnostic criteria for temporomandibular disorders (DC/TMD) for clinical and research applications: Recommendations of the International RDC/TMD Consortium Network and Orofacial Pain Special Interest Group. Journal of Oral & Facial Pain and Headache. 2014;**28**:6-27. DOI: 10.11607/jop.1151

[6] Sangani D, Suzuki A, VonVille H, Hixson JE, Iwata J. Gene mutations associated with temporomandibular joint disorders: A systematic review. OAlib. 2015;**2**:e1583. DOI: 10.4236/oalib.1101583

[7] de Boever JA, Carlsson GE, Klineberg IJ. Need for occlusal therapy and prosthodontic treatment in the management of temporomandibular disorders. Part I. Occlusal interferences and occlusal adjustment. Journal of Oral Rehabilitation. 2000;**27**:367-379. DOI: 10.1046/j.1365-2842.2000.00574.x

[8] Patil AS, Bindra GK. Morphology of the temporomandibular joint (TMJ) of sheep (*Ovis aries*). Open Journal of Veterinary Medicine. 2012;**2**:242-244. DOI: 10.4236/ojvm.2012.24039

[9] Alomar X, Medrano J, Cabratosa J, Clavero JA, Lorente M, Serra I, Monill JM, Salvador A. Anatomy of the temporomandibular joint. Seminars in Ultrasound, CT, and MR. 2007;**28**:170-183. DOI: 10.1053/j.sult.2007.02.002

[10] Maynard SJ, Savage RJG. The mechanics of mammalian jaws. The School Science Review. 1959;**40**:289-301

[11] Fanghänel J, Gedrange T. On the development, morphology and function of the temporomandibular joint in the light of the orofacial system. Annals of Anatomy—Anatomischer Anzeiger. 2007;**189**:314-319

[12] Xiong H, Rabie ABM, Hagg U. Mechanical strain leads to condylar growth in adult rats. Frontiers in Bioscience. 2005;**10**:65-73

[13] Gray H. Anatomy of the Human Body. 20th ed. Philadelphia: Lea & Febiger; 1918. 1396 p

[14] Leander D. Role of growth factors in the development of mandible. The Journal of Indian Orthodontic Society. 2011;**45**:51-60. DOI: 10.5005/jp-journals-10021-1010

[15] Kantomaa T, Ronning O. Growth mechanisms of the mandible. Dixon AD, Hoyte DA, Ronning O, editors. In: Fundamentals of Craniofacial Growth. New York: CRC Press; 1997. pp. 189-204

[16] Nakano H, Watahiki J, Kubota M, Maki K, Shibasaki Y, Hatcher D, Miller AJ. Micro X-ray computed tomography analysis for the evaluation of asymmetrical condylar growth in the rat. Orthodontics & Craniofacial Research. 2003;**6**:Suppl 1:168-172; discussion: 179-182

[17] Shen G, Rabie B, Hägg U. Neovascularization in the TMJ in response to mandibular protrusion. Chinese Journal of Dental Research. 2003;**6**:28-38

[18] Luder H. Frequency and distribution of articular tissue features in adult human mandibular condyles: A semiquantitative light microscopic study. The Anatomical Record. 1997;**248**:18-28. DOI: 10.1002/(SICI)1097-0185(199705)248:1<18::AID-AR3>3.0.CO;2-B

[19] Luder H. Age changes in the articular tissue of human mandibular condyles from adolescence to old age: A semiquantitative light microscopic study. The Anatomical Record. 1998;**251**:439-447. DOI: 10.1002/(SICI)1097-0185(199808)251:4<439::AID-AR3>3.0.CO;2-N

[20] Shen G, Hägg U, Rabie AB, Kaluarachchi K. Identification of temporal pattern of mandibular condylar growth: A molecular and biochemical experiment. Orthodontics & Craniofacial Research. 2005;**8**:114-122. DOI: 10.1111/j.1601-6343.2005.00316.x

[21] Van Lam S, Rabie AB. Mechanical strain induces Cbfa1 and type X collagen expression in mandibular condyle. Frontiers in Bioscience. 2005;**10**:2966-2971

[22] She TT, Rabie ABM. Expression of SOX9 in the mandibular condyle. Lecture presented at: 77th European orthodontic society congress; Ghent, Belgium: June 19-23. 2001

[23] Shen G, Zhao Z, Kaluarachchi K, Rabie AB. Expression of type X collagen and capillary endothelium in condylar cartilage during osteogenic transition — A comparison between adaptive remodelling and natural growth. European Journal of Orthodontics. 2006;**28**:210-216. DOI: 10.1093/ejo/cji123

[24] Rabie AB, Hägg U. Factors regulating mandibular condylar growth. American Journal of Orthodontics and Dentofacial Orthopedics. 2002;**122**:401-409. DOI: 10.1067/mod.2002.125713

[25] Yang YQ, Tan YY, Wong R, Wenden A, Zhang LK, Rabie AB. The role of vascular endothelial growth factor in ossification. International Journal of Oral Science. 2012;**4**:64-68. DOI: 10.1038/ijos.2012.33

[26] Bruder SP, Jaiswal N, Haynesworth SE. Growth kinetics, self-renewal, and the osteogenic potential of purified human mesenchymal stem cells during extensive subcultivation and following cryopreservation. Journal of Cellular Biochemistry. 1997;**64**:278-294. DOI: 10.1002/(SICI)1097-4644(199702)64:2<278::AID-JCB11>3.0.CO;2-F

[27] Rabie AB, Wong L, Tsai M. Replicating mesenchymal cells in the condyle and the glenoid fossa during mandibular forward positioning. American Journal of Orthodontics and Dentofacial Orthopedics. 2003;**123**:49-57. DOI: 10.1067/mod.2003.46

[28] Rabie AB, Leung FY, Chayanupatkul A, Hägg U. The correlation between neovascularization and bone formation in the condyle during forward mandibular positioning. The Angle Orthodontist. 2002;**72**:431-438. DOI: 10.1043/0003-3219(2002)072<0431:TCBNAB>2.0.CO;2

[29] Gerstenfeld LC, Shapiro FD. Expression of bone-specific genes by hypertrophic chondrocytes: Implication of the complex functions of the hypertrophic chondrocyte during endochondral bone development. Journal of Cellular Biochemistry 1996;**62**:1-9. DOI: 10.1002/(SICI)1097-4644(199607)62:1<1::AID-JCB1>3.0.CO;2-X

[30] Hashimoto S, Setareh M, Ochs RL, Lotz M. Fas/Fas ligand expression and induction of apoptosis in chondrocytes. Arthritis and rheumatism. 1997;**40**:1749-1755. DOI: 10.1002/1529-0131(199710)40:10<1749::AID-ART4>3.0.CO;2-D

[31] Garant PR. Oral Cells and Tissues. Quintessence: Illinois; 2003. 400 p. DOI: 10.1016/j.oraloncology.2004.06.001

[32] Chung U-I, Schipani E, McMahon AP, Kronenberg HM. Indian hedgehog couples chondrogenesis to osteogenesis in endochondral bone development. Journal of Clinical Investigation. 2001;**107**:295-304. DOI: 10.1172/JCI11706

[33] Rabie AB, Tang GH, Xiong H, Hägg U. PTHrP regulates chondrocyte maturation in condylar cartilage. Journal of Dental Research. 2003;**82**:627-631. DOI: 10.1177/154405910308200811

[34] Ng TC, Chiu KW, Rabie AB, Hägg U. Repeated mechanical loading enhances the expression of Indian hedgehog in condylar cartilage. Frontiers in Bioscience. 2006;**11**:943-948. DOI: 10.2741/1851

[35] Maor G, Hochberg Z, Silbermann M. Insulin-like growth factor I accelerates proliferation and differentiation of cartilage progenitor cells in cultures of neonatal mandibular condyles. Acta Endocrinologica. 1993;**128**:56-64. DOI: 10.1530/acta.0.1280056

[36] Fuentes MA, Opperman LA, Bellinger LL, Carlson DS, Hinton RJ. Regulation of cell proliferation in rat mandibular condylar cartilage in explant culture by insulin-like growth factor-I and fibroblast growth factor-2. Archives of Oral Biology. 2002;**47**:643-654. DOI: 10.1016/S0003-9969(02)00052-3

[37] Itoh K, Suzuki S, Kuroda T. Effects of local administration of insulin-like growth factor-I on mandibular condylar growth in rats. Journal of Medical and Dental Sciences. 2003;**50**:79-85. DOI: 10.11480/jmds.500111

[38] Dai J, Rabie AB. VEGF: An essential mediator of both angiogenesis and endochondral ossification. Journal of Dental Research. 2007;**86**:937-950. DOI: 10.1177/154405910708601006

[39] Ivkovic S, Yoon BS, Popoff SN, Safadi FF, Libuda DE, Stephenson RC, Daluiski A, Lyons KM. Connective tissue growth factor coordinates chondrogenesis and angiogenesis during skeletal development. Development. 2003;**130**:2779-2791. DOI: 10.1242/dev.00505

[40] Horner A, Kemp P, Summers C, Bord S, Bishop NJ, Kelsall AW, Coleman N, Compston JE. Expression and distribution of transforming growth factor-β isoforms and their signaling receptors in growing human bone. Bone. 1998;**23**:95-102. DOI: 10.1016/S8756-3282(98)00080-5

[41] Fukumura K, Matsunaga S, Yamamoto T, Nagamine T, Ishidou Y, Sakou T. Immunolocalization of transforming growth factor-betas and type I and type II receptors in rat articular cartilage. Anticancer Research. 1998;**18**:4189-4193

[42] Crabb ID, O'Keefe RJ, Puzas JE, Rosier RN. Synergistic effect of transforming growth factor β and fibroblast growth factor on DNA synthesis in chick growth plate chondrocytes. Journal of Bone and Mineral Research. 1990;**11**:1105-1112. DOI: 10.1002/jbmr.5650051103

[43] O'Keefe RJ, Crabb ID, Puzas JE, Rosier RN. Effects of transforming growth factor-β1 and fibroblast growth factor on DNA synthesis in growth plate chondrocytes are enhanced

by insulin-like growth factor-1. Journal of Orthopaedic Research. 1994;**12**:299-310. DOI: 10.1002/jor.1100120302

[44] Grimaud E, Heymann D, Redini F. Recent advances in TGF-β effects on chondrocyte metabolism. Potential therapeutic roles of TGF-β in cartilage disorders. Cytokine & Growth Factor Reviews. 2002;**13**:241-257. DOI: 10.1016/S1359-6101(02)00004-7

[45] Ballock RT, Heydemann A, Wakefield LM, Flanders KC, Roberts AB, Sporn MB. TGF-beta-1 prevents hypertrophy of epiphyseal chondrocytes: Regulation of gene expression for cartilage matrix proteins and metalloproteases. Developmental Biology. 1993;**158**:414-429. DOI: 10.1006/dbio.1993.1200

[46] Bohme K, Winterhalter KH, Bruckner P. Terminal differentiation of chondrocytes in culture is a spontaneous process and is arrested by transforming growth factor-β2 and basic fibroblast growth factor in synergy. Experimental Cell Research. 1995;**216**:191-198

[47] Ferguson CM, Schwarz EM, Reynolds PR, Puzas JE, Rosier RN, O'Keefe RJ. Smad2 and 3 mediate transforming growth factor-βl-induced inhibition of chondrocyte maturation. Endocrinology. 2000;**141**:4728-4735. DOI: 10.1210/endo.141.12.7848

[48] Ueno T. Kagawa T. Kanou M, Fujii T, Kukunaga J, Mizukawa N, Sugahara T, Yamamoto T. Immunohistochemical observations of cellular differentiation and proliferation in endochondral bone formation from grafted periosteum: Expression and localization of BMP-2 and -4 in the grafted periosteum. Journal of Craniomaxillofacial Surgery. 2003;**31**:356-361. DOI: 10.1016/j.jcms.2003.07.006

[49] Salo LA. Raustia AM. Type II and type III collagen in mandibular condylar cartilage of patients with temporomandibular joint pathology. Journal of Oral and Maxillofacial Surgery. 1995;**53**:39-45. DOI: 10.1016/0278-2391(95)90498-0

[50] Vu TH, Shipley JM, Bergers G, Berger JE, Helms JA, Hanahan D, Shapiro SD, Senior RM, Werb Z. MMP-9/gelatinase B is a key regulator of growth plate angiogenesis and apoptosis of hypertrophic chondrocytes. Cell. 1998;**93**:411-422. DOI: 10.1016/S0092-8674(00)81169-1

[51] Zheng LW, Ma L, Rabie AB, Cheung LK. Effect of recombinant human tissue inhibitor of matrix metalloproteinase-1 in rabbit mandibular distraction osteogenesis: A histological and immunohistochemical study. Journal of Cranio-Maxillo-Facial Surgery. 2006;**34**:277-282. DOI: 10.1016/j.jcms.2006.02.005

[52] Rabie AB, Shum L, Chayanupatkul A. VEGF and bone formation in the glenoid fossa during forward mandibular positioning. American Journal of Orthodontics and Dentofacial Orthopedics. 2002;**122**:202-209. DOI: 10.1067/mod.2002.125991

[53] Xiong H, Rabie AB, Hagg U. Neovascularization and mandibular condylar bone remodeling in adult rats under mechanical strain. Frontiers in Bioscience. 2005;**10**:74-82

[54] Gracia-Ramirez M, Toran N, Andaluz P, Carrascosa A, Audi L. Vascular endothelial growth factor is expressed in human fetal growth cartilage. Journal of Bone and Mineral Research. 2000;**15**:534-540. DOI: 10.1359/jbmr.2000.15.3.534

[55] Dai J, Bakr A, Rabie M. Gene therapy to enhance condylar growth using rAAV-VEGF. The Angle Orthodontist. 2008;**78**:89-94. DOI: 10.2319/102606-441.1

[56] Triffitt JT, Joyner CJ, Oreffo RO, Virdi AS. Osteogenesis: Bone development from primitive progenitors. Biochemical Society Transactions. 1998;**26**:21-27. DOI: 10.1042/bst0260021

[57] Leung FY, Rabie AB, Hagg U. Neovascularization and bone formation in the condyle during stepwise mandibular advancement. European Journal of Orthodontics. 2004;**26**:137-141. DOI: 10.1093/ejo/26.2.137

[58] Rabie AB. Vascular endothelial growth pattern during demineralized bone matrix induced osteogenesis. Connective Tissue Research. 1997;**36**:337-345. DOI: 10.3109/03008209709160232

[59] Lee K, Lanske B, Karaplis AC, Deeds JD, Kohno H, Nissenson RA, Kronenberg HM, Segre GV. Parathyroid hormone-related peptide delays terminal differentiation of chondrocytes during endochondral bone development. Endocrinology. 1996;**137**:5109-5118. DOI: 10.1210/endo.137.11.8895385

[60] Stevens DA, Williams GR. Hormone regulation of chondrocyte differentiation and endochondral bone formation. Molecular and Cellular Endocrinology. 1999;**151**:195-204. DOI: 10.1016/S0303-7207(99)00037-4

[61] de Crombrugghe B, Lefebvre V, Nakashima K. Regulatory mechanisms in the pathways of cartilage and bone formation. Current Opinion in Cell Biology. 2001;**13**:721-727. DOI: 10.1016/S0955-0674(00)00276-3

[62] Wu Q, Zhang Y, Chen Q. Indian hedgehog is an essential component of mechanotransduction complex to stimulate chondrocyte proliferation. The Journal of Biological Chemistry. 2001;**276**:35290-35296. DOI: 10.1074/jbc.M101055200

[63] Shibukawa Y, Young B, Wu C, Yamada S, Long F, Pacifi M, Koyama E. Temporomandibular joint formation and condyle growth require Indian hedgehog signaling. Developmental Dynamics. 2007;**236**:426-434. DOI: 10.1002/dvdy.21036

[64] Song Y, Wu C, Wing R, Wong K, Rabie ABM. Identification of the chondrogenic pathway in the mandibular condylar cartilage. Frontiers in Bioscience. 2009;**14**:1932-1938

[65] Long F, Zhang XM, Karp S, Yang Y, McMahon AP. Genetic manipulation of hedgehog signaling in the endochondral skeleton reveals a direct role in the regulation of chondrocyte proliferation. Development. 2001;**128**:5099-5108

[66] Kronenberg HM. Developmental regulation of the growth plate. Nature. 2003;**423**:332-336. DOI: 10.1038/nature01657

[67] Twyman R. Advanced Molecular Biology. Singapore: Springer; 1998. 510 p

[68] Rabie AB, Tang GH, Hagg U. Cbfa1 couples chondrocytes maturation and endochondral ossification in rat mandibular condylar cartilage. Archives of Oral Biology. 2004;**49**: 109-118. DOI: 10.1016/j.archoralbio.2003.09.006

[69] Tang GH, Rabie AB. Runx2 regulates endochondral ossification in condyle during mandibular advancement. Journal of Dental Research. 2005;**84**:166-171. DOI: 10.1177/154405910508400211

[70] Zelzer E, Glotzer DJ, Hartmann C, Thomas D, Fukai N, Soker S, Olsen BR. Tissue specific regulation of VEGF expression during bone development requires Cbfa1/Runx2. Mechanisms of Development. 2001;**106**:97-106. DOI: 10.1016/S0925-4773(01)00428-2

[71] Akiyama H, Chaboissier M-C, Martin JF, Schedl A, de Crombrugghe B. The transcription factor Sox9 has essential roles in successive steps of the chondrocyte differentiation pathway and is required for expression of Sox5 and Sox6. Genes & Development. 2002;**16**:2813-2828. DOI: 10.1101/gad.1017802

[72] Al-kalaly A, Wu C, Wong R, Rabie AB. The assessment of cell cycle genes in the rat mandibular condyle. Archives of Oral Biology. 2009;**54**:470-478. DOI: 10.1016/j.archoralbio.2009.01.020

[73] Rudnicki JA, Brown AM. Inhibition of chondrogenesis by Wnt gene expression in vivo and in vitro. Developmental Biology. 1997;**185**:104-118. DOI: 10.1006/dbio.1997.8536

[74] Church V, Nohno T, Linker C, Marcelle C, Francis-West P. Wnt regulation of chondrocyte differentiation. Journal of Cell Science. 2002;**115**:4809-4818. DOI: 10.1242/jcs.00152

[75] Nowak-Soliska E, Bakr A, Rabie M, Wong RWK, Lei SWY. The effect of naringin on early growth and development of the spheno-occipital synchondrosis as measured by the expression of PTHrP and Sox9—An in vitro model. European Journal of Orthodontics. 2013;**35**:826-831. DOI: 10.1093/ejo/cjs089

[76] Rabie AB, She TT, Harley VR. Forward mandibular positioning up-regulates SOX9 and type II collagen expression in the glenoid fossa. Journal of Dental Research. 2003;**82**:725-730. DOI: 10.1177/154405910308200913

[77] Cendekiawan T, Wong RW, Rabie AB. Temporal expression of SOX9 and type II collagen in spheno-occipital synchondrosis of mice after mechanical tension stimuli. The Angle Orthodontist. 2008;**78**:83-88. DOI: 10.2319/012507-36.1

[78] Zhao Q, Eberspaecher H, Lefebvre V, de Crombrugghe B. Parallel expression of Sox9 and Col2a1 in cells undergoing chondrogenesis. Developmental Dynamics. 1997;**209**:377-386. DOI: 10.1002/(SICI)1097-0177(199708)209:4<377::AID-AJA5>3.0.CO;2-F

[79] Rabie A, Dai J, Xu R. Recombinant AAV-mediated VEGF gene therapy induces mandibular condylar growth. Gene Therapy. 2007;**14**:972-980. DOI: 10.1038/sj.gt.3302943

[80] Dai J, Rabie AB. The use of recombinant adeno-associated virus for skeletal gene therapy. Orthodontics Craniofacial Research. 2007;**10**:1-14. DOI: 10.1111/j.1601-6343.2007.00381.x

[81] Dai J, Rabie AB. Recombinant adeno-associated virus vector hybrids efficiently target different skeletal cells. Frontiers in Bioscience. 2007;**12**:4280-4287. DOI: 10.2741/2387

[82] Street J, Bao M, deGuzman L, Bunting S, Peale Jr FV, Ferrara N, Steinmetz H, Hoeffel J, Cleland JL, Daugherty A, van Bruggen N, Redmond HP, Carano RA, Filvaroff EH. Vascular endothelial growth factor stimulates bone repair by promoting angiogenesis and bone turnover. Proceedings of the National Academy of Sciences of the United States of America. 2002;**99**:9656-9661. DOI: 10.1073/pnas.152324099

[83] Tarkka T, Sipola A, Jamsa T, Soini Y, Yla-Herttuala S, Tuukkanen J, Hautala T. Adenoviral VEGF-A gene transfer induces angiogenesis and promotes bone formation in healing osseous tissues. The Journal of Gene Medicine. 2003;**5**:560-566. DOI: 10.1002/jgm.392

[84] Rabie AB, Zhao Z, Shen G, Hägg EU, Robinson W. Osteogenesis in the glenoid fossa in response to mandibular advancement. American Journal of Orthodontics and Dentofacial Orthopedics. 2001;**119**:390-400. DOI: 10.1067/mod.2001.112875

[85] Ruf S, Pancherz H. Temporomandibular joint remodeling in adolescent and young adult during Herbst treatment: A prospective longitudinal magnetic resonance imaging and cephalometric radiographic investigation. American Journal of Orthodontics and Dentofacial Orthopedics. 1999;**115**:607-618. DOI: 10.1016/S0889-5406(99)70285-4

[86] Hansen K, Pancherz H, Hagg U. Long-term effects of the Herbst appliance in relation to the treatment growth period: A cephalometric study. European Journal of Orthodontics. 1991;**13**:471-481. DOI: 10.1093/ejo/14.4.285

[87] Von Bremen J, Pancherz H. Efficiency of class II, division 1 therapy in relation to treatment timing and modality. American Journal of Orthodontics and Dentofacial Orthopedics. 2002;**121**:31-37

[88] Pancherz H. Treatment of class II malocclusions by jumping the bite with the Herbst appliance: A cephalometric investigation. American Journal of Orthodontics and Dentofacial Orthopedics. 1979;**76**:423-442. DOI: 10.1016/0002-9416(79)90227-6

[89] Weislander L. Intensive treatment of severe class II malocclusion with a headgear-Herbst appliance in the early mixed dentition. American Journal of Orthodontics and Dentofacial Orthopedics. 1984;**86**:1-13. DOI: 10.1016/0002-9416(84)90271-9

[90] Pancherz H. The Herbst appliance—its biological effects and clinical use. American Journal of Orthodontics and Dentofacial Orthopedics. 1985;**87**:1-20. DOI: 10.1016/0002-9416(85)90169-1

[91] Hagg U, Du X, Rabie ABM. Growth modification of severe skeletal class II malocclusions by dentofacial orthopedics. Lecture presented at: 77th European Orthodontic Society Congress; Ghent, Belgium: June 19-23. 2001

[92] Wey MC, Bendeus M, Peng L, Hägg U, Rabie AB, Robinson W. Stepwise advancement versus maximum jumping with headgear activator. European Journal of Orthodontics. 2007;**29**:283-293. DOI: 10.1093/ejo/cjm018

[93] Hägg U, Du X, Rabie AB. Initial and late treatment effects of headgear-Herbst appliance with mandibular step- by-step advancement. American Journal of Orthodontics and Dentofacial Orthopedics. 2002;**122**:477-485. DOI: 10.1067/mod.2002.128218

[94] Phan KL, Bendeus M, Hägg U, Hansen K, Rabie AB. Comparison of the headgear activator and Herbst appliance--effects and post-treatment changes. European Journal of Orthodontics. 2006;**28**:594-604. DOI: 10.1093/ejo/cjl052

[95] Du X, Hägg U, Rabie AB. Effects of headgear Herbst and mandibular step-by-step advancement versus conventional Herbst appliance and maximal jumping of the mandible. European Journal of Orthodontics. 2002;**24**:167-174. DOI: 10.1067/mod.2002.127476

[96] Petrovic A, Stutzmann J, Gasson N. The final length of the mandible: Is it genetically predetermined? In: Craniofacial Biology. Craniofacial Growth Series. 2nd ed. The University of Michigan, Ann Arbor: 1981. p.105-126

[97] Rabie ABM, Al-Kalaly A. Does the degree of advancement during functional appliance therapy matter? European Journal of Orthodontics. 2008;**30**:274-282. DOI: 10.1093/ejo/cjm129

[98] Rabie AB, Wong L. Hägg U 2003c correlation of replicating cells and osteogenesis in the glenoid fossa during stepwise advancement. American Journal of Orthodontics and Dentofacial Orthopedics. 2003;**123**:521-526. DOI: 10.1016/S0889-5406(02)57033-5

[99] Ng AF, Yang YO, Wong RW, Hägg EU, Rabie AB. Factors regulating condylar cartilage growth under repeated load application. Frontiers in Bioscience. 2006;**11**:949-954

[100] Shum L, Rabie AB, Hägg U. Vascular endothelial growth factor expression and bone formation in posterior glenoid fossa during stepwise mandibular advancement. American Journal of Orthodontics and Dentofacial Orthopedics. 2004;**125**:185-190. DOI: 10.1016/S0889540603007194

[101] Rabie AB, Tsai MJ, Hägg U, Du X, Chou BW. The correlation of replicating cells and osteogenesis in the condyle during stepwise advancement. The Angle Orthodontist. 2003;**73**:457-465. DOI: 10.1043/0003-3219(2003)073<0457:TCORCA>2.0.CO;2

[102] Rabie AB, Xiong H, Hägg U. Forward mandibular positioning enhances condylar adaptation in adult rats. European Journal of Orthodontics. 2004;**26**:353-358. DOI: 10.1093/ejo/26.4.353

[103] Chayanupatkul A, Rabie AB, Hägg U. Temporomandibular response to early and late removal of bite-jumping devices. European Journal of Orthodontics. 2003;**25**:465-470. DOI: 10.1093/ejo/25.5.465

[104] Rabie AB, She TT, Hägg U. Functional appliance therapy accelerates and enhances condylar growth. American Journal of Orthodontics and Dentofacial Orthopedics. 2003;**123**:40-48. DOI: 10.1067/mod.2003.45

[105] Haijar D, Santos MF, Kimura ET. Propulsive appliance stimulates the synthesis of insulin-like growth factors I and II in the mandibular condylar cartilage of young rats. Archives of Oral Biology. 2003;**48**:635-642. DOI: 10.1016/S0003-9969(03)00128-6

[106] Rabie ABM, Shen G, Hägg U, Kalurachchi T. Type X collagen—A marker for endochondral ossification of the mandibular condyles. Quintessence orthodontics year book. Tokyo. 2000;**2000**:50-58

[107] Tang GH, Rabie ABM, Hagg U. Indian hedgehog: A mechanotransduction mediator in condylar cartilage. Journal of Dental Research. 2004;**83**:434-438. DOI: 10.1177/154405910408300516

[108] McNamara JA Jr, Hinton RJ, Hoffman DL. Histologic analysis of temporomandibular joint adaptation to protrusive function in young adult rhesus monkeys (*Macaca mulatta*). American Journal of Orthodontics and Dentofacial Orthopedics. 1982;**82**:288-298. DOI: 10.1016/0002-9416(82)90463-8

[109] Hinton RJ, McNamara JA Jr. Temporal bone adaptations in response to protrusive function in juvenile and young adult rhesus monkeys (*Macaca mulatta*). European Journal of Orthodontics. 1984;**6**:155-174. DOI: 10.1016/0002-9416(85)90183-6

[110] Woodside DG, Metaxas A, Altuna G. The influence of functional appliance therapy on glenoid fossa remodeling. American Journal of Orthodontics and Dentofacial Orthopedics. 1987;**92**:181-198. DOI: 10.1016/0889-5406(87)90411-2

[111] Raab-Cullen DM, Akhter MP, Kimmel DB, Recker RR. Periosteal bone formation stimulated by externally induced bending strains. Journal of Bone and Mineral Research. 1994;**9**:1143-1152. DOI: 10.1002/jbmr.5650090803

[112] Xiong H, Hägg U, Tang GH, Rabie ABM. The effect of continuous bite-jumping in adult rats: A morphological study. The Angle Orthodontist. 2004;**74**:86-92. DOI: 10.1043/0003-3219(2004)074<0086:TEOCBI>2.0.CO;2

9

Osteoarthritis of the Temporomandibular Joint: Clinical and Imagenological Diagnosis, Pathogenic Role of the Immuno-Inflammatory Response, and Immunotherapeutic Strategies Based on T Regulatory Lymphocytes

Gustavo Monasterio, Francisca Castillo, Daniel Betancur, Arnoldo Hernández, Guillermo Flores, Walter Díaz, Marcela Hernández and Rolando Vernal

Abstract

Osteoarthritis is a degenerative disease affecting the TMJ. It is the most common TMJ disorder and shows a higher prevalence in women and older people. TMJ osteoarthritis (TMJ-OA) is characterized by variable degrees of inflammation, destruction of the articular cartilage, and sub-chondral bone resorption. In this context, diverse pro-inflammatory cytokines, chemokines, enzymes, and bone-resorptive associated factors have been considered as possible markers of active TMJ-OA. The molecular balance is determinant not only for initiation and progression, but also for the clinical expression of the disease. Recent advances in the biochemical analysis of synovial fluid from affected patients have provided new insights into the patho-physiology of the TMJ-OA; however, its molecular pathogenesis still remains unclear. Recently, a Th1 and Th17-dominated immune response has been associated with the inflammatory and destructive events characteristic of TMJ-OA and, in particular, the Th17 lymphocyte pathway has a pivotal role in the increased production of RANKL, which is involved in osteoclast activation and subsequent sub-chondral bone resorption. Understanding the TMJ physiology and pathogenesis of the TMJ-OA, together with the key molecular determinants of the TMJ tissue destruction, will enable the development of new chair-side point of care diagnostics and more conservative treatment modalities with minimal complications.

Keywords: osteoarthritis, temporomandibular joint, pathogenesis, diagnosis, immunotherapy, Treg cells

1. Introduction

The temporomandibular joint (TMJ) is the movable articulation of the bone head. Its structure and morphology share common features with other synovial joints; however, it also presents particularities that make it unique. In fact, deep knowledge of the anatomy and function of the TMJ is a central challenge for clinicians and scientists, since many of the pathological conditions that affect this articulation can be explained based on its morphological and physiological aspects.

2. Temporomandibular joint: anatomical characteristics

The TMJ is a synovial joint composed of two articular surfaces [1–4] (**Figure 1**). The inferior articular surface is given by the mandibular articular surface, which is part of the mandibular head. Structurally, the mandibular head is formed by two surfaces, anterior and posterior, both separated by a ridge that follows the same axis of the mandibular head [5–7]. The anterior portion of the mandibular head is relatively convex in contrast with the posterior surface which is characterized for being flat and vertical [7, 8] (**Figure 2**). On the other hand, the superior articular surface of the TMJ is given by the horizontal portion of the squama of the temporal bone, which is organized forming two highly relevant structures: the mandibular fossa and the articular eminence of the temporal, also called temporal condyle [1, 2, 7–11]. The mandibular fossa corresponds to a concave surface with its greater axis in the transverse diameter [2, 7, 8, 12] and the temporal condyle corresponds to a convex bony elevation with its major dimension at the transverse axis, formed by an anterior and posterior surfaces without a clear boundary between the two of them [8, 9, 11]. Additionally, in the TMJ, it is possible

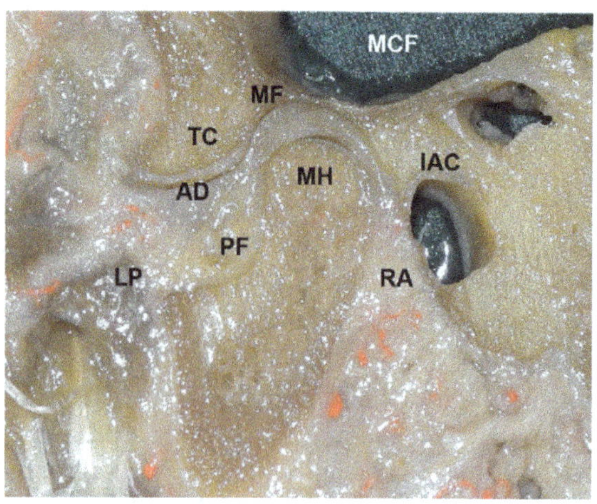

Figure 1. Anatomical characteristics of the temporomandibular joint (TMJ). Sagittal section of TMJ. Mandibular head (MH) articulating with temporal condyle (TC) and mandibular fossa (MF). Between the two joint surfaces the articular disc (AD) is interposed. The middle portion of the thinner disc portion being located in the work area; the anterior articular disc is continuous with the fibers of the lateral pterygoid muscle (LP), which is also inserted into the pterygoid fossa (PF) of the mandibular condyle neck; the back of the disc is related to the vascularized tissue in the retrodiscal area (RA). TMJ localizes superior to the middle cranial fossa (MCF) and posterior to the internal auditory canal (IAC).

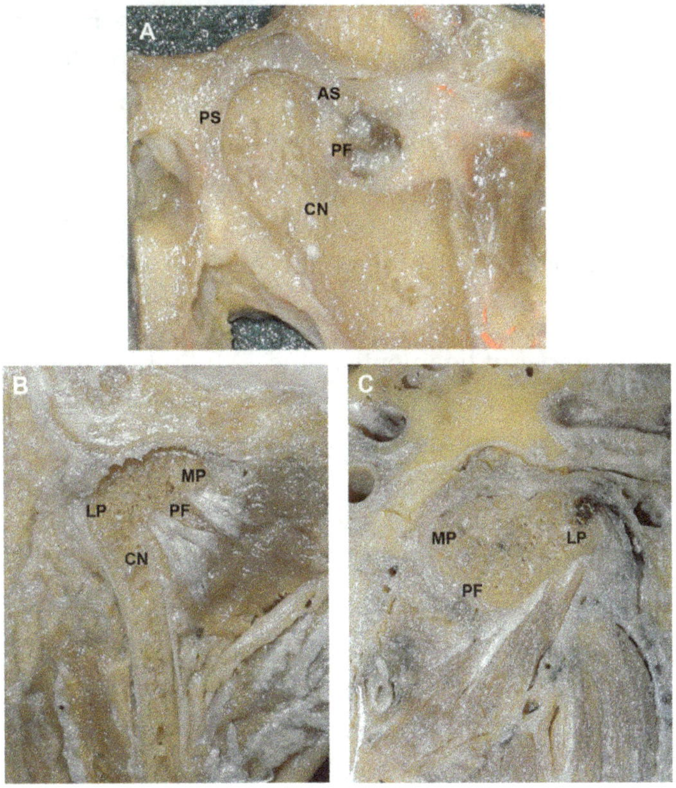

Figure 2. Anatomical characteristics of the temporomandibular joint. (A) Lateral, (B) frontal, and (C) superior view of the mandibular head. This is formed by two poles, the lateral pole (LP) and the medial pole (MP), the latter being larger. In a side view, it is possible to observe the morphology of the anterior surface (AS) (convex) and posterior surface (PS) (flat) of the mandibular head. In the lower portion of the mandibular head at its point of junction with the condylar neck (CN), the pterygoid fossa can be seen (PF), where the lateral pterygoid muscle is inserted.

to observe an articular disc, which allows fitting the temporal condyle and the mandibular head [1, 5]. It is avascular and not innervated at its center, which coincides with the area of greatest work [2, 6, 8, 13]. Like the mandibular fossa and head, its greater dimension is at the transverse axis and adapts closely to the adjacent surfaces [2, 6–8].

3. Temporomandibular joint: physiological characteristics

Mandibular movements are limited by a number of structures, which actively or passively avoid excessive mandibular displacement and consequently limit the movements within the joint. The main protective and customizing element of the joint complex relates to the joint capsule. This structure consists of thick organized bundles of collagen fibers that are upholstered with several proprioceptors that report changes in mandibular dynamics, thereby limiting the mandibular border movements [6]. Anteriorly, the capsule is inserted in the articular eminence [7, 8]. Laterally, the capsule strongly adheres to the longitudinal root of the zygoma and is continued backwards in tympanosquamous fissure [7, 8, 14]. The medial insertion is less extensive, inserted mainly in the sphenoid spine. The inferior insertion of the capsule extends along the condyle neck as a ring that is down on the backside of condylar process neck [7, 8, 14].

There is a set of ligaments that meet a similar role to the capsule, functionally and structurally reinforcing the TMJ [6–8]. The main reinforcement ligament capsule corresponds to temporomandibular ligament which is located lateral to it. From this point of insertion the temporomandibular ligament lateral band descends obliquely and posteriorly, and finally inserts onto the posterior surface of condylar neck [7]. The medial band is horizontal, presenting a similar cranial origin to the lateral band, and is inserted into the lateral side of the mandibular head [11]. Portions of the temporomandibular ligament execute a different role within the mandibular dynamics [6].

Additionally, there are a number of ligaments in the TMJ that are not structural or for its reinforcement, however limit the mandibular dynamics and hence the joint function. The stylomandibular, sphenomandibular, pterygomandibular and pterygospinous ligaments meet this role [7, 14]. The stylomandibular ligament is a segment of the muscular structures and it is originated in the styloid process forming the styloid bouquet [7]. Since its origin, the stylomandibular ligament descends obliquely to finally insert on the posterior and inferior border of the ramus. In the case of the sphenomandibular ligament, this appears as a thickening of the interpterygoid fascia, which inserts cranially into the sphenoid spine and in the mandibular lingula [7, 14, 15]. Its thickness and extent varies between the individuals and in its upper portion penetrates into the middle ear throughout the petrotympanic fissure being continued as the anterior ligament of the malleus [10, 16–18]. The pterigomandibular ligament originates from the pterygoid hamulus of the medial lamina of the pterygoid process of the sphenoid bone and from that point is inserted into the lateral lip of the mandibular retromolar trigone [7]. It is inserted in the buccinator muscles anteriorly and the superior constrictor muscle of the pharynx posteriorly. Finally, the pterygoespinous ligament, like the sphenomandibular, corresponds to a thickening of the interpterygoid fascia. It is reported that this ligament may undergo calcifications, which could produce alterations in the transmission of the mandibular nerve, because of its intimate relationship with the mandibular foramen determining nerve compression [19].

4. TMJ-OA: clinical classification and diagnosis

Temporomandibular disorders (TMDs) are the most widely accepted term to designate the musculoskeletal alterations of the TMJs. All TMDs share similar signs and symptoms, traditionally described as a triad of pain (TMJs, muscles, and tooth pain), interferences during mandibular movement (frequently associated with joint noises), and/or movement range limitation [20]. Bell developed the first classification of TMDs in 1986, and it was based on an orthopedic-mechanical model [21]. This classification was composed of four major categories (masticatory pain, restriction of mandibular movements, joint interference during mandibular movements, and acute malocclusion) and identified five muscular processes (myositis, muscle spasm, myofascial pain, late-onset muscle irritation, and protective co-contraction or protective stiffness). However, it was not until 1990 that the American Academy of Craniomandibular Disorders (AACD), along with the International Headache Society (IHS), developed the first taxonomic system of classification [22]. The main contributions were the distinction of two major categories (joint disorders and muscle disorders) and the possibility of establishing multiple diagnoses.

In 1992, a new taxonomic classification system was developed and termed "The Research Diagnostic Criteria for Temporomandibular Disorders (RDC/TMD)" [23]. This system was based on the biopsychosocial model of pain, and included the Axis I (physical assessment using reliable and well-operationalized diagnostic criteria), and Axis II (assessment of psychosocial status and pain-related disability) [23]. The main purpose of this classification system was to establish standardized criteria for research, and to provide simultaneously a physical diagnosis in order to identify other patients' characteristics that could modify the expression and eventually the management of their TMD [22].

Since 2014, the new DC/TMD Axis I and Axis II provide an evidence-based assessment protocol also based on the biopsychosocial model (**Figure 3**) that can be directly applied in the clinical and research setting [24]. In this consensus, the information required for fulfilling the Axis I diagnostic criteria is obtained from a specified examination protocol in conjunction with the core self-report instruments that assess pain symptoms involving the jaw, jaw noise and locking, and headache. Axis II core assessment instruments assess pain disability, pain intensity, jaw functioning, parafunctional behaviors, psychosocial distress, and widespread pain. All of these incorporations and changes in the core patient assessment instrument set serve as a broad foundation for patient assessment and further research [24].

The DC/TMD also includes changes to original RDC/TMD TMJ diagnoses. An important consideration was the low sensitivity for the diagnostic algorithms for disc displacement (DD) and degenerative joint disease (DJD) (osteoarthritis and osteoarthrosis) in RDC/TMD that can provide only provisional diagnoses [24]. This is due to the fact that some DD with reduction do not have clinically detectable noise, and the disorder will not be diagnosed using the clinical criteria

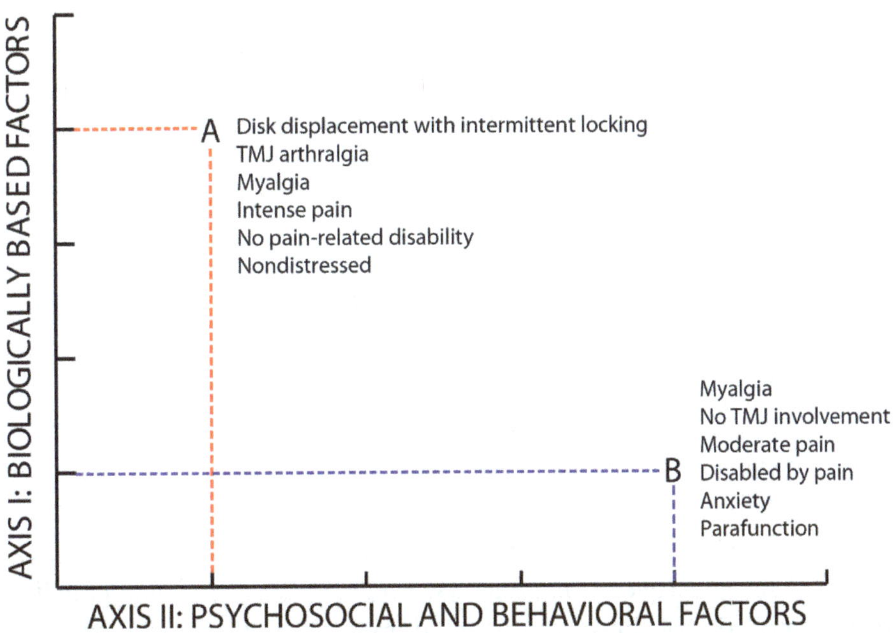

Figure 3. Biopsychosocial model of disease applied to temporomandibular disorders. Axis I refers to the severity of the patient's biological factors, including physical disorders. Axis II refers to the severity of psychosocial and behavioral factors, including interference in functioning because of pain. Two possible types of patients are depicted, each situated according to disease severity on the respective axes: Patient A has a mechanical temporomandibular joint (TMJ) disorder without secondary factors; and patient B has a pain diagnosis and clinically significant disruption in overall function and mood.

(positive history of noise and the presence of clicking noises) [25]. DD with reduction is highly prevalent, and crescent data suggest that internal derangement, such as DD with reduction, is likely to progress to osteoarthritis [20, 26, 27]. However, based on the evidence, DD with reduction is probably without clinical consequences unless pain occurs with noises or functional limitations, such as limited opening or interference in mastication. Nonetheless, the DC/TMD suggests that imaging using MRI is required for a definitive diagnosis of TMJ DD [24].

The differential diagnosis with the other TTMs is very important in the clinical assessment. The DC/TMD taxonomic classification for TMDs is divided in four major groups: temporomandibular joint disorders, masticatory muscle disorders, headache, and associated structures. Of these, the temporomandibular joint disorders main group includes two subtypes of joint pain, three subtypes of joint disorders, and seven different subtypes of joint disease (**Table 1**). The clinical procedures to evaluate DD with reduction, DD without reduction without limited opening, and DJD lead to clinical diagnoses based on procedures that exhibit low sensitivity but well to excellent specificity. Thus, for treatment decision in selective cases, confirmation of presumptive diagnostic requires imaging. In contrast, clinical algorithm for assessing DD without reduction with limited opening has good sensitivity and specificity (80 and 97%, respectively) [28], being enough with the clinical evaluation for the initial working diagnosis [24].

DC/TMD made some changes to the diagnostic procedures of RDC/TMD for DD and DJD. TMJ noise by history is one of the recommended criteria for the intra-articular disorders of DD with reduction and DJD. The patient's report of any joint noise (click or crepitus) during the 30 days prior to examination should be met by the history criterion or the patient's detection of any joint noise with jaw movements during the clinical examination. Furthermore, DD with reduction diagnosis requires examiner detection of clicking, popping, or snapping noises during examination. In DJD diagnosis requires examiner detection of crepitus (e.g., crunching, grinding, or grating noises) during the examination, and distinction between fines versus coarse crepitus is not necessary. For DD without reduction, the subtype depends on an assisted opening measurement (including the amount of vertical incisal overlap): if is <40 mm it is "with limited opening" subtype, and if is ≥40 mm it is "without limited opening" subtype. In this category, joint noise does not affect the diagnosis of DD without reduction as long as the required criteria for DD without reduction are met (**Table 2**) [24].

The DJD includes osteoarthritis and osteoarthrosis (**Table 1**). While the DD with reduction was described as "*An intracapsular biomechanical disorder involving the condyle-disc complex. In the closed mouth position, the disc is in an anterior position relative to the condylar head and the disc reduces upon opening of the mouth. Medial and lateral displacement of the disc may also be present. Clicking, popping, or snapping noises may occur with disc reduction. A history of prior locking in the closed position coupled with interference in mastication precludes this diagnosis*," the description given by the DC/TMD to DJD is "*A degenerative disorder involving the joint characterized by deterioration of articular tissue with concomitant osseous changes in the condyle and/or articular eminence*" [24]. The diagnostic criteria for these conditions demand a meticulous anamnesis and clinical examination. The DJD diagnosis is considered positive when either the patient reports any TMJ noise in the last 30 days (during mastication or any jaw movement) or the clinician detects any noise during mandibular movements. In addition, the DJD diagnosis is associated with clinical detection of TMJ crepitus during palpation, when patient is doing opening, closing, lateral, or protrusive mandibular movements. These important differences along exploration

I. Temporomandibular joint disorders

a. Joint Pain
   - i. Arthralgia
   - ii. Arthritis

b. Joint Disorders
   - i. Disc disorders
     - 1. Disc displacement with reduction
     - 2. Disc displacement with reduction with intermittent locking
     - 3. Disc displacement without reduction with limited opening
     - 4. Disc displacement without reduction without limited opening
   - ii. Hypomobility disorders other than disc disorders
     - 1. Adhesions/adherence
     - 2. Ankylosis
       - a. Fibrous
       - b. Osseous
   - iii. Hypermobility disorders
     - 1. Dislocations
       - a. Subluxation
       - b. Luxation

c. Joint diseases
   - i. Degenerative joint disease
     - 1. Osteoarthrosis
     - 2. Osteoarthritis
   - ii. Systemic arthritides
   - iii. Condylysis/idiopathic condylar resorption
   - iv. Osteochondritis dissecans
   - v. Ostronecrosis
   - vi. Neoplasm
   - vii. Synovial chondromatosis

d. Fractures

e. Congenital/developmental disorders
   - i. Aplasia
   - ii. Hypoplasia
   - iii. Hyperplasia

Table 1. DC/TMD taxonomic classification for temporomandibular disorders (only TMJ disorders).

History

a. In last 30 days, any noise present" applicable to disc displacement with reduction with and without intermittent locking, and degenerative joint disease.

b. In last 30 days, jaw locks with limited mouth opening and then unlocks" applicable to disc displacement with reduction with intermittent locking.

c. "Ever has jaw lock or catch so that it would not open all the way" and "interfered with eating" applicable to disc displacement without reduction with and without limited opening.

d. In last 30 days, when you opened your mouth wide, jaw locked or caught so that it would not close all the way" applicable to subluxation.

Examination

i. Disc displacement with reduction.

1. Report by patient of any joint noise (click or crepitus).
2. Click detection (# of opening/closing cycles required for click) (1 of 3).
3. Click detection during lateral and protrusive movements.

ii. Disc displacement with reduction with intermittent locking.

iii. Disc displacement without reduction with limited opening.

1. Assisted opening* < 40 mm.

iv. Disc displacement without reduction without limited opening.

1. Assisted opening* ≥ 40 mm.

v. Degenerative joint disease.

1. Report by patient of any joint noise (click or crepitus).
2. Crepitus (either fine or coarse) with palpation.

*Measurement of opening includes interincisal opening plus vertical incisal overlap.

Table 2. DC/TMD diagnostic procedures for disc displacements and degenerative joint disease with new history-based diagnosis of subluxation.

were not reported in the RDC/TMD previous consensus, which only included coarse crepitus detected by the examiner's palpation. Nevertheless, the sensitivity and specificity of these criteria are 55 and 61%, respectively, being the imaging the reference standard for this diagnosis. In particular, the diagnosis confirmation suggest by DC/TMD is with TMJ CT [24].

In summary, the DC/TMD assessment protocol has both screening and confirmatory tests for the most common Axis I physical diagnoses and for Axis II contributing factors (**Table 3**). However, an important remark is the poor diversity of diagnostic tools available until now. The DC/TMD raise a useful systematic imagenological and clinical diagnostic tool, but with no usefulness in the study of disease progression and/or prediction. Several studies suggest some biological markers of degenerative joint disease, such as certain cytokines or proinflammatory mediators [29–42], and could be useful in the elaboration of complementary tools for diagnostic purposes with potential in the study of disease prediction/progression. Thereby, the development of diagnostic/prognostic devices based on these molecular markers is an interesting research field that could significantly improve the precision of osteoarthritis diagnosis.

	Axis I: Physical diagnosis		**Axis II: Psychosocial status**	
	Pain diagnoses	Joint diagnoses	Distress and pain disability	
Application	Clinical or research		Clinical	Clinical or research
Screening test	TMD pain screener	DC/TMD for disc displacements, degenerative joint disease, and subluxation	PHQ-4 and GCPS	PHQ-9, GAD-7, PHQ-15, and GCPS
Confirmatory test	DC/TMD for myalgia, arthralgia, and headache attributed to TMD	Imaging: MRI for disc displacements, CT for degenerative joint disease, and panoramic radiographs, MRI, or CT for subluxation	Consultation with mental health provider	Structured psychiatric or behavioral medicine interview

Patient Health Questionnaire-4 (PHQ-4), Graded Chronic Pain Scale (GCPS), Patient Health Questionnaire-9 (PHQ-9), Generalized Anxiety Disorder-7 (GAD-7), and Patient Health Questionnaire-15 (PHQ-15).

Table 3. Clinical and research applications of selected DC/TMD Axis I and Axis II tests.

5. TMJ-OA: imagenological characteristics

Computed tomography (CT) and magnetic resonance (MRI) are widely useful tools for imaging the TMJ region of TMD patients, in particular for assessing degenerative bony changes, disc position and configuration, inflammatory pathological changes in the posterior disc attachment, the presence of effusion in joint spaces, and bone marrow edematous involvement [43]. Cone beam computed tomography (CBCT) allows the visualization of the TMJ in all three planes with high resolution, minimal distortion, and great precision for identifying condylar cortical changes [44]. The TMJ imaging by CBCT also allows the evaluation of the integrity of the bony structures when a degenerative disease is suspected, and to confirm the extent and progression of any bony changes [45].

The degenerative changes of bone in DJD are more frequent in the mandibular condyle than in the mandibular fossa or the articular eminence, and the characteristic pathological bony changes are erosion, osteophytes, and deformity; and adaptive bony changes are marginal proliferation, flattening, concavity, sclerosis, and sub-chondral cyst [46–49]. All of these anomalies are considered, for diagnostic purposes, as signs of osteoarthritis and frequently are observed in joints with long-standing DD without reduction [47].

Some imaging technologies such as CT [49–51], CBCT [46, 52, 53], and MR [47, 54–56] have been widely used for diagnosing DJD such as TMJ osteoarthritis. However, is CBCT, a fairly new imaging technology, that has the possibility to create images of high diagnostic quality using lower radiation doses than CT [53]. CBCT imaging has shown to be very helpful for depicting abnormal bony changes such as the cortical margin of the surface and sub-chondral cancellous trabecular structure present in the mandibular condyle, where the conventional radiography has shown difficulties to analyze successfully [30]. Conventional tomography also has difficulties in detailed assessment of changes in the surface morphology of the condyle and fossa, due to the thickness of the slices (1.0–3.0 mm) [57].

Another interesting imaging technique for the diagnosis of TMJ osteoarthritis evaluated in the evidence is the bone scintigraphy [58–61]. This technique shows a correlation with signs and symptoms with very good sensitivity, specificity, and accuracy (100, 90.91, and 96.97%, respectively) [59]. Interestingly, some radiographic changes seen by follow-up CBCT, MRI, and scintigraphy suggested that osteonecrosis may be the initial phase of an osteoarthritic process [30]. Thus, knowing all the potential imaging findings of every imaging modality is very important to make right imaging diagnostics (**Table 4**).

Imaging modality	**Imaging findings**
Medical CT and cone beam CT	Pathological bony changes such as erosion, osteophyte and deformity
	Osteochondritis disseccans
Static MR imaging	Disc positional abnormalities
	(1) DD without reduction
	(2) DD with reduction
	(3) Sideways disc displacement
	Joint effusion presence of marked effusion
	A higher T2 signal of the posterior disc attachment
	Bone marrow abnormalities
	(1) Bone marrow edema
	(2) Bone marrow osteonecrosis
	Tumor involvement and inflammatory diseases into the TMJ
	region and the surrounding structures
	Autoimmune processes such as rheumatoid arthritis
	A closer proximity between the TMJ disc and the mandibular nerve
Dynamic MR imaging with contrast material	Prominent contrast enhancement of the posterior disc attachment
	Contrast enhancement of effusion
Magnetization transfer contrast imaging	Detection for the edematous and ischemic changes in the muscles
Magnetic resonance spectroscopy	Ascending of insular glutamine levels by 1H MRS
Functional MR imaging	The regions and the network of brain activation associated with TMD
Ultrasonography	Muscular edema by low-level contraction
Bone scintigraphy	Detection for early changes on the osseous reaction of OA

TMJ, temporomandibular joint; MM, masticatory muscle; DD, disc displacement; TMD, temporomandibular disorders; OA, osteoarthritis.

Table 4. A rating of the usefulness of each imaging modality related to TMJ pain, MM pain and fatigue.

When the clinical diagnosis of DD with reduction or with reduction with intermittent locking needs imaging confirmation, the DC/TMD suggests positive detection of the following: "(1) *in the maximum intercuspal position, the posterior band of the disc is located anterior to the 11:30 position and the intermediate zone of the disc is anterior to the condylar head;* and (2) *on full opening, the intermediate zone of the disc is located between the condylar head and the articular eminence*" [24]. Otherwise, the imaging confirmation criteria by TMJ MRI of DD without reduction with/without limited opening clinical diagnosis are: "(1) *in the maximum intercuspal position, the posterior band of the disc is located anterior to the 11:30 position and the intermediate zone of the disc is anterior to the condylar head;* and (2) *on full opening, the intermediate zone of the disc is located anterior to the condylar head (Note: Maximum assisted opening of* < 40 *or* ≥ 40 *mm is determined clinically)*" [24].

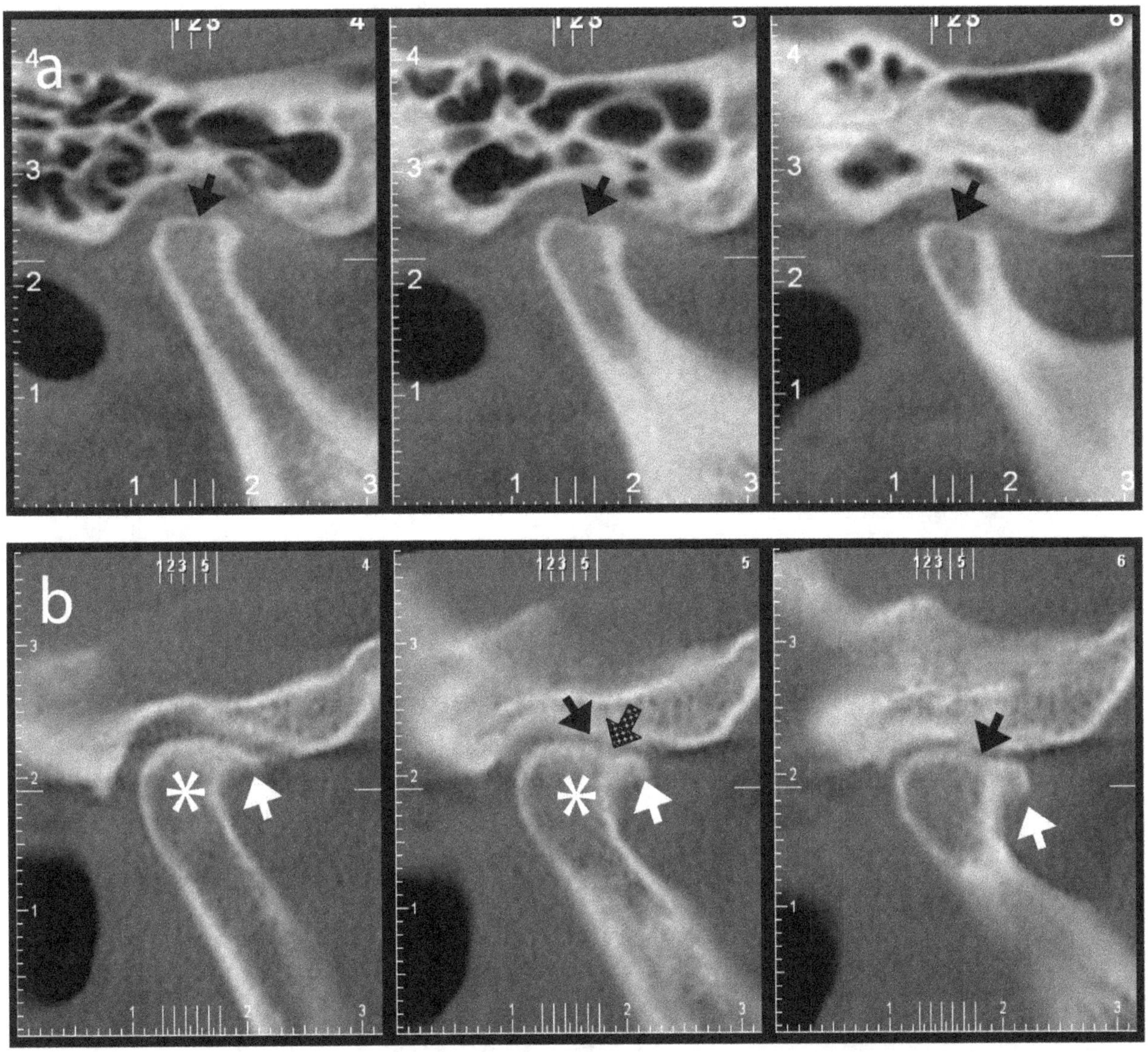

Figure 4. Imagenological characteristics of the temporomandibular joint affected with osteoarthritis. (A) Sagittal CBCT images of a TMJ of a patient with DC/TMD diagnosis of osteoarthritis but without bony osteoarthritic changes (erosions and osteophytes). (B) Sagittal CBCT images of a TMJ of a patient with a DC/TMD diagnosis of osteoarthritis and with bony osteoarthritic changes (erosions and osteophyte). CBCT: Cone beam computed tomography, TMJ: temporomandibular joint, DC/TMD: diagnostic criteria for temporomandibular joint. White arrow: osteophyte; black arrow: flattening; dot pattern arrow: erosion; asterisk: sclerosis.

The DC/TMD criteria consider a positive diagnostic of DJD when the TMJ-CBCT is positive for at least one of the following: sub-chondral cyst(s), erosion(s), generalized sclerosis, or osteophyte(s). An important difference between RDC/TMD and DC/TMD is in flattening and/or cortical sclerosis, because while the first consider as positive findings, the second consider indeterminate findings and possible sign of normal variation, aging, remodeling, or a precursor to frank DJD [24].

The great sensitivity and specificity of TMJ-CBCT in the DJD diagnoses compared with the clinical assessment was well demonstrated in the work of Bakke et al., that shows 21 TMJ-CBCTs positive for osteoarthrosis while only two were clinically positive for the disease [62]. The high frequencies of bony changes in the CBCT images of pain-free subjects in this study were in accordance with the findings of Krisjane et al. indicating that radiographic signs of osteoarthritis are a poor indicator of pain [63]. Furthermore, several studies have demonstrated that there is a poor correlation between condylar bony changes including pathological changes, adaptive changes and/or remodeling and pain symptoms in TMJ osteoarthritis [55, 56, 64–66]. These results support the idea that many times the bony changes are not associated with the clinical diagnoses (**Figure 4**), and that good diagnoses comprehend history of the patient, and clinical/imaging diagnostic, although, new assessment tools are necessary for accuracy of the diagnoses.

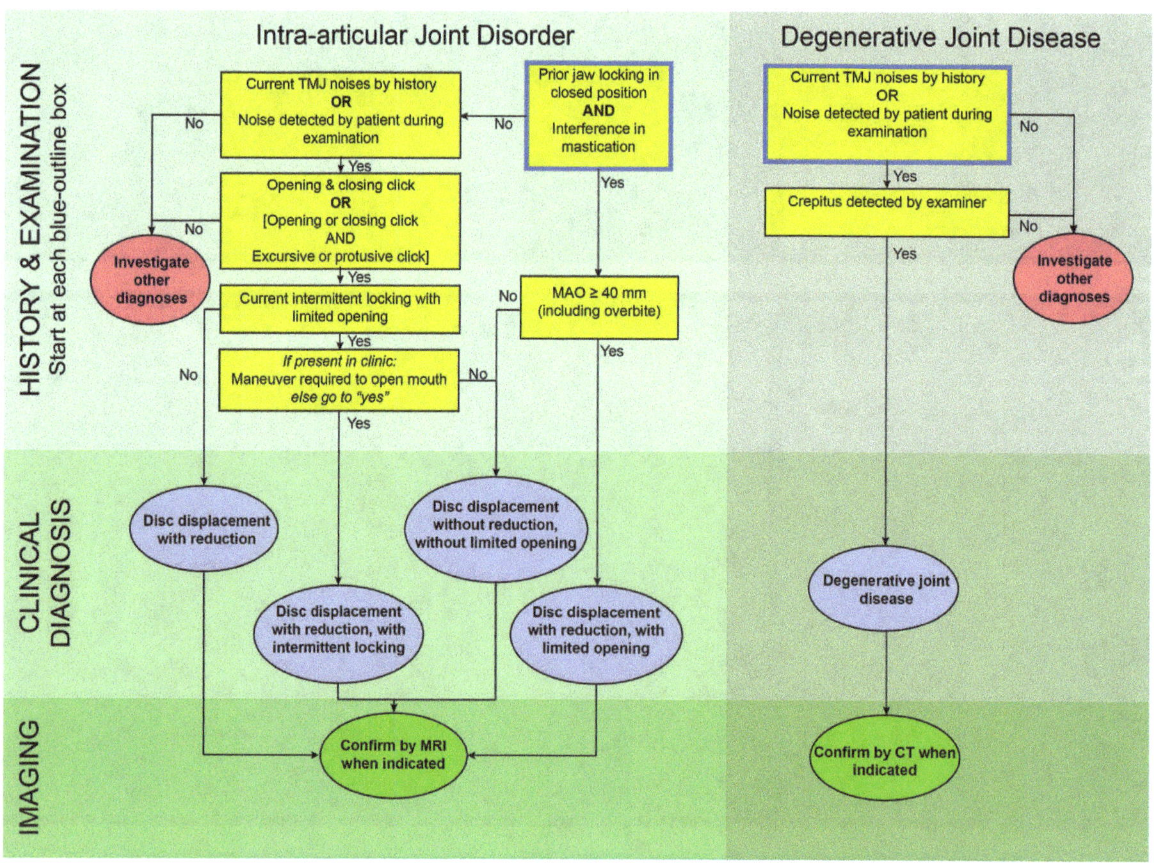

Figure 5. Diagnostic criteria for temporomandibular disorders (DC/TMD): diagnostic decision tree. Schematic diagnostic decision tree made to summarize the algorithm of diagnostic for intra-articular disorders (disc displacement with reduction, disc displacement with reduction with intermittent locking, disc displacement without reduction with limited opening, or disc displacement without reduction without limited opening), or degenerative joint disease (osteoarthritis or osteoarthrosis), including history, clinical examination, and imaging.

Finally, **Figure 5** shows the decision tree made in the DC/TMD consensus summarizes the algorithm made for the diagnosis of degenerative joint disease and intra-articular joint disorders with history, clinical, and imagenological features.

6. Role of the immuno-inflammatory response in the pathogenesis of the TMJ-OA

TMJ-OA is a disease having a great deal of variation in progression, symptoms, epidemiology, pathophysiology, and presentation. The rate of progression from a healthy joint to a severe TMJ-OA can vary from weeks to decades and TMJ-OA affects all of the tissues of the joint, including the articular cartilage, synovium, sub-chondral bone, capsule, ligaments, peri-articular muscles, and the sensory nerves innervating the tissues.

Many factors have been proposed as responsible for the TMJ-OA development, such as genetic factors, over-loading, unilateral chewing, bruxism, and internal derangement; however, the molecular basis of the TMJ-OA aetio-pathogenesis remains unclear [67–70].

During TMJ-OA, a complex inflammatory response is developed, involving the synthesis of different cytokines by resident cells (e.g., synovial fibroblast, chondrocytes, and macrophages) and inflammatory cells that infiltrate the joint tissues [71, 72]. This inflammatory response could be triggered as result of the tissue breakdown and the consequent release of damage-associated molecular patterns (DAMPs), such as low molecular weight hyaluronan (LMW-HA), high-mobility group protein 1 (HMGB1), and S100 proteins [73, 74], activating resident inflammatory cells, including dendritic cells and macrophages [75]. At initial stages of the disease, functional overload induces oxidative stress that initiates cartilage disruption [76, 77] and activation of MMPs and aggrecanases, promoting the secretion of DAMPs and the activation of the immune response [75]. During the disease progression, there is a local imbalance between the expression of specific cytokines, their receptors, and regulatory soluble receptors, which may be critical in the biological activity of the cytokine network [35]. Under these conditions, both fibroblast and synovial cells are activated to express MMPs and bone-associated cytokines that control the formation/destruction of articular cartilage and bone, determining the clinical outcome of the OA-TMJ (**Figures 6** and **7**). In fact, higher levels of interleukin (IL)-1β, IL-6, IL-17, interferon (IFN)-γ, tumor necrosis factor (TNF)-α, prostaglandin E_2 (PGE_2), matrix metalloproteinase (MMP)-2, MMP-9, aggrecanase-1, superoxide dismutase, substance P, and receptor-activator of nuclear factor-κB ligand (RANKL) have been detected in synovial fluid from TMJ-OA patients as compared with disc displacement with reduction (DDWR), disc displacement without reduction (DDWOR), or healthy subjects **Table 5** [35, 40, 42, 68, 69, 78–86].

Certain cytokines such as IL-1β, IL-6, and TNF-α has been associated with signs and symptoms of TMJ-OA, in particular, synovitis and arthralgia [39]. In addition, TNF-α and IL-6 have been described as markers of pain and successful clinical outcomes in TMDs [87, 88]. However, a study assessing the relation between the scores from a visual analog scale of pain and the levels of IL-1β, IL-6, and TNF-α reported no positive correlation [35]. Differences among different studies results could be due to variability in the selection criteria of subjects, sampling techniques, and/or analysis methods.

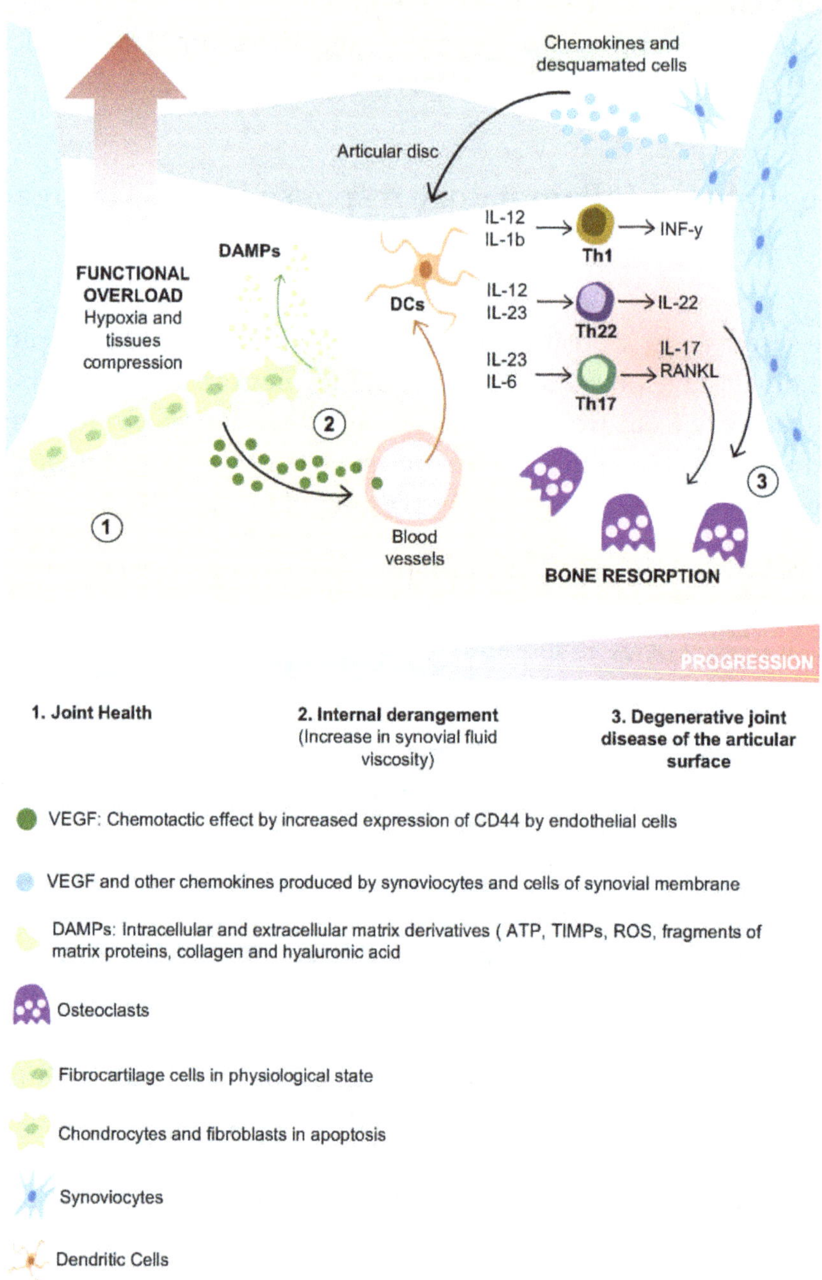

Figure 6. Phases in progression of the degenerative joint disease of the temporomandibular joint. (1) Fibrocartilage and bone tissue in physiological state, (articular disc in correct position). (2) The presence of functional overload or individual susceptibility generates hypoxia and compression of the articular tissues, resulting in apoptosis of chondrocytes and fibroblasts of the fibrocartilage, and DAMP's release, such as ATP, ROS, TIMPs, fragments of collagen and low molecular weight hyaluronic acid. In addition to cytokines and chemokines, these molecules produced by synoviocytes allow the migration of immune cells into the joint, such as dendritic cells that generate the environment leading to the polarization of T cell populations towards Th1, Th22, and Th17 phenotypes. These polarized cells in turn will allow the differentiation and activation of osteoclasts that will degrade the articular surface establishing the degenerative and destructive pathology (3).

IL-17 plays a key role in the pathogenesis of rheumatoid arthritis by inducing the synoviocyte-dependent IL-6 secretion [89]. In addition, TNF-α and IFN-γ augment the IL-17 activity and IL-17 activity has been associated with synovitis, chondral degradation, and inhibition of chondrocyte proliferation [89]. The presence of IL-17 in the TMJ synovial

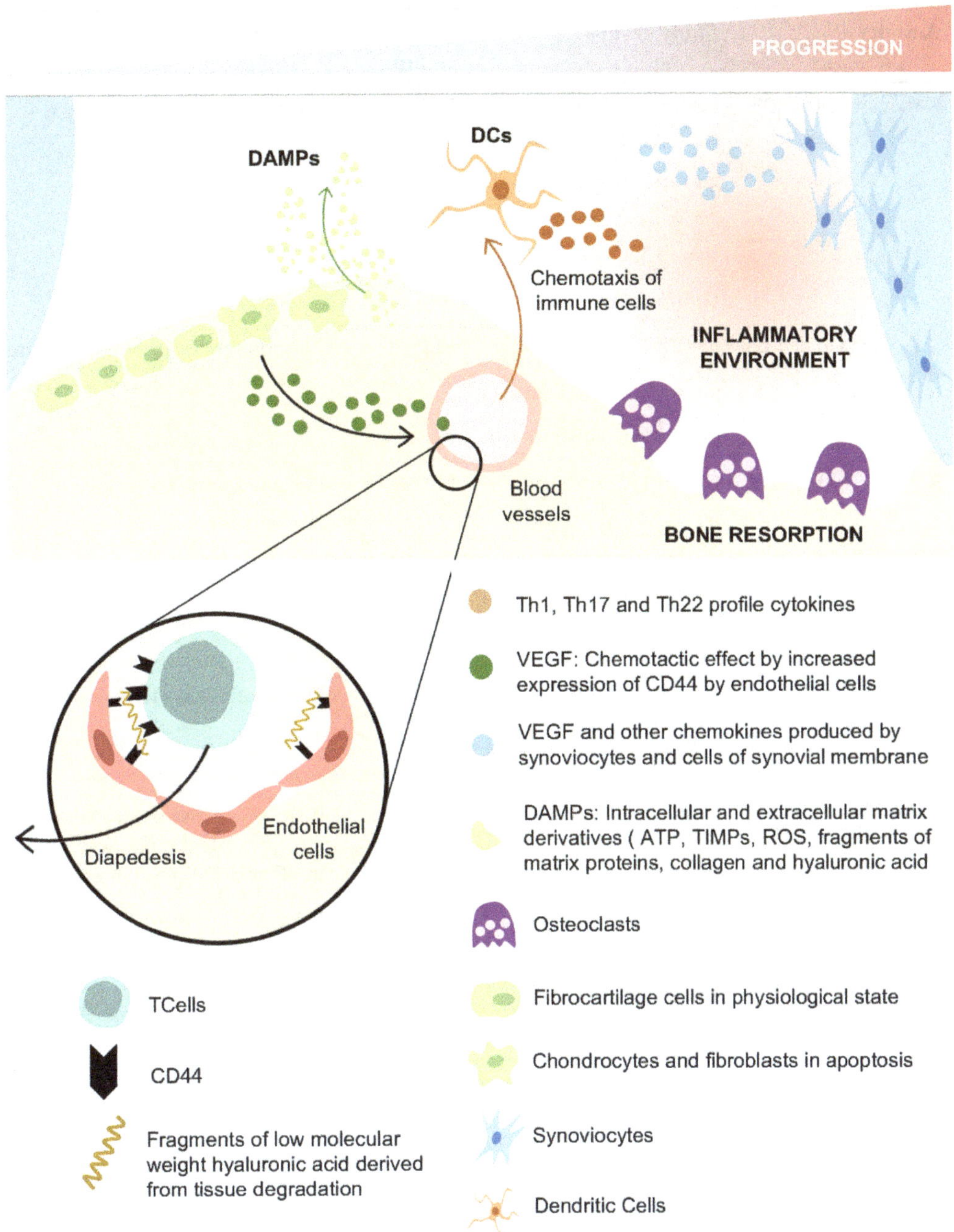

Figure 7. Chemotaxis of immune cells to the subarticular space. Synoviocytes, fibroblasts and chondrocytes produce cytokines, chemokines, intracellular DAMPs, and extracellular matrix derivatives that facilitate the migration of immune cells from the bloodstream into the joint. VEGF and CCL5 facilitate the overexpression of CD44 in endothelial cells and T cells. These molecules, together with low molecular weight hyaluronic acid fragments (sandwich effect), facilitate the diapedesis of lymphocytes through the vessels, enhancing the inflammatory stage of the disease in progress.

fluid could be an important pathophysiological biomarker of TMJ-OA [40]. In fact, bone resorption associated with an increased osteoclast activity is a central phenomenon in the pathophysiology of autoimmune and inflammatory arthritis, and it is also related to IL-17 presence, mainly through T lymphocyte-associated direct and indirect regulation [90, 91]. RANKL is the main molecule involved in the direct regulation of osteoclast activity, through the direct activation of osteoclast precursors [92]. Conversely, the indirect regulation depends on the secretion of IL-17, IL-1β, and TNF-α by synoviocytes, cytokines that in

Cytokine studied	Authors	Study groups	Measuring technique	Outcomes of study
IL-1β	Kaneyama et al. [33]	Group 1: DID with clicking. (n = 8)	**ELISA**	Groups 1, 2 and 3 > Group 4.
		Group 2: DID with locking. (n = 52)		
		Group 3: OA. (n = 57)		
		Group 4: Control. (n = 7)		
	Kaneyama et al. [32]	Group 1: DID (n = 24)	**ELISA**	No differences among the groups.
		Group 2: OA (n = 26)		
		Group 3: Control (n = 5)		
	Kaneyama et al. [35]	Group 1: Control (n = 5)	**ELISA**	Groups 2, and 3 > Group 1.
		Group 2: DID (n = 41)		
		Group 3: OA (n = 14)		
	Kubota et al. [36]	Group 1: DID and OA (n = 22)	**ELISA**	Groups 1 > Group 2.
		Group 2: Control (n = 12)		TMJs with OA > TMJs with DID.
		Group 3: OA of Knee (n = 10)		
	Takahashi et al. [39]	Group 1: DID with clicking (n = 8)	**ELISA**	IL-1β presented the higher incidence. Strong correlation between the presence of IL-1β and TMJ pain in groups 1, 2, and 3.
		Group 2: DID with locking (n = 25)		No cytokines were detected in Group 4.
		Group 3: OA (n = 18)		
		Group 4: Control (n = 6)		
	Vernal et al. [40]	Group 1: OA (n = 12)	**RT-qPCR**	Group 1 > Group 2.
		Group 2: Control (n = 6)		
TNF-α	Kaneyama et al. [33]	*	**ELISA**	Groups 1, 2 and 3 > Group 4.
	Kaneyama et al. [32]	*	**ELISA**	No differences among the groups.
	Kaneyama et al. [35]	*	**ELISA**	Groups 2, and 3 > Group 1.
				TNF-α level was positively correlated with those of IL-6, sTNFR-I and s TNFR-II.
	Takahashi et al. [39]	*	**ELISA**	TNF-α presented the lower incidence.
				No cytokines were detected in Group 4.
	Vernal et al. [40]	*	**RT-qPCR**	Group 1 > Group 2.
IL-6	Kaneyama et al. [33]	*	**ELISA**	Groups 1, 2 and 3 > Group 4.
	Kaneyama et al. [34]	Group 1: Control (n = 7)	**ELISA**	In groups 2 and 3 was significantly higher in joints with osseous changes in the condyle.
		Group 2: DID (n = 39)		No cytokines detected in group 1.
		Group 3: OA (n = 22)		

Cytokine studied	Authors	Study groups	Measuring technique	Outcomes of study
	Kubota et al. [36]	*	ELISA	Groups 1 > Group 2.
				TMJs with OA > TMJs with DID.
	Takahashi et al. [39]	*	ELISA	Group 1, 2 and 3 presented at least 1 of the cytokines in 64.5% of the cases.
	Vernal et al. [40]	*	RT-qPCR	Group 1 > Group 2.
IL-17	Kaneyama et al. [34]	*	ELISA	Detection rate of IL-17 was low, and there was no association between the concentration of IL-17 and the presence or absence of osseous changes.
	Vernal et al. [40]	*	RT-qPCR	Group 1 > Group 2.
IL-8	Kaneyama et al. [33]	*	ELISA	Groups 1, 2 and 3 > Group 4.
	Takahashi et al. [39]	*	ELISA	Group 1, 2 and 3 presented at least 1 of the cytokines in 64.5% of the cases.
TGF-β1	Fang et al. [29]	Group 1: DID (n = 12)	ELISA	Group 2 > Group 1.
		Group 2: OA (n = 15)		
		Group 3: Control (n = 4)		
IL-11	Kaneyama et al. [34]	*	ELISA	In groups 2 and 3 was significantly higher in joints with osseous changes in the condyle.
RANKL	Wakita et al. [42]	Group 1: DID with reduction (n = 25)	ELISA	No significance difference in RANKL concentration between group 4 compared to the rest of groups.
		Group 2: DID without reduction (n = 39)		RANKL/ OPG ratio in group 3 was increased.
		Group 3: OA (n = 53)		
		Group 4: Control (n = 13)		
IL-10	Fang et al. [29]	*	ELISA	Undetectable in all the groups.
	Vernal et al. [40]	*	RT-qPCR	Group 2 > Group 1.
OPG	Kaneyama et al. [32]	*	ELISA	Group 3 > Group 2.
	Wakita et al. [42]	*	ELISA	Group 4 > Groups 1, 2, and 3.
				RANKL/OPG ratio in group 3 was increased.

Table 5. Molecular mediators proposed as associated with signs and symptoms of TMJ disorders.

turn induce the RANKL expression on synovial fibroblast and osteoblasts [92]. Recently, it has been reported that IL-17, rather than IL-12 or IFN-γ, is critical for the onset of autoimmune arthritis [91, 92]. Thereby, the role of IL-17 in bone metabolism-associated diseases has been extensively defined, and this role is mainly associated with the induction of proinflammatory cytokines, chemokines, and matrix metalloproteinases that leads pathological bone and/or cartilage damage [89, 93, 94].

Our recent data revealed that higher levels of IL-1β, IL-17, and IL-22, associated with the Th1, Th17, and Th22-pattern of immuno-inflammatory response, were detected in TMJ-OA as compared with DDWR. Increased cytokine levels significantly correlated with an enhancement of RANKL expression and the detection of imagenological signs of articular bone degeneration [95]. IL-22 plays a proinflammatory role through the synergistic activity with IL-1β and TNF-α [96–98] and IL-22 can indirectly induce osteoclastogenesis and bone resorption by the induction of Th17 lymphocyte activity and IL-17 production [99]. In fact, previous reports have detected over-expressed levels of IL-22 in rheumatoid arthritis synovial fibroblasts, demonstrating a pathogenic role of IL-22 in the rheumatic joint inflammation and destruction through the modulation of the IL-1β and IL-17R expression [100, 101]. In general terms, we believe that the Th1/Th17/Th22 immuno-inflammatory cell pathways, associated with the production of IL-1β, IL-17, and IL-22, play a central role in the pathogenesis of the TMJ-OA. Similarly, the role of the Th2/Th9/T regulatory cell pathways, responsible for the production of IL-4, IL-9, and TGF-β1, respectively, could be associated with TMJ-OA disease healing.

7. Therapeutic potential of T regulatory lymphocytes in TMJ-OA

At the beginning of 1980s, the existence of a suppressor T cell population was proposed, suggesting that these T cells restrict the induction or expression of effector T cells and thereby prevent and control exaggerated immune response and autoimmune disease development [102]. The modern view of suppressor cells began with the observation that the transfer of T cells depleted of the IL-2Rα$^+$ (CD25$^+$) cell subpopulation induced multiorgan autoimmunity in recipient mice [103]. Nowadays, suppressor T cells have been renamed and are currently known as T regulatory cells (Tregs). These cells have been isolated from mice and humans and their regulatory functions have been demonstrated not only *in vitro* but also *in vivo*. It has also been established that several types of cells carry out regulatory activities. These include IL-10-secreting CD4$^+$ T regulatory-1 (Tr1) cells, TGF-β1-secreting CD4$^+$ Th3 cells, NKT cells, CD8$^+$CD28$^-$Foxp3$^+$ cells, γ/δ TCR cells, and CD4$^+$CD25^{high}Foxp3$^+$ T cells, the last one widely accepted as "professional Tregs" or naturally occurring Tregs [104, 105].

Natural Tregs are CD4$^+$ T cells that develop and mature in the thymus carry out their regulatory function during normal surveillance of self-antigens [106]. On normal individuals, they represent 5–10% of the peripheral CD4$^+$ T cell population and are characterized by the constitutive expression of high levels of CD25 and low levels of CD45RB [107]. In turn, adaptive Tregs represent CD4$^+$ T cells that acquire their regulatory activity during activation [106]. Unlike natural Tregs, which came out from the thymus as CD4$^+$CD25$^+$ cells, adaptive Tregs originate from peripheral naïve T cells [106]. They are derived from CD4$^+$CD25$^-$ T cells and show variable expression of CD25 during their mature phenotype, depending on the disease and the site of regulatory activity [108] Induced Tregs require TCR stimulation for induction of regulatory functions and have demonstrated limited proliferation *in vitro* [109].

Although induced Tregs and effector Th17 cells play different roles during the immunity, reciprocal developmental pathways have been demonstrated for their generation. Naïve T cells exposed to TGF-β1 up-regulate Foxp3 and become induced Tregs; however, when cultured with TGF-β1 and IL-6, naïve T cells generate IL-17 secreting Th17 cells with pathologic activities [110, 111]. Thus, when the immune response is not activated, TGF- β1 favors the generation of induced Tregs, which suppress inflammation; however, when the inflammatory process is established, IL-6 is synthesized during the innate immune response, inhibiting the generation of Tregs and inducing the differentiation of proinflammatory of Th17 cells in presence of TGF-β1 [112]. Thus, induced Tregs and Th17 lymphocytes may arise from the same precursor cell and selective differentiation would depend on the local cytokine milieu, which would determine the predominance of either Tregs with suppressor activity or Th17 cells with pathologic activities, determining the outcome of the disease [112].

8. Conclusion

The therapeutic potential of Tregs has created a lot of expectations and a large number of publications have assayed their properties either *in vitro* or in experimental models. Tregs suppress *in vitro* proliferation and cytokine production from co-cultured effector T cells [113]. Tregs suppressed autoimmune diabetes and altered the course of lupus in a TGF-β1-dependent manner [114]. Additionally, induced Tregs have been successfully used to prevent organ graft rejection [115]. A model of Treg therapy aimed to induce tolerance and restoration of function might show promising results during treatment of TMJ-OA, but additional research is necessary for a better understanding of Treg physiology and to solve several yet unanswered aspects associated to their therapeutic potential in humans.

Author details

Gustavo Monasterio[1], Francisca Castillo[1], Daniel Betancur[2], Arnoldo Hernández[3], Guillermo Flores[4], Walter Díaz[4], Marcela Hernández[1,5] and Rolando Vernal[1,6*]

*Address all correspondence to: rvernal@uchile.cl

1 Periodontal Biology Laboratory, Faculty of Dentistry, Universidad de Chile, Chile

2 Molecular Immunology Laboratory, Faculty of Biological Sciences, Universidad de Concepción, Chile

3 Anatomy and Biology Program, Faculty of Medicine, Universidad de Chile, Chile

4 Department of Prosthesis, Faculty of Dentistry, Universidad de Chile, Chile

5 Department of Pathology and Oral Medicine, Faculty of Dentistry, Universidad de Chile, Chile

6 Department of Conservative Dentistry, Faculty of Dentistry, Universidad de Chile, Chile

References

[1] Stankovic S, Vlajkovic S, Boskovic M, Radenkovic G, Antic V, Jevremovic D. Morphological and biomechanical features of the temporomandibular joint disc: An overview of recent findings. Archives of Oral Biology. 2013;**58**(10):1475-1482. DOI: 10.1016/j.archoralbio.2013.06.014

[2] Bag AK, Gaddikeri S, Singhal A, Hardin S, Tran BD, Medina JA, et al. Imaging of the temporomandibular joint: An update. World Journal of Radiology. 2014;**6**(8):567-582. DOI: 10.4329/wjr.v6.i8.567

[3] Siessere S, Vitti M, Semprini M, Regalo SC, Iyomasa MM, Dias FJ, et al. Macroscopic and microscopic aspects of the temporomandibular joint related to its clinical implication. Micron. 2008;**39**(7):852-858. DOI: 10.1016/j.micron.2007.12.006

[4] Kuroda S, Tanimoto K, Izawa T, Fujihara S, Koolstra JH, Tanaka E. Biomechanical and biochemical characteristics of the mandibular condylar cartilage. Osteoarthritis and Cartilage. 2009;**17**(11):1408-1415. DOI: 10.1016/j.joca.2009.04.025

[5] Davies JC, Charles M, Cantelmi D, Liebgott B, Ravichandiran M, Ravichandiran K, et al. Lateral pterygoid muscle: A three-dimensional analysis of neuromuscular partitioning. Clinical Anatomy. 2012;**25**(5):576-583. DOI: 10.1002/ca.21298

[6] Wurgaft RaM MA. Desarrollo y estructura de la articulación témporomandibular. 1st ed. Servimpres Ltda: Santiago, Chile; 2003. DOI: 10.4067/S0717-95022006000300020

[7] Rouvière HD. A. Anatomía Humana descriptiva, topografica y funcional. 11th ed. Barcelona, España: Editorial Masson; 2005

[8] Garino F. Anatomía odontológica funcional y aplicada. 2nd ed. Buenos Aires-Argentina, El Ateneo; 2010

[9] Ilguy D, Ilguy M, Fisekcioglu E, Dolekoglu S, Ersan N. Articular eminence inclination, height, and condyle morphology on cone beam computed tomography. ScientificWorld Journal. 2014;**2014**:761714. DOI: 10.1155/2014/761714

[10] Rodriguez-Vazquez JF, Murakami G, Verdugo-Lopez S, Abe S, Fujimiya M. Closure of the middle ear with special reference to the development of the tegmen tympani of the temporal bone. Journal of Anatomy. 2011;**218**(6):690-698. DOI: 10.1111/j.1469-7580.2011.01378.x

[11] Lang. Clinical Anatomy of the Masticatory Apparatus and Peripharyngeal Spaces. Stuttgart: G Thieme Co; 1995

[12] Arai H, Sato I. Anatomical study of the human discomallear ligament using cone beam computed tomography imaging and morphological observations. Okajimas Folia Anatomica Japonica. 2011;**88**(3):89-101. DOI: 10.2535/ofaj.88.89

[13] Asaki S, Sekikawa M, Kim YT. Sensory innervation of temporomandibular joint disk. Journal of Orthopaedic Surgery (Hong Kong). 2006;**14**(1):3-8. DOI: 10.1177/230949900601400102

[14] Lataryet MRL. A. Anatomia Humana. 4th ed. Buenos Aires, Argentina: Ed. Medica Panamericana; 2004

[15] Shiozaki H, Abe S, Tsumori N, Shiozaki K, Kaneko Y, Ichinohe T. Macroscopic anatomy of the sphenomandibular ligament related to the inferior alveolar nerve block. Cranio. 2007;**25**(3):160-165. DOI: 10.1179/crn.2007.025

[16] Sencimen M, Varol A, Baykal B, Altug HA, Dogan N, Sahin S, et al. Histological characteristics of ligaments between middle ear and temporomandibular joint. European Journal of Dentistry. 2009;**3**(4):280-284. DOI: 10.1016/j.bjoms.2009.06.203

[17] Anagnostopoulou S, Venieratos D, Antonopoulou M. Temporomandibular joint and correlated fissures: Anatomical and clinical consideration. Cranio. 2008;**26**(2):88-95. DOI: 10.1179/crn.2008.013

[18] Monteiro JC, Ennes JP, Zorzatto JR. Ossification of the petrotympanic fissure: Morphological analysis and clinical implications. Cranio. 2011;**29**(4):284-290. DOI: 10.1179/crn.2011.042

[19] Saran RS, Ananthi KS, Subramaniam A, Balaji MT, Vinaitha D, Vaithianathan G. Foramen of civinini: A new anatomical guide for maxillofacial surgeons. Journal of Clinical and Diagnostic Research. 2013;**7**(7):1271-1275. DOI: 10.7860/JCDR/2013/5100.3115

[20] Stegenga B. Osteoarthritis of the temporomandibular joint organ and its relationship to disc displacement. Journal of Orofacial Pain. 2001;**15**(3):193-205

[21] Bell WE. Temporomandibular Disorders: Classification, Diagnosis, Management: Year Book Medical; 1986. DOI: 10.1016/0300-5712(88)90071-1

[22] Poveda Roda R, Bagan JV, Diaz Fernandez JM, Hernandez Bazan S, Jimenez Soriano Y. Review of temporomandibular joint pathology. Part I: Classification, epidemiology and risk factors. Medicina Oral, Patología Oral y Cirugía Bucal. 2007;**12**(4):E292-E298

[23] Dworkin SF, LeResche L. Research diagnostic criteria for temporomandibular disorders: Review, criteria, examinations and specifications, critique. Journal of Craniomandibular Disorders. 1992;**6**(4):301-355

[24] Schiffman E, Ohrbach R, Truelove E, Look J, Anderson G, Goulet JP, et al. Diagnostic criteria for temporomandibular disorders (DC/TMD) for clinical and research applications: Recommendations of the international RDC/TMD consortium network and Orofacial pain special interest Groupdagger. Journal of Oral & Facial Pain and Headache. 2014; **28**(1):6-27. DOI: 10.11607/jop.1151

[25] Okeson JP. Critical commentary 1: Evaluation of the research diagnostic criteria for temporomandibular disorders for the recognition of an anterior disc displacement with reduction. Journal of Orofacial Pain. 2009;**23**(4):312-315; author reply 323-314. DOI: 10.1038/sj.bdj.2010.128

[26] de Leeuw R, Boering G, Stegenga B, de Bont LG. Temporomandibular joint osteoarthrosis: Clinical and radiographic characteristics 30 years after nonsurgical treatment: A preliminary report. Cranio. 1993;**11**(1):15-24. DOI: 10.1080/08869634.1993.11677936

[27] Wilkes CH. Internal derangements of the temporomandibular joint. Pathological variations. Archives of Otolaryngology – Head & Neck Surgery. 1989;**115**(4):469-477. DOI: 10.1001/archotol.1989.01860280067019

[28] Schiffman E, Ohrbach R. Executive summary of the diagnostic criteria for temporomandibular disorders for clinical and research applications. Journal of the American Dental Association (1939). 2016;**147**(6):438-445. DOI: 10.1016/j.adaj.2016.01.007

[29] Fang PK, Ma XC, Ma DL, Fu KY. Determination of interleukin-1 receptor antagonist, interleukin-10, and transforming growth factor-β1 in synovial fluid aspirates of patients with temporomandibular disorders. Journal of Oral and Maxillofacial Surgery. 1999; **57**(8):922-928; discussion 928-929. DOI: 10.1016/s0278-2391(99)90009-5

[30] KY F, Li YW, Zhang ZK, Ma XC. Osteonecrosis of the mandibular condyle as a precursor to osteoarthrosis: A case report. Oral Surgery, Oral Medicine, Oral Pathology, Oral Radiology, and Endodontics. 2009;**107**(1):e34-e38. DOI: 10.1016/j.tripleo.2008.09.013

[31] Herr MM, Fries KM, Upton LG, Edsberg LE. Potential biomarkers of temporomandibular joint disorders. Journal of Oral and Maxillofacial Surgery. 2011;**69**(1):41-47. DOI: 10.1016/j.joms.2010.05.013

[32] Kaneyama K, Segami N, Nishimura M, Sato J, Suzuki T, Fujimura K. Osteoclastogenesis inhibitory factor/osteoprotegerin in synovial fluid from patients with temporomandibular disorders. International Journal of Oral and Maxillofacial Surgery. 2003;**32**(4):404-407. DOI: 10.1054/ijom.2002.0363

[33] Kaneyama K, Segami N, Nishimura M, Suzuki T, Sato J. Importance of proinflammatory cytokines in synovial fluid from 121 joints with temporomandibular disorders. The British Journal of Oral & Maxillofacial Surgery. 2002;**40**(5):418-423. DOI: 10.1016/S0266-4356(02)00215-2

[34] Kaneyama K, Segami N, Sato J, Nishimura M, Yoshimura H. Interleukin-6 family of cytokines as biochemical markers of osseous changes in the temporomandibular joint disorders. The British Journal of Oral & Maxillofacial Surgery. 2004;**42**(3):246-250. DOI: 10.1016/S0266-4356(03)00258-4

[35] Kaneyama K, Segami N, Sun W, Sato J, Fujimura K. Analysis of tumor necrosis factor-alpha, interleukin-6, interleukin-1β, soluble tumor necrosis factor receptors I and II, interleukin-6 soluble receptor, interleukin-1 soluble receptor type II, interleukin-1 receptor antagonist, and protein in the synovial fluid of patients with temporomandibular joint disorders. Oral Surgery, Oral Medicine, Oral Pathology, Oral Radiology, and Endodontics. 2005;**99**(3):276-284. DOI: 10.1016/j.tripleo.2004.06.074

[36] Kubota E, Kubota T, Matsumoto J, Shibata T, Murakami KI. Synovial fluid cytokines and proteinases as markers of temporomandibular joint disease. Journal of Oral and Maxillofacial Surgery. 1998;**56**(2):192-198. DOI: 10.1016/s0278-2391(98)90868-0

[37] Lee JK, Cho YS, Song SI. Relationship of synovial tumor necrosis factor alpha and interleukin 6 to temporomandibular disorder. Journal of Oral and Maxillofacial Surgery. 2010;**68**(5):1064-1068. DOI: 10.1016/j.joms.2009.08.007

[38] Shinoda C, Takaku S. Interleukin-1β, interleukin-6, and tissue inhibitor of metalloproteinase-1 in the synovial fluid of the temporomandibular joint with respect to cartilage destruction. Oral Diseases. 2000;**6**(6):383-390. DOI: 10.1111/j.1601-0825.2000.tb00131.x

[39] Takahashi T, Kondoh T, Fukuda M, Yamazaki Y, Toyosaki T, Suzuki R. Proinflammatory cytokines detectable in synovial fluids from patients with temporomandibular disorders. Oral Surgery, Oral Medicine, Oral Pathology, Oral Radiology, and Endodontics. 1998;**85**(2):135-141. DOI: 10.1016/s1079-2104(98)90415-2

[40] Vernal R, Velasquez E, Gamonal J, Garcia-Sanz JA, Silva A, Sanz M. Expression of proinflammatory cytokines in osteoarthritis of the temporomandibular joint. Archives of Oral Biology. 2008;**53**(10):910-915. DOI: 10.1016/j.archoralbio.2008.04.004

[41] Wake M, Hamada Y, Kumagai K, Tanaka N, Ikeda Y, Nakatani Y, et al. Up-regulation of interleukin-6 and vascular endothelial growth factor-a in the synovial fluid of temporomandibular joints affected by synovial chondromatosis. The British Journal of Oral & Maxillofacial Surgery. 2013;**51**(2):164-169. DOI: 10.1016/j.bjoms.2012.03.004

[42] Wakita T, Mogi M, Kurita K, Kuzushima M, Togari A. Increase in RANKL:OPG ratio in synovia of patients with temporomandibular joint disorder. Journal of Dental Research. 2006;**85**(7):627-632. DOI: 10.1177/154405910608500709

[43] Suenaga S, Nagayama K, Nagasawa T, Indo H, Majima HJ. The usefulness of diagnostic imaging for the assessment of pain symptoms in temporomandibular disorders. Japanese Dental Science Review. 2016;**52**(4):93-106. DOI: 10.1016/j.jdsr.2016.04.004

[44] Honey OB, Scarfe WC, Hilgers MJ, Klueber K, Silveira AM, Haskell BS, et al. Accuracy of cone-beam computed tomography imaging of the temporomandibular joint: Comparisons with panoramic radiology and linear tomography. American Journal of Orthodontics and Dentofacial Orthopedics. 2007;**132**(4):429-438. DOI: 10.1016/j.ajodo.2005.10.032

[45] Wiese M, Wenzel A, Hintze H, Petersson A, Knutsson K, Bakke M, et al. Influence of cross-sectional temporomandibular joint tomography on diagnosis and management decisions of patients with temporomandibular joint disorders. Journal of Orofacial Pain. 2011;**25**(3):223-231

[46] Talaat W, Al Bayatti S, Al Kawas S. CBCT analysis of bony changes associated with temporomandibular disorders. Cranio. 2015:1-7. DOI: 10.1080/08869634.2015.1097323

[47] Campos MI, Campos PS, Cangussu MC, Guimaraes RC, Line SR. Analysis of magnetic resonance imaging characteristics and pain in temporomandibular joints with and without degenerative changes of the condyle. International Journal of Oral and Maxillofacial Surgery. 2008;**37**(6):529-534. DOI: 10.1016/j.ijom.2008.02.011

[48] Cho BH, Jung YH. Osteoarthritic changes and condylar positioning of the temporomandibular joint in Korean children and adolescents. Imaging Science in Dentistry. 2012;**42**(3): 169-174. DOI: 10.5624/isd.2012.42.3.169

[49] Koyama J, Nishiyama H, Hayashi T. Follow-up study of condylar bony changes using helical computed tomography in patients with temporomandibular disorder. Dento Maxillo Facial Radiology. 2007;**36**(8):472-477. DOI: 10.1259/dmfr/28078357

[50] Cevidanes LH, Walker D, Schilling J, Sugai J, Giannobile W, Paniagua B, et al. 3D osteoarthritic changes in TMJ condylar morphology correlates with specific systemic and local biomarkers of disease. Osteoarthritis and Cartilage. 2014;**22**(10):1657-1667. DOI: 10.1016/j.joca.2014.06.014

[51] Lim MJ, Lee JY. Computed tomographic study of the patterns of oesteoarthritic change which occur on the mandibular condyle. Journal of Cranio-Maxillo-Facial Surgery. 2014;**42**(8):1897-1902. DOI: 10.1016/j.jcms.2014.07.009

[52] Cevidanes LH, Hajati AK, Paniagua B, Lim PF, Walker DG, Palconet G, et al. Quantification of condylar resorption in temporomandibular joint osteoarthritis. Oral Surgery, Oral Medicine, Oral Pathology, Oral Radiology, and Endodontics. 2010;**110**(1):110-117. DOI: 10.1016/j.tripleo.2010.01.008

[53] Tsiklakis K, Syriopoulos K, Stamatakis HC. Radiographic examination of the temporomandibular joint using cone beam computed tomography. Dento Maxillo Facial Radiology. 2004;**33**(3):196-201. DOI: 10.1259/dmfr/27403192

[54] Bertram S, Rudisch A, Innerhofer K, Pumpel E, Grubwieser G, Emshoff R. Diagnosing TMJ internal derangement and osteoarthritis with magnetic resonance imaging. Journal of the American Dental Association (1939). 2001;**132**(6):753-761. DOI: 10.14219/jada.archive.2001.0272

[55] Schmitter M, Essig M, Seneadza V, Balke Z, Schroder J, Rammelsberg P. Prevalence of clinical and radiographic signs of osteoarthrosis of the temporomandibular joint in an older persons community. Dento Maxillo Facial Radiology. 2010;**39**(4):231-234. DOI: 10.1259/dmfr/16270943

[56] Takatsuka S, Yoshida K, Ueki K, Marukawa K, Nakagawa K, Yamamoto E. Disc and condyle translation in patients with temporomandibular disorder. Oral Surgery, Oral Medicine, Oral Pathology, Oral Radiology, and Endodontics. 2005;**99**(5):614-621. DOI: 10.1016/j.tripleo.2004.08.024

[57] Ikeda K, Kawamura A. Assessment of optimal condylar position with limited cone-beam computed tomography. American Journal of Orthodontics and Dentofacial Orthopedics. 2009;**135**(4):495-501. DOI: 10.1016/j.ajodo.2007.05.021

[58] Ahn BC, Kim HJ, Lee SW, Yoo J, Choi JK, Lee J. New quantitative method for bone tracer uptake of temporomandibular joint using Tc-99m MDP skull SPECT. Annals of Nuclear Medicine. 2009;**23**(7):651-656. DOI: 10.1007/s12149-009-0287-8

[59] Coutinho A, Fenyo-Pereira M, Dib LL, Lima EN. The role of SPECT/CT with 99mTc-MDP image fusion to diagnose temporomandibular dysfunction. Oral Surgery, Oral Medicine, Oral Pathology, Oral Radiology, and Endodontics. 2006;**101**(2):224-230. DOI: 10.1016/j.tripleo.2005.03.018

[60] Hersek N, Canay S, Caner B, Ulutuncel N. Bone SPECT imaging of patients with internal derangement of temporomandibular joint before and after splint therapy. Oral Surgery, Oral Medicine, Oral Pathology, Oral Radiology, and Endodontics. 2002;**94**(5):576-580. DOI: 10.1067/moe.2002.124855

[61] Kim JH, Kim YK, Kim SG, Yun PY, Kim JD, Min JH. Effectiveness of bone scans in the diagnosis of osteoarthritis of the temporomandibular joint. Dento Maxillo Facial Radiology. 2012;**41**(3):224-229. DOI: 10.1259/dmfr/83814366

[62] Bakke M, Petersson A, Wiesel M, Svanholt P, Sonnesen L. Bony deviations revealed by cone beam computed tomography of the temporomandibular joint in subjects without ongoing pain. Journal of Oral & Facial Pain and Headache. 2014;**28**(4):331-337. DOI: 10.11607/ofph.1255

[63] Krisjane Z, Urtane I, Krumina G, Neimane L, Ragovska I. The prevalence of TMJ osteoarthritis in asymptomatic patients with dentofacial deformities: A cone-beam CT study. International Journal of Oral and Maxillofacial Surgery. 2012;**41**(6):690-695. DOI: 10.1016/j.ijom.2012.03.006

[64] Ha MH, Kim YI, Park SB, Kim SS, Son WS. Cone-beam computed tomographic evaluation of the condylar remodeling occurring after mandibular set-back by bilateral sagittal split ramus osteotomy and rigid fixation. Korean Journal of Orthodontics. 2013;**43**(6):263-270. DOI: 10.4041/kjod.2013.43.6.263

[65] Honda K, Natsumi Y, Urade M. Correlation between MRI evidence of degenerative condylar surface changes, induction of articular disc displacement and pathological joint sounds in the temporomandibular joint. Gerodontology. 2008;**25**(4):251-257. DOI: 10.1111/j.1741-2358.2008.00219.x

[66] Palconet G, Ludlow JB, Tyndall DA, Lim PF. Correlating cone beam CT results with temporomandibular joint pain of osteoarthritic origin. Dento Maxillo Facial Radiology. 2012;**41**(2):126-130. DOI: 10.1259/dmfr/60489374

[67] Berenbaum F. Osteoarthritis year 2010 in review: Pharmacological therapies. Osteoarthritis and Cartilage. 2011;**19**(4):361-365. DOI: 10.1016/j.joca.2011.01.019

[68] Kellesarian SV, Al-Kheraif AA, Vohra F, Ghanem A, Malmstrom H, Romanos GE, et al. Cytokine profile in the synovial fluid of patients with temporomandibular joint disorders: A systematic review. Cytokine. 2016;**77**:98-106. DOI: 10.1016/j.cyto.2015.11.005

[69] Li C, Long X, Deng M, Li J, Cai H, Meng Q. Osteoarthritic changes after superior and inferior joint space injection of hyaluronic acid for the treatment of temporomandibular joint osteoarthritis with anterior disc displacement without reduction: A cone-beam computed tomographic evaluation. Journal of Oral and Maxillofacial Surgery. 2015;**73**(2):232-244. DOI: 10.1016/j.joms.2014.08.034

[70] Liu F, Steinkeler A. Epidemiology, diagnosis, and treatment of temporomandibular disorders. Dental Clinics of North America. 2013;**57**(3):465-479. DOI: 10.1016/j.cden.2013.04.006

[71] de Bont LG, Boering G, Liem RS, Eulderink F, Westesson PL. Osteoarthritis and internal derangement of the temporomandibular joint: A light microscopic study. Journal of Oral and Maxillofacial Surgery. 1986;**44**(8):634-643. DOI: 10.1016/s0278-2391(86)80075-1

[72] Yamada K, Saito I, Hanada K, Hayashi T. Observation of three cases of temporomandibular joint osteoarthritis and mandibular morphology during adolescence using helical CT. Journal of Oral Rehabilitation. 2004;**31**(4):298-305. DOI: 10.1046/j.1365-2842.2003.01246.x

[73] Foell D, Wittkowski H, Roth J. Mechanisms of disease: A 'DAMP' view of inflammatory arthritis. Nature Clinical Practice. Rheumatology. 2007;**3**(7):382-390. DOI: 10.1038/ncprheum0531

[74] Jiang W, Pisetsky DS. Mechanisms of disease: The role of high-mobility group protein 1 in the pathogenesis of inflammatory arthritis. Nature Clinical Practice. Rheumatology. 2007;**3**(1):52-58. DOI: 10.1038/ncprheum0379

[75] Nefla M, Holzinger D, Berenbaum F, Jacques C. The danger from within: Alarmins in arthritis. Nature Reviews Rheumatology. 2016;**12**(11):669-683. DOI: 10.1038/nrrheum.2016.162

[76] Milam SB, Zardeneta G, Schmitz JP. Oxidative stress and degenerative temporomandibular joint disease: A proposed hypothesis. Journal of Oral and Maxillofacial Surgery. 1998;**56**(2):214-223

[77] Kawai Y, Kubota E. Oxidative stress and temporomandibular joint disorders. Japanese Dental Science Review. 2008;**44**(2):145-150

[78] Guo H, Fang W, Li Y, Ke J, Deng M, Meng Q, et al. Up-regulation of proteoglycan 4 in temporomandibular osteoarthritic synovial cells by hyaluronic acid. Journal of Oral Pathology & Medicine. 2015;**44**(8):622-627. DOI: 10.1111/jop.12273

[79] Lim WH, Toothman J, Miller JH, Tallents RH, Brouxhon SM, Olschowka ME, et al. IL-1β inhibits TGFβ in the temporomandibular joint. Journal of Dental Research. 2009;**88**(6):557-562. DOI: 10.1177/0022034509336823

[80] Long E, Motwani R, Reece D, Pettit N, Hepworth J, Wong P, et al. The role of TGF-β1 in osteoarthritis of the temporomandibular joint in two genetic mouse models. Archives of Oral Biology. 2016;**67**:68-73. DOI: 10.1016/j.archoralbio.2016.03.004

[81] Lu L, Zhang X, Zhang M, Zhang H, Liao L, Yang T, et al. RANTES and SDF-1 are keys in cell-based therapy of TMJ osteoarthritis. Journal of Dental Research. 2015;**94**(11):1601-1609. DOI: 10.1177/0022034515604621

[82] Ferreira LM, Moura ÁFB, Barbosa GAS, Pereira HSG, dos Santos Calderon P. Do matrix metalloproteinases play a role in degenerative disease of temporomandibular joint? A systematic review. Cranio. 2016;**34**(2):112-117. DOI: 10.1179/2151090314Y.0000000034

[83] Luo S, Deng M, Long X, Li J, Xu L, Fang W. Association between polymorphism of MMP-1 promoter and the susceptibility to anterior disc displacement and temporomandibular joint osteoarthritis. Archives of Oral Biology. 2015;**60**(11):1675-1680. DOI: 10.1016/j.archoralbio.2015.08.001

[84] Sato J, Segami N, Yoshitake Y, Kaneyama K, Yoshimura H, Fujimura K, et al. Specific expression of substance P in synovial tissues of patients with symptomatic, non-reducing internal derangement of the temporomandibular joint: Comparison with clinical findings. The British Journal of Oral & Maxillofacial Surgery. 2007;**45**(5):372-377. DOI: 10.1016/j.bjoms.2006.09.011

[85] Tanaka A, Kumagai S, Kawashiri S, Takatsuka S, Nakagawa K, Yamamoto E, et al. Expression of matrix metalloproteinase-2 and -9 in synovial fluid of the temporomandibular joint accompanied by anterior disc displacement. Journal of Oral Pathology & Medicine. 2001;**30**(1):59-64. DOI: 10.1034/j.1600-0714.2001.300110.x

[86] Yoshida K, Takatsuka S, Tanaka A, Hatada E, Nakamura H, Nakagawa K, et al. Aggrecanase analysis of synovial fluid of temporomandibular joint disorders. Oral Diseases. 2005;**11**(5):299-302. DOI: 10.1111/j.1601-0825.2005.01120.x

[87] Fu K, Ma X, Zhang Z, Pang X, Chen W. Interleukin-6 in synovial fluid and HLA-DR expression in synovium from patients with temporomandibular disorders. Journal of Orofacial Pain. 1995;**9**(2):131-137

[88] Shafer DM, Assael L, White LB, Rossomando EF. Tumor necrosis factor-alpha as a biochemical marker of pain and outcome in temporomandibular joints with internal derangements. Journal of Oral and Maxillofacial Surgery. 1994;**52**(8):786-791; discussion 791-782. DOI: 10.1016/0278-2391(94)90217-8

[89] Fossiez F, Banchereau J, Murray R, Van Kooten C, Garrone P, Lebecque S. Interleukin-17. International Reviews of Immunology. 1998;**16**(5-6):541-551. DOI: 10.3109/08830189809043008

[90] Sato K, Suematsu A, Okamoto K, Yamaguchi A, Morishita Y, Kadono Y, et al. Th17 functions as an osteoclastogenic helper T cell subset that links T cell activation and bone destruction. The Journal of Experimental Medicine. 2006;**203**(12):2673-2682. DOI: 10.1084/jem.20061775

[91] Nakae S, Nambu A, Sudo K, Iwakura Y. Suppression of immune induction of collagen-induced arthritis in IL-17-deficient mice. Journal of Immunology. 2003;**171**(11):6173-6177. DOI: 10.4049/jimmunol.171.11.6173

[92] Sato K, Takayanagi H. Osteoclasts, rheumatoid arthritis, and osteoimmunology. Current Opinion in Rheumatology. 2006;**18**(4):419-426. DOI: 10.1097/01.bor.0000231912.24740.a5

[93] Gravallese EM. Bone destruction in arthritis. Annals of the Rheumatic Diseases. 2002;**61**(Suppl 2):ii84-ii86. DOI: 10.1136/ard.61.suppl_2.ii84

[94] Vernal R, Dutzan N, Chaparro A, Puente J, Antonieta Valenzuela M, Gamonal J. Levels of interleukin-17 in gingival crevicular fluid and in supernatants of cellular cultures of gingival tissue from patients with chronic periodontitis. Journal of Clinical Periodontology. 2005;**32**(4):383-389. DOI: 10.1111/j.1600-051X.2005.00684.x

[95] Monasterio G, Castillo F, Pujol M, Rojas L, Alvarez C, Carvajal P, et al. Variability in the Th1/Th17/Th22 and Th2/Th9/Treg-type of immuno-inflammatory responses and their association with joint pain, imagenological bone degeneration, Rankl expression, and osteoclast-induced bone resorption in temporomandibular joint osteoarthritis and disk displacement with reduction. Journal of Orofacial Pain. 2017:Submitted

[96] Kim KW, Kim HR, Park JY, Park JS, HJ O, Woo YJ, et al. Interleukin-22 promotes osteoclastogenesis in rheumatoid arthritis through induction of RANKL in human synovial fibroblasts. Arthritis and Rheumatism. 2012;**64**(4):1015-1023. DOI: 10.1002/art.33446

[97] Elyaman W, Bradshaw EM, Uyttenhove C, Dardalhon V, Awasthi A, Imitola J, et al. IL-9 induces differentiation of TH17 cells and enhances function of FoxP3+ natural regulatory T cells. Proceedings of the National Academy of Sciences of the United States of America. 2009;**106**(31):12885-12890. DOI: 10.1073/pnas.0812530106

[98] Marijnissen RJ, Koenders MI, Smeets RL, Stappers MH, Nickerson-Nutter C, Joosten LA, et al. Increased expression of interleukin-22 by synovial Th17 cells during late stages of murine experimental arthritis is controlled by interleukin-1 and enhances bone degradation. Arthritis and Rheumatism. 2011;**63**(10):2939-2948. DOI: 10.1002/art.30469

[99] Zhang L, Li JM, Liu XG, Ma DX, NW H, Li YG, et al. Elevated Th22 cells correlated with Th17 cells in patients with rheumatoid arthritis. Journal of Clinical Immunology. 2011;**31**(4):606-614. DOI: 10.1007/s10875-011-9540-8

[100] Carrion M, Juarranz Y, Martinez C, Gonzalez-Alvaro I, Pablos JL, Gutierrez-Canas I, et al. IL-22/IL-22R1 axis and S100A8/A9 alarmins in human osteoarthritic and rheumatoid arthritis synovial fibroblasts. Rheumatology (Oxford, England). 2013;**52**(12):2177-2186. DOI: 10.1093/rheumatology/ket315

[101] Pinto LG, Talbot J, Peres RS, Franca RF, Ferreira SH, Ryffel B, et al. Joint production of IL-22 participates in the initial phase of antigen-induced arthritis through IL-1β production. Arthritis Research & Therapy. 2015;**17**:235. DOI: 10.1186/s13075-015-0759-2

[102] Green DR, Flood PM, Gershon RK. Immunoregulatory T-cell pathways. Annual Review of Immunology. 1983;**1**:439-463. DOI: 10.1146/annurev.iy.01.040183.002255

[103] Sakaguchi S, Toda M, Asano M, Itoh M, Morse SS, Sakaguchi N. T cell-mediated maintenance of natural self-tolerance: Its breakdown as a possible cause of various autoimmune diseases. Journal of Autoimmunity. 1996;**9**(2):211-220. DOI: 10.1006/jaut.1996.0026

[104] Pillai V, Karandikar NJ. Human regulatory T cells: A unique, stable thymic subset or a reversible peripheral state of differentiation? Immunology Letters. 2007;**114**(1):9-15. DOI: 10.1016/j.imlet.2007.08.012

[105] Sakaguchi S. Regulatory T cells in the past and for the future. European Journal of Immunology. 2008;**38**(4):901-937. DOI: 10.1002/eji.200890012

[106] Bluestone JA, Abbas AK. Natural versus adaptive regulatory T cells. Nature Reviews. Immunology. 2003;**3**(3):253-257. DOI: 10.1038/nri1032

[107] McGuirk P, Mills KH. Pathogen-specific regulatory T cells provoke a shift in the Th1/Th2 paradigm in immunity to infectious diseases. Trends in Immunology. 2002;**23**(9):450-455. DOI: 10.1016/s1471-4906(02)02288-3

[108] Gonzalez A, Andre-Schmutz I, Carnaud C, Mathis D, Benoist C. Damage control, rather than unresponsiveness, effected by protective DX5+ T cells in autoimmune diabetes. Nature Immunology. 2001;**2**(12):1117-1125. DOI: 10.1038/ni738

[109] Mittrucker HW, Kaufmann SH. Mini-review: Regulatory T cells and infection: Suppression revisited. European Journal of Immunology. 2004;**34**(2):306-312. DOI: 10.1002/eji.200324578

[110] Bettelli E, Carrier Y, Gao W, Korn T, Strom TB, Oukka M, et al. Reciprocal developmental pathways for the generation of pathogenic effector TH17 and regulatory T cells. Nature. 2006;**441**(7090):235-238. DOI: 10.1038/nature04753

[111] Yamazaki S, Bonito AJ, Spisek R, Dhodapkar M, Inaba K, Steinman RM. Dendritic cells are specialized accessory cells along with TGF- for the differentiation of Foxp3$^+$ CD4$^+$ regulatory T cells from peripheral Foxp3 precursors. Blood. 2007;**110**(13):4293-4302. DOI: 10.1182/blood-2007-05-088831

[112] Bettelli E, Oukka M, Kuchroo VK. T (H)-17 cells in the circle of immunity and autoimmunity. Nature Immunology. 2007;**8**(4):345-350. DOI: 10.1038/ni0407-345

[113] Brusko T, Bluestone J. Clinical application of regulatory T cells for treatment of type 1 diabetes and transplantation. European Journal of Immunology. 2008;**38**(4):931-934. DOI: 10.1002/eji.200738108

[114] You S, Leforban B, Garcia C, Bach JF, Bluestone JA, Chatenoud L. Adaptive TGF-β-dependent regulatory T cells control autoimmune diabetes and are a privileged target of anti-CD3 antibody treatment. Proceedings of the National Academy of Sciences of the United States of America. 2007;**104**(15):6335-6340. DOI: 10.1073/pnas.0701171104

[115] Horwitz DA, Zheng SG, Wang J, Gray JD. Critical role of IL-2 and TGF-β in generation, function and stabilization of Foxp3$^+$CD4$^+$ Treg. European Journal of Immunology. 2008;**38**(4): 912-915. DOI: 10.1002/eji.200738109

10

JVA, Mastication and Digital Occlusal Analysis in Diagnosis and Treatment of Temporomandibular Disorders

Serdar Gözler

Abstract

Temporomandibular joint disorder (TMJ) is a complex and multifactorial functional disorder. Best approach in the treatment of TMJ disorders needs in detail proper diagnostic study. Joint vibration analysis (JVA) device, a new age technology and one of the most important diagnostic tools, is used for detecting intra-articular sound vibrations. Every type of vibration in different frequencies shows us the status of joint. Evaluation can be made after analyzing the results applying to a diagram. Like Combining of the sound vibration diagnostic techniques with other examination methods may be very meaningful in efforts of treating TMJ problems. Another diagnosis method is the evaluation of chewing movements. Best chewing efficiency is the most important purpose of masticatory system. Final product is a very important indicator for the efficiency of the mastication, and chewing pattern. T-Scan digital occlusal analyzing system is another important occlusal diagnostic instrument. Digital occlusal analysis system is currently the most powerful method of TMD clinics for treatment of patients with muscle pain dysfunction syndrome. Digital occlusal analysis system allows us to perform the MPDS treatments, splint and occlusal rehabilitation. The three important diagnostic systems are described in this chapter.

Keywords: JVA, T-Scan, chewing pattern, mastication, temporomandibular disorders, MPDS

1. Introduction

Temporomandibular joint disorders (TMD) is one of the highly complicated fields in dentistry [1, 2]. It can emerge in various manners at any time during human life with symptoms such as limited mouth opening, pain at TMJ area, pain in masticatory muscles, headache specially around anterior temporal area, sounds emerging from temporomandibular joints, morning soreness, bruxism, clenching, head and neck pains, attrition and/or abfraction of teeth, internal derangement of temporomandibular disks, decreasing of volume in the synovial liquid. Temporomandibular joint disorder is a functional disturbance. Temporomandibular joints, masticatory muscles, teeth, bones and the central nerve system are all involved in TMJ pathology [3–6]. For many years, clinicians have employed various mechanical tools for diagnosis and to understand the reasons for the problem [7]. Due to the development of the chipset technology and software programming, we have now device-based diagnostic tools, joint vibration analysis, joint tracking measuring mastication analysis, computer-based occlusal analysis devices, and so on [8–10] available. However, there are still many questions and discussion points about some of the device-based diagnostic techniques [9]. These kind of device-based technologies require studying with a new methodology. Joint vibration analysis, joint tracker and mastication analysis, electromyography, tens devices and finally digital occlusal analysis systems all need new methodologies. That is to say if you have enough knowledge on how to conduct a joint vibration analysis or a digital occlusal analysis, it is possible to collect a lot of useful information with these devices [11–14].

All these symptoms are assembled under TMJ pathology [10, 15–19]. In dentistry, there is no other problem that must be managed in a multidisciplinary fashion like TMJ disorders.

Occlusal trauma that may occur after restorations is one of the biggest causes of temporomandibular disorders [20–23]. Dental extraction and orthodontic restorations are also important conditions that cause this discomfort [22, 24–27].

A large number of devices and methods are used for diagnosis and treatment of temporomandibular disorder. The reason for this is not only the complexity of the problem but also the demand for the use of noninvasive methods [10, 28–31].

For example, if you have enough knowledge about the joint vibration analysis or if you can use digital occlusal analysis properly, you can access very important information about the temporomandibular disorder [17, 32–34]. In addition, you may also have the opportunity to see and avoid pathology that may be related to joints according to the course of the treatment of the initial chewing pattern of orthodontic treatments [35–37]. However, it is very important to know how to use these devices, what their capabilities are, and how effective they can be so that it can be done. The predisposing factors of temporomandibular joint disorders can be eliminated before presenting whether all these devices are professionally used [28, 38–40].

Nowadays, one of the most widely used diagnostic tools in the examination of the pathology of temporomandibular joints is magnetic resonance imaging (MRI) technique [4, 11, 15]. MRI represents the golden standard among the temporomandibular diagnostic tools [41]. However, its acquisition is more difficult and costly than other diagnostic tools. Moreover, MRI examination of children is very difficult and complicated.

Craniomandibular dysfunctions are often multistructural [42] and intracapsular problems are one of the most important subjects that have been studied by dentists for a long time [33, 40, 43]. Normally, if there is no problem in a joint, no sound comes from that joint. There is no distortion in the relationship between joint-disk-articular surface. Joint is lined with synovium secreted for lubrication and nutrition. Joints are connected to a common bone, and therefore, they function together. Normal joints produce very little friction and vibration. If there is degeneration in the joint, there is sound in the joint [44–47]. The sound spectrum may be bigger or less than the human hearing limits. Scientific research has shown that TMJ sounds have been well categorized. Every TMJ sound is like a signature to a problem [48]. Since sound is a pressure energy, it has a particular frequency.

Another kind of useful information source is spectrum of TMJ sound. TMJ sounds have distinctive characteristics in clinical diagnosis efforts. Additionally, clinical-arthrographic investigations correlate arthrographic characteristics of intracapsular dysfunction of the temporomandibular joint with sound analysis. Sound patterns are reproducible and provide a noninvasive tool for diagnosis and treatment [14, 49].

In **Figure 1**, a graphic illustration screen shows the results of a clinical software that recorded and analyzed sounds emitted from the temporomandibular joint (TMJ) during simple function as a means for differentially diagnosing disorders of the joint. The patient's mouth opening distance is measured as 45 mm max. The repeated sounds emitted from the left joint peaks at around 43 mm. Spectral analysis of the same patient is shown in **Figure 2**.

Generally, spectral analysis considers the problem of determining the spectral content (i.e., the distribution of power over frequency) of a time series from a finite set of measurements, by

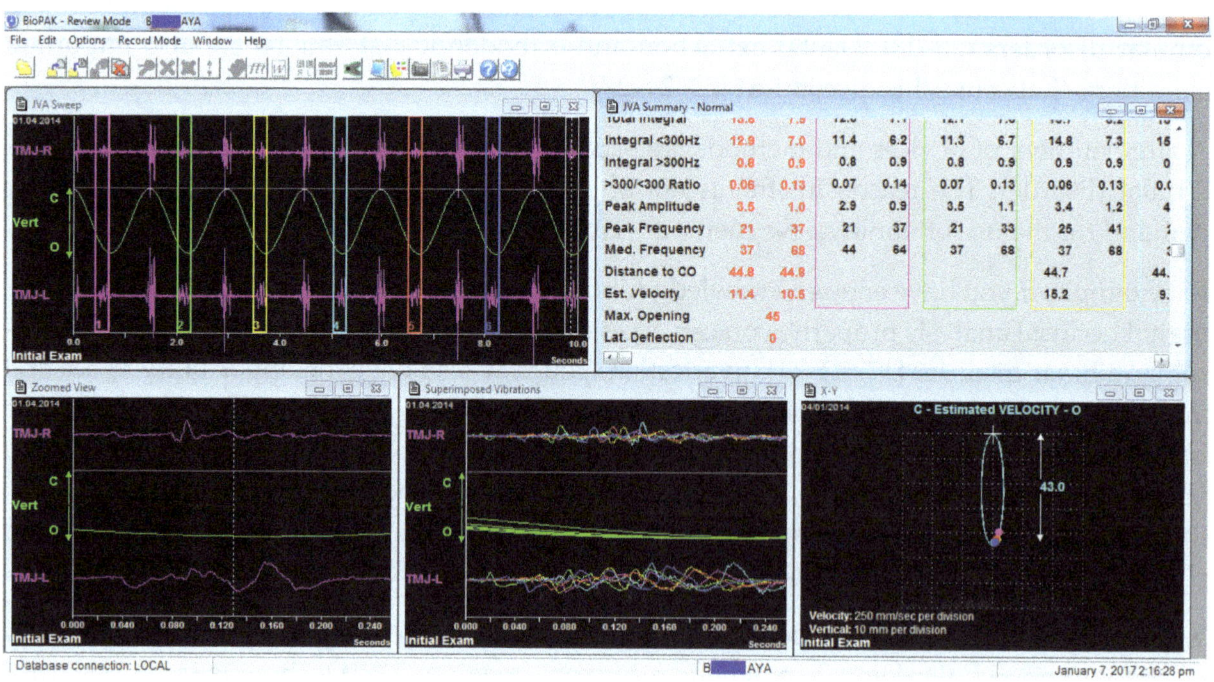

Figure 1. Maximum opening of the mouth is marked as 45 mm; however, there is a crepitation sound in the left joint at 43 mm of opening of the mouth. The crepitation sound was detected at this level in which head of the condyle is almost at the end of the protrusion. The condyle condition may be considered as only some ligament laxity.

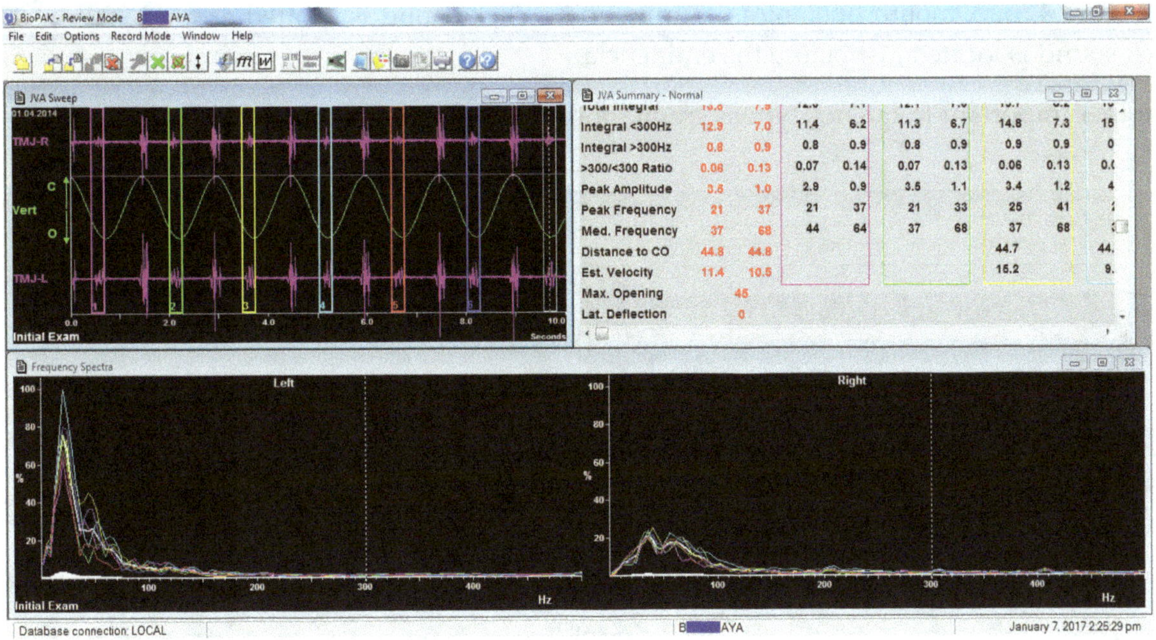

Figure 2. Spectral analysis considers the problem of determining the spectral content. Differences between energies of left and right joints are very clear. In this case, aggregation place of peak frequency is very close to the max opening limit, intracapsular deterioration has just started and it is only the beginning phase. We may consider this finding as only an MPD syndrome.

means of either nonparametric or parametric techniques. At JVA Sweep window of **Figure 2**, sound energy frequencies of left joint are shown on a time line.

Sounds due to temporomandibular joint disorders have been studied for a long time and are classified to the particular groups [45, 47, 50–52]. Very well-known sound frequencies belong to the "click" sound energy (**Figure 3**). A 2x zoom view of the click sound is shown in **Figure 3**.

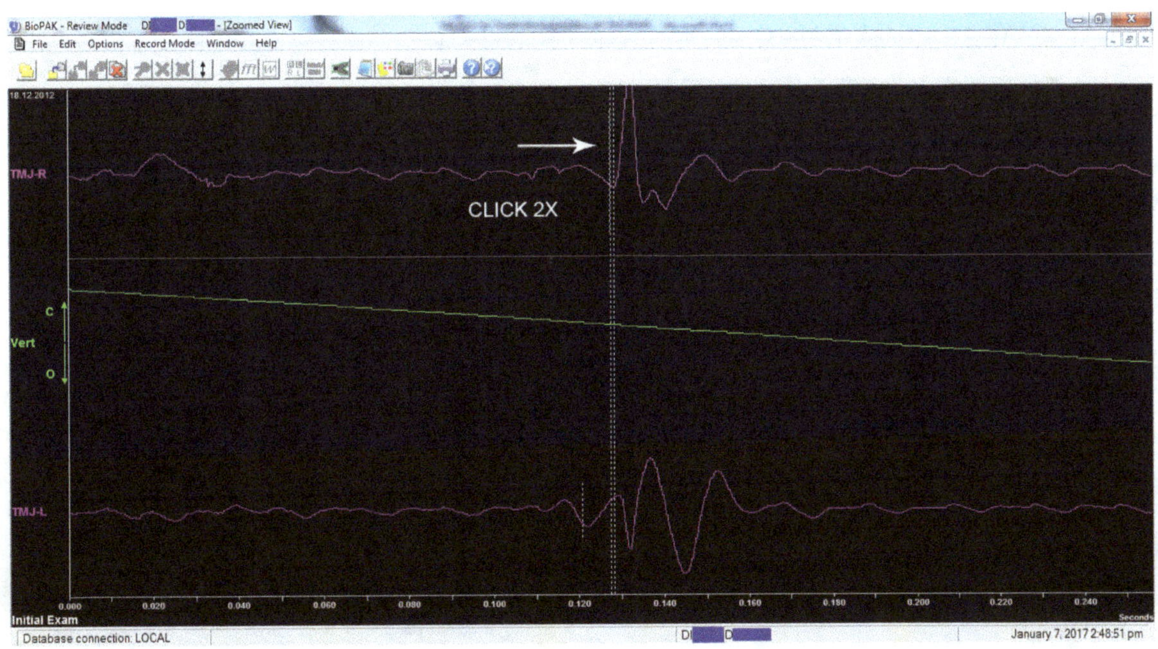

Figure 3. Click-type TMJ signal, TMJ signal (by) frequency of click sound followed by crepitation sound starts. Crepitation wave is shown on the left TMJ.

In **Figure 4**, max mouth opening is 45 mm, and a click sound is spotted around 30 mm. The click sound is located just before the eminencia.

Another important frequency type is crepitation: (**Figure 5**).

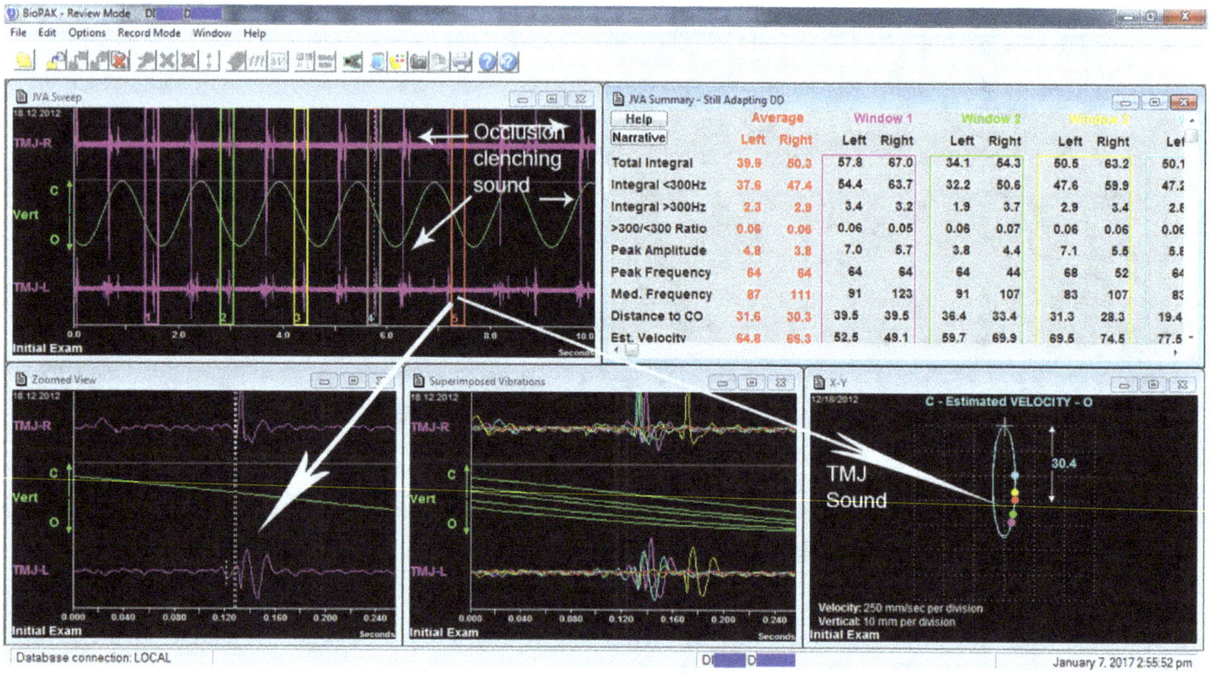

Figure 4. After six cycles of frequencies, average level of the click sound is around 30.4 mm of this patient who has a mouth opening of 45 mm. Location of the click sound is around the anterior part of the glenoid fossa. In this case, crepitation wave followed by the click sound must be considered an aggravation of the problem.

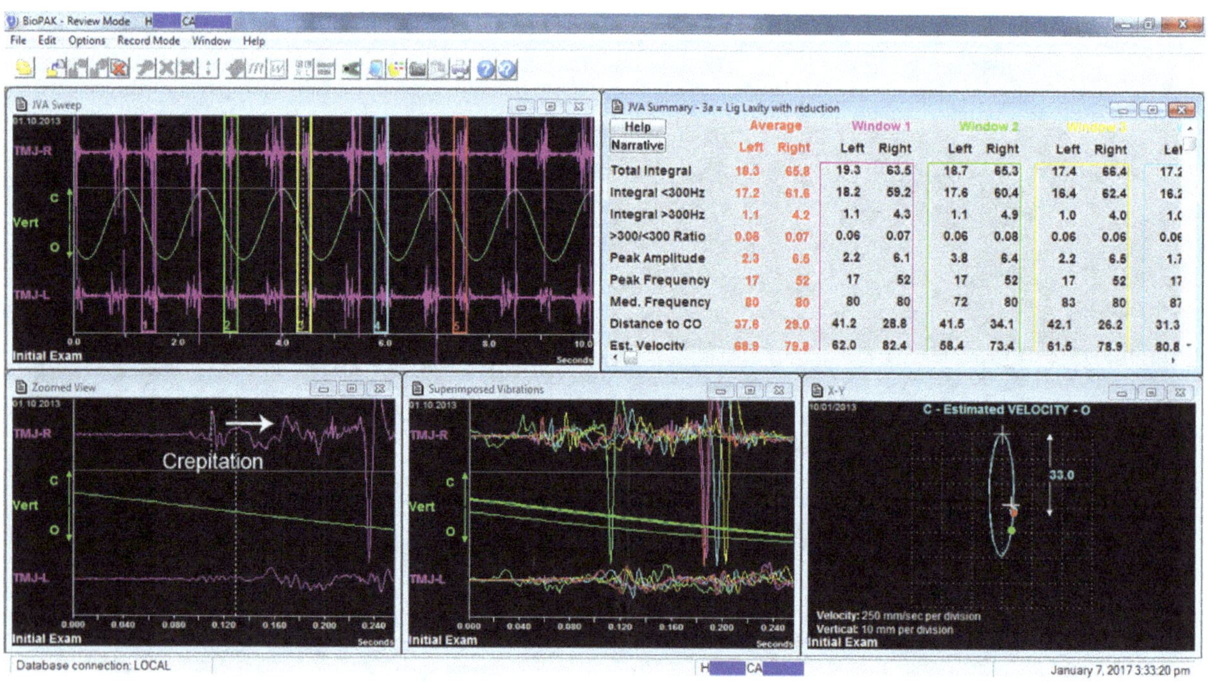

Figure 5. Crepitation wave is located just before a click frequency. It is located at the opening distance of 33.0 mm, where the patient's maximum opening distance is 49 mm.

2. How can we detect Temporomandibular joint sounds?

We can detect the temporomandibular joint sounds using frequency accelerators. An accelerator is neither a microphone nor an ultrasound; it is a typical sound receptor. In **Figure 6**, a typical sound accelerator is shown designed by Bioresearch Inc. (Milwaukee, USA).

The overall accuracy of clinical testing for TMD, using both auscultation and palpation, is 43% [53]. Vibration sound analysis procedure aids in diagnosis and thus can be helpful in treatment decisions (**Figure 7**).

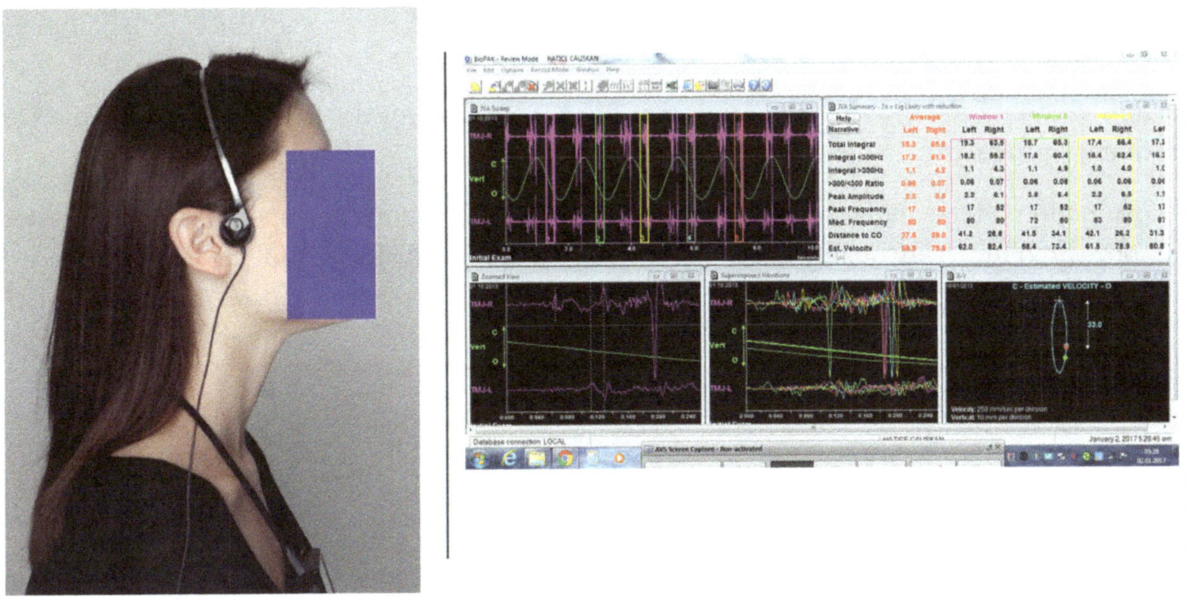

Figure 6. Research shows that experienced clinicians correctly diagnose the status of the TMJ less than 50% of the time. Inexperience can only increase this margin for error.

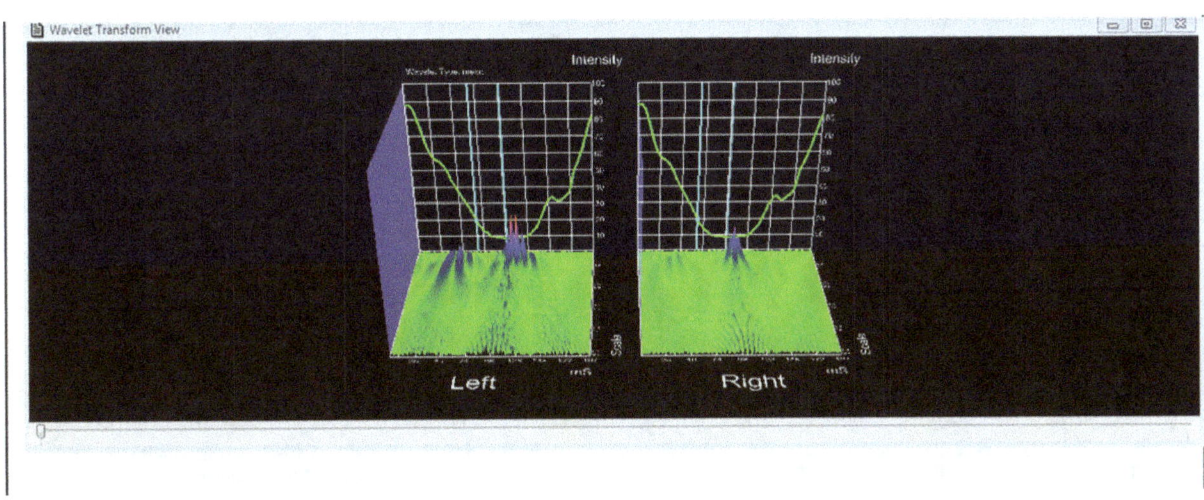

Figure 7. Wavelet transform viewer of a patient.

3. Clinical application of the joint vibration analysis

Condylar pathology is linked to articular surface degenerations [54]. Joint vibration analysis tests are helpful for the evaluation of the significance of joint sounds and can help us decide whether the condition is a progressive or degenerative one. Research shows that experienced clinicians correctly diagnose the status of the TMJ less than 50% of the time [53].

According to the Akin et al. [51],

1. Click: very short duration with high amplitude peaks,
2. Click with crepitation: a short duration click followed by multiple low amplitude peaks,
3. Hard crepitation: short duration, medium or high amplitude multiple peaks in low-frequency range,
4. Soft crepitation: long duration, low amplitude, multiple peaks that cover the whole frequency range.

The evaluation can be made according to the data mentioned above or a special table (suggested by Bioresearch Inc., Milwaukee, USA) is shown in **Figure 8**, which is useful in clinical practice.

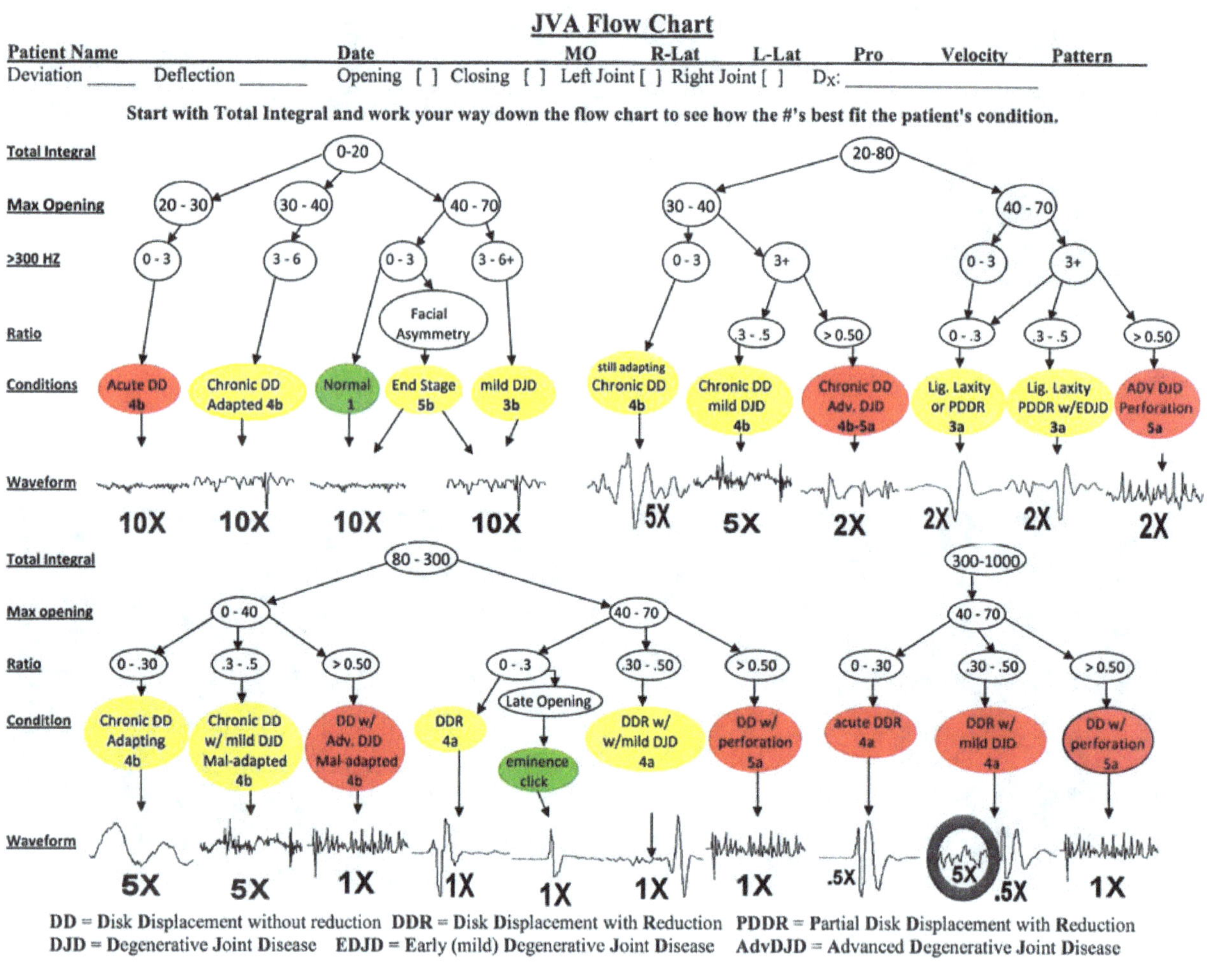

Figure 8. Clinical evaluation chart suggested by Bioresearch Inc., Milwaukee, USA.

The following evaluations can be made with the JAVA analysis data:

1. DD = Disk displacement without reduction,
2. DDR = Disk displacement with reduction,
3. PDDR = Partial disk displacement with reduction,
4. EDJD = Early degenerative joint disease,
5. ADvDJD = Advanced degenerative joint disease.

Subgroups of these main groups can also be reached with the help of additional clinical findings.

Evaluation study must start with a total integral value found in the chart. Second stage is the maximum mouth opening value of the patient, measured between the distance of anterior lower and upper teeth. Overbite distance must be added to the measured mouth opening value. Lateral deviation distance also must be measured, as it will be evaluated in the examination. To properly assess temporomandibular sounds, joint vibration sounds should be assessed with the patient's mouth opening and closing movements.

Joints are located in the glenoid fossa at the maximum occlusion position of mandible and during the opening of the mouth, translation movement is accompanied by rotation movement. Joint vibration analysis must be calibrated with other clinical findings, such as the

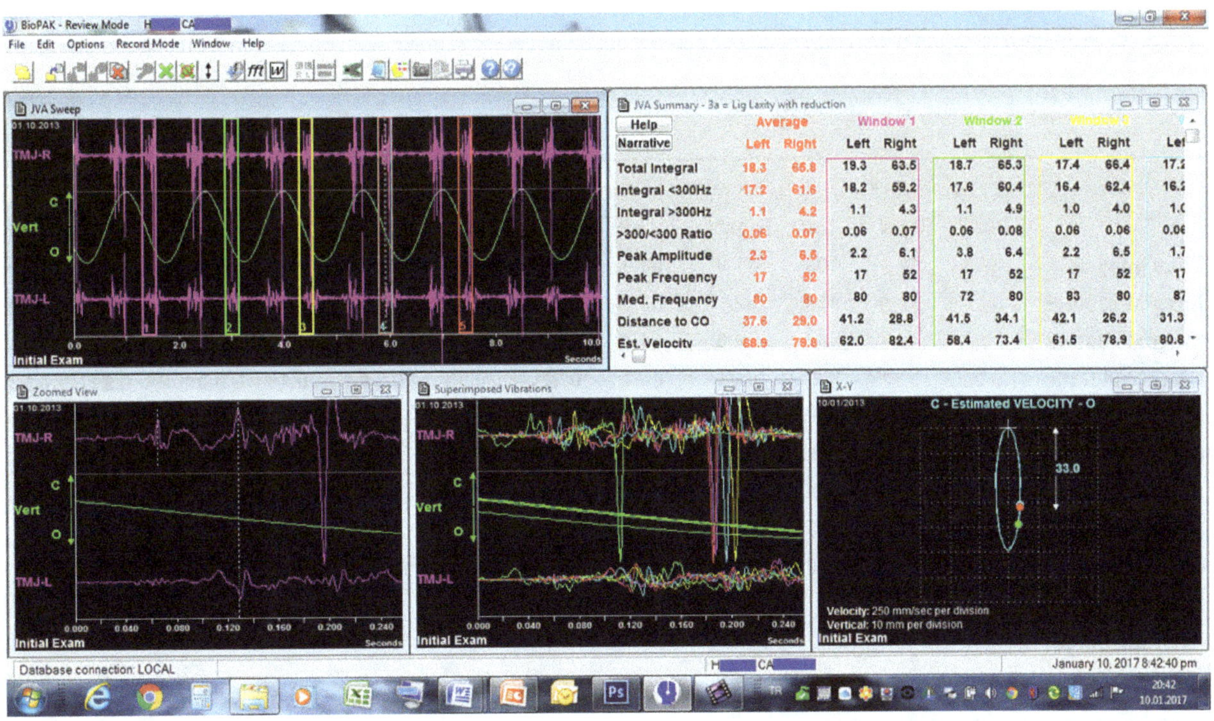

Figure 9. A patient's JVA record, total integral value has been found after capturing the frequencies of pathological sounds. According to the value of maximum opening distance, total integral value, integral >300 Hz and ratio of >300/<300 Hz value; in this case, "ligament laxity situation" may be considered.

maximum occlusion position. The patient is said to strike his teeth strongly, so at this moment a big and equal frequency in both side scan be spotted. This is the maximum occlusion position, and other intermediate frequencies indicate deterioration in the joint (**Figure 9**).

Case No.1.

Patient D.Y. 24 years old, Female *(History of the Patient, translation from her voice record).*

My name is D...Y.... Sounds coming from my joint, especially after lunches .... it started 4 months ago, a tooth extracted from here (*showing left side her face*), I think this is the reason of my problem ... I had it treated, because of a problem here..... Dr. xxxx made the extraction procedure, after the extraction great possible, I heard some cracking sounds. I cannot eat. When I eat something I hear a click sounds, I also have headaches.

"Clinician's Question: When you have your headache?"

Around afternoons, but not too strong, I mean I hear only click sound. It comes from my left side, from my left joint; tooth extraction was made on that side. I have no more pain, only there is click sound *"**click** (click sound)"*. Oh! I want to add something more, I am in orthodontic treatment since the last year.

The patient's JVA record results as follows (**Figures 10** and **11**):

We must consider the **Left Joint** as problem. If we apply the numerical data to JVA flow chart as follows:

	Average		Window 1		Window 2		Window 3		Window 4		Window 5	
	Left	Right	Left	Right	Left	Right	Left	Right	Left	Right	Left	Right
Total Integral	47.3	39.8	50.6	41.9	63.9	54.9	49.2	33.4	35.7	26.2	33.4	32.2
Integral <300Hz	39.4	31.5	42.2	32.0	52.8	43.0	41.3	25.0	30.2	20.1	27.7	26.2
Integral >300Hz	7.8	8.4	8.3	9.9	11.1	11.9	8.0	8.4	5.5	6.1	5.7	6.1
>300/<300 Ratio	0.20	0.27	0.20	0.31	0.21	0.28	0.19	0.34	0.18	0.30	0.21	0.23
Peak Amplitude	2.52	4.04	2.81	4.61	3.44	5.52	2.93	3.53	1.98	3.21	1.94	3.30
Peak Frequency	100	56	124	56	85	56	85	51	100	51	95	56
Med. Frequency	134	100	139	95	139	100	139	114	134	109	134	95
Distance to CO	22.2	22.2	37.0	37.0	26.2	26.2	7.2	7.2	1.0	1.0	38.9	38.9
Est. Velocity	39.0	40.3	36.0	37.9	77.2	80.3	60.9	63.7	-25.6	-25.6	10.0	10.0
Max. Opening	39											
Lat. Deflection	0											
Initial Exam 2												
JVA Summary - Still Adapting Chronic DD / 4b												

Figure 10. The patient's JVA data show that the total integral value of the left joint is bigger than the right joint. This value is 47.3 and indicates a problem. Integral>300 Hz value is 7.8 and ratio value is 0.20.

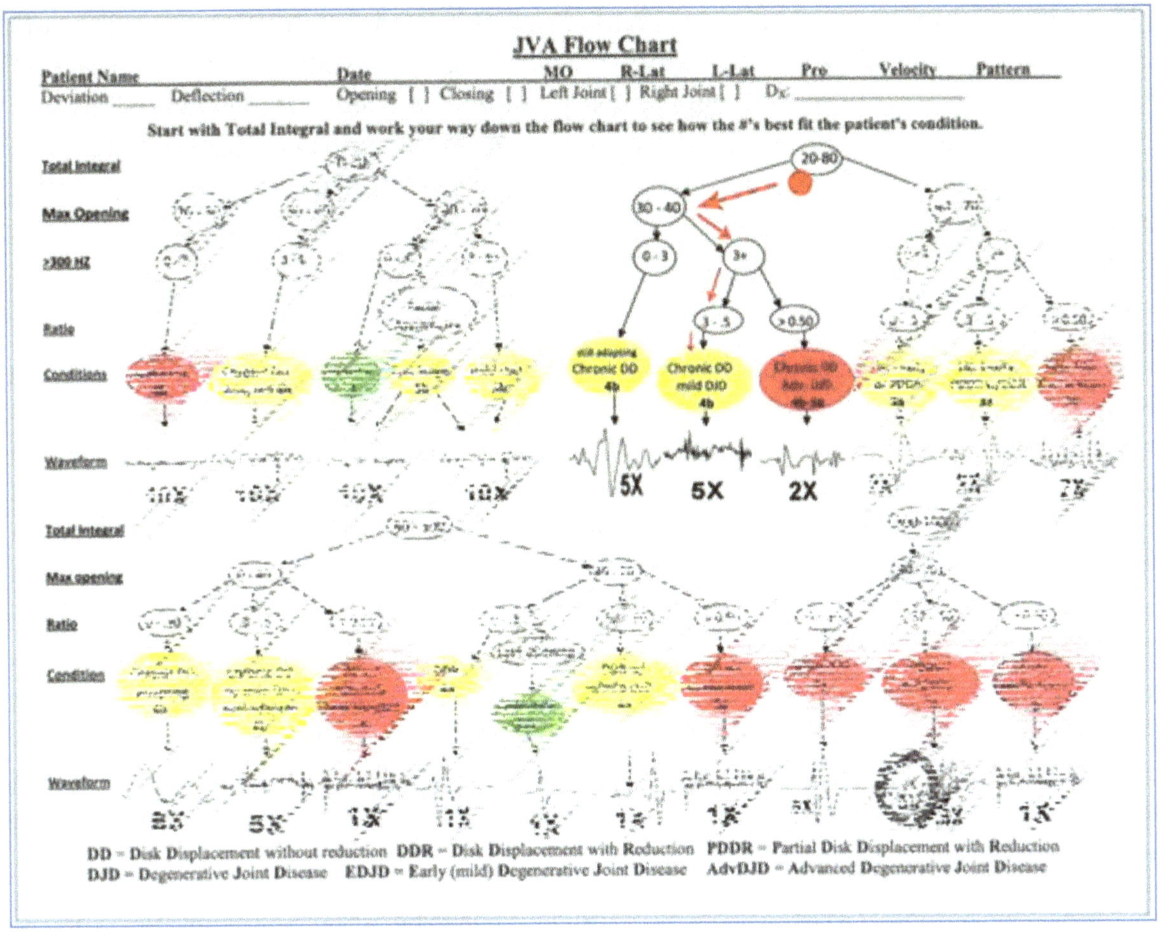

Figure 11. Total integral value is 47.3 (see **Figure 10**), and this value places between the range of 20 and 80. Second step maximum opening mouth is 39 mm, and this value is between the range of 30 and 40. Third step is "integral >300 Hz" value which is 7.8, and it is located in the 3+ area. Finally, we look the value of "ratio" which is 0.20 of this patient, and it is located in the range of 3–5. As a result, "Chronic disk displacement or mild degenerative joint disease (Piper's 4b)" must be considered for this patient. Other clinical examination results (extra-oral examination, radiographic findings, etc.) must be combined with the result of JVA.

4. JT mastication analysis

Chronic temporomandibular disorder (TMD) patients, specifically those with severe symptomatology, shows a reorganized activity, mainly resulting in worsening functional performances [55]. Mastication is one of the most important vital functions of human being. Occlusal disorders can cause people to swallow food without chewing enough. Shimshak and DeFuria showed that TMD patients have, on average, 112% more digestive complaints (in terms of the cost of medical treatment) than a comparable normal group [56]. High-level masticatory performance is the main purpose of dental restorative studies. Chewing pattern is linked to occlusal relationship, it may vary with the occlusal model [57, 58]. Studies have focused on two main types of motions:

- physiologic (functional) movements which occur during chewing
- nonphysiologic movements such as maximal opening/closing or lateral excursions.

Nonphysiologic movements can be difficult to reproduce (due to conscious actions of the patient) and are questionable indicators of the functional state of the stomatognathic system. During mastication, the angle of the mandible as it approaches occlusion is quite different from that occurring with lateral excursions from centric occlusion. Interferences identified in lateral excursions may or may not represent functional interferences during mastication. For these reasons, chewing motions (which are subconscious, physiologic, and reproducible) are considered to be the most applicable for a clinical classification of TMD [59].

The fundamental quantity in mastication analysis is the chewing cycle, representing the motion of the mandible from occlusion to open and from open back to occlusion. The turning point (*TP*) is defined to be the most open position of the mandible in the middle of a chewing cycle. It averages about 2 mm laterally toward the working (chewing) side and normally 16 mm open from centric occlusion. The terminal chewing position (*TCP*) is defined as the most closed position of the mandible as it approaches occlusion during mastication. There may be a difference between TCP and maximum intercuspal position of between 0 and 5 mm, default value being 0.3 mm. This number determines the vertical thresholds of each chewing cycle in relation to the *TCP* of each cycle. For example, a value of 2 will cause the start of opening and ending of closing of a given cycle to be positioned a distance of 2 mm below the TCP. The value can range from 0.0 to 5.0 mm (default is 0.3). Swallowing occurs after every 5–10 chewings approximately. Mandible is in maximum intercuspal position during swallowing.

There are great differences between orthodontically Class I normal occlusion type and Class II malocclusion or Class III malocclusion chewing patterns. When we look at the breakdown of treatments, we can see many changes in the magnitude of chewing. The analysis of the patterns of chewing in the onset of treatment and later in the course of treatment will provide us concrete information on the success of the treatment [59–61]. Nowadays, though not routinely used, especially the measurement of chewing performance is important in terms of trying to measure the success of the treatment by comparing the values before and after treatment.

A classic pattern of chewing is basically examined in three parts [62, 63] (**Figure 12**):

1. Opening phase,
2. Closing phase, and
3. Occlusal phase.

There are various methods and tools for the examination of masticatory movements [34, 48, 64]. These methods can be grouped under three main headings [65]:

1. Masticatory movement analysis,
2. Masticatory muscles analysis,
3. Analysis of mastication product (analysis of the food).

However, chewing movements may also be useful in investigating temporomandibular disorders [66]. Masticatory analysis history is based on the beginning time of modern dentistry. In early studies, a video recorder has been used for taking serial pictures of chewing pattern. A rounded white paper part was attached to the patient's chin, and serial pictures were taken from front of the face of the patient. In this system, a magnet attached onto the lower anterior teeth (**Figure 13**) and using a software, record video movie of movements of the magnet together with the mandible (**Figure 14**).

To record chewing patterns, a small magnet is placed on the vestibular side of the lower anterior teeth using a sticky wax (**Figure 13**). A headgear containing bilateral electromagnetic

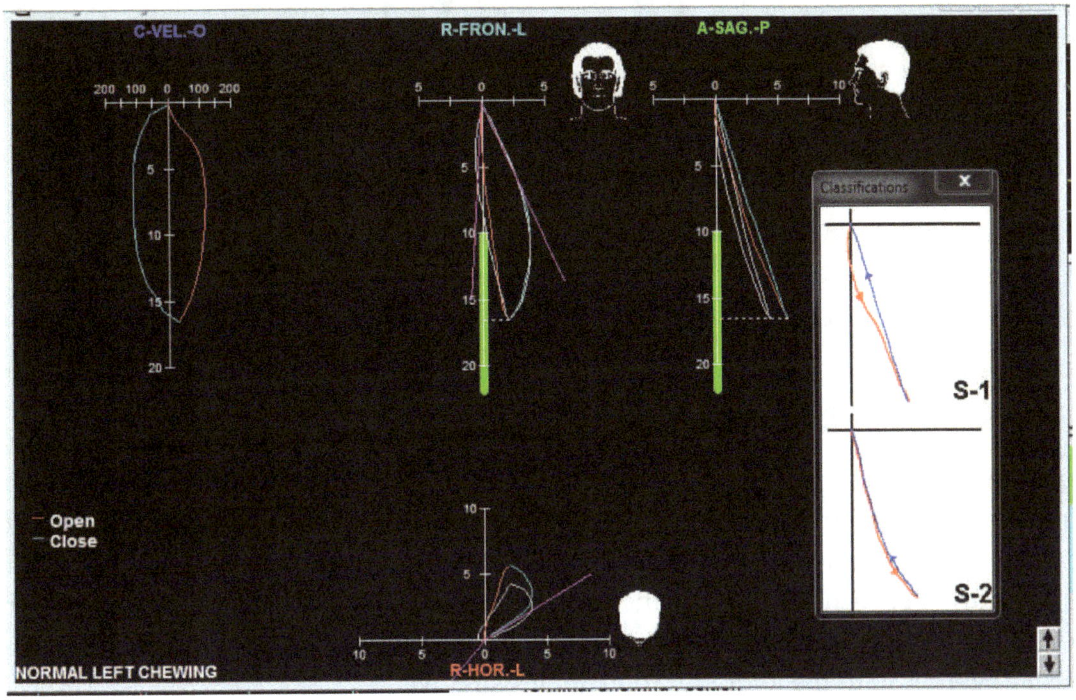

Figure 12. A chewing pattern consists of three different phases: Opening(red), closing (blue) and occlusal phase (0 point in the diagram). From the opening phase to the closing phase, basically there are three parts in one cycle of mastication. Returning from opening phase is called a "turning point."

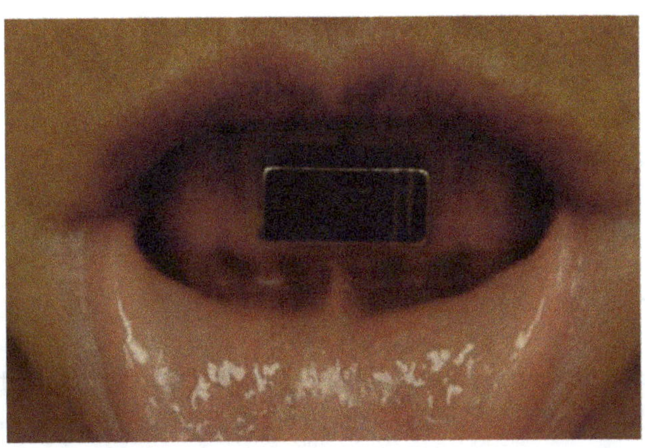

Figure 13. Placing of magnet.

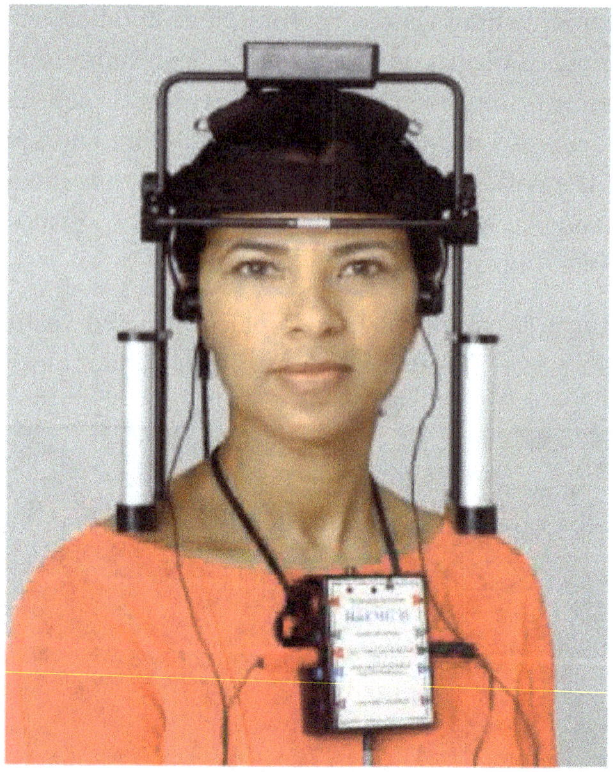

Figure 14. Head parts of Bio-JT (Bioresearch Inc., USA).

controller mechanism senses "xyz" position of the magnet within an accuracy of 0.1 mm. After aligning headgear, using its screw movements of the magnet is recorded (**Figure 14**). Besides the analysis of mastication, this gear can be used to measure and record the range of motions of the jaw during speech, distance of the freeway space (with extreme accuracy), velocity and bite registrations. We can see exact positions of the mandible if we use this equipment simultaneously together with the joint vibration analysis (JVA).

The basic parameters of mastication analysis are given as follows:

5. Starting cycle

This is the first chewing cycle to display and analyze. The cycles before the designated starting cycle are neglected. Starting cycle is the default cycle. The first few cycles may be disregarded as they are more often inconsistent.

5.1. Maximum number of cycles to analyze

The maximum number of chewing cycles are averaged to calculate the average CP. It also determines how many cycles will be taken into account in the sweep and segmented XY views. Maximum number of cycles are variable between 10 and 30 (default value of number of cycles is 15).

5.2. Occlusal threshold (OT)

This number determines the vertical thresholds of each chewing cycle in relation to the *TCP* of each cycle. Occlusal threshold is the start and the end point of a cycle. For example, a value of 1.0 will cause the start of opening and end of closing of a given cycle to be positioned a distance of 1.0 mm below the TCP. The value can range from 0.0 to 5.0 mm. (default is 0.3 mm).

5.3. Standard deviation limit

The number of standard deviations is used as a limit when validating cycles. If a given cycle differs from the average of all cycles by more than this amount, it is marked as deviated and not correct. The value can range from 1.0 to 3.0 mm (default is 2.0).

5.4. What can be read from masticatory analysis?

There is a sample screen (the record has been taken from the sample record of User Manual of Bioresearch Inc., USA) [94] in **Figure 15**:

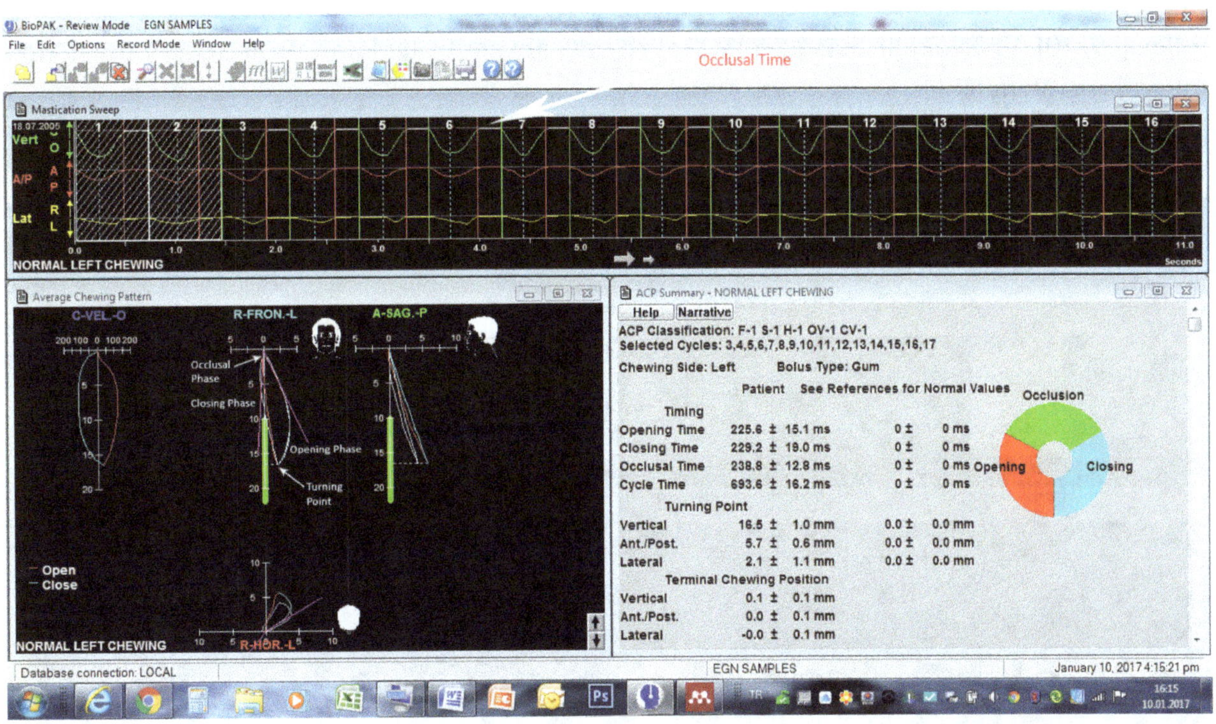

Figure 15. Mastication narrative: The patient chewed a bolus(gum) on the left side, and 15 chewing cycles were used to average the chewing pattern. The average opening time was consistently short at 225 ± 16 ms. The average closing time was consistently short at 232 ± 20 ms. The average occlusal time was consistently short at 240 ± 13 ms. The average cycle time was consistently short at 697 ± 17 ms. The average vertical turning point consistently occurred at 16.5 ± 1.0 mm from centric occlusion. The average anteroposterior turning point consistently occurred at 5.7 ± 0.6 mm from centric occlusion. The average lateral turning point consistently occurred at 2.1 ± 1.1 mm from centric occlusion. The average maximum lateral width of the chewing cycles was consistent at 4.2 ± 0.6 mm.

The following record is taken from a patient using full denture in the TMD Clinic of Istanbul Aydin University Dentistry Faculty (**Figure 16**):

In the research, studies of masticatory movements have been focused on following the two main types of motions:

- physiologic (functional) movements which occur during chewing
- nonphysiologic movements such as maximal opening/closing or maximum lateral excursions-border movements.

Average physiologic pattern of masticatory movements (**Figures 15** and **16**) is produced by a healthy stomathognathic system. It is result of a reflex mechanism and controlled by mechanoreseptors and proprioceptors located in periodontal ligaments [67]. Moreover, premature contact in masticatory occlusion may stimulate neural mechanisms in masticatory system (**Figure 17**).

The production of nonphysiologic movements otherwise is very difficult. There is also a quite difference between approaching angle of mandible in mastication and the angle of lateral excursion to the maximum intercuspal position. For these reasons, subconscious, physiologic and reflex chewing motions are considered to be the most applicable for a clinical classification of TMD. Mastication is a physiologic movement, but grinding of an empty mouth is a parafunctional movement. Masticatory movements start as a conscious movement and continue as reflex [69, 70]. Physiologic masticatory movements are controlled and protected by the neuromuscular system [67].

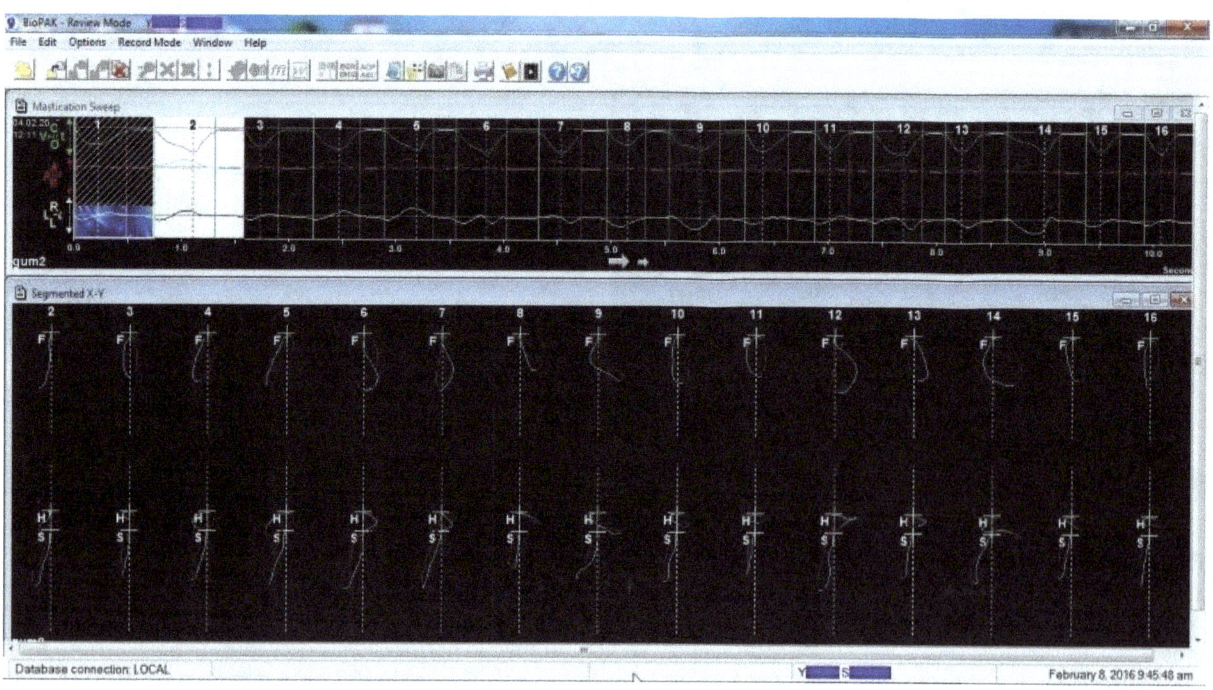

Figure 16. Chewing patterns of a CAD-CAM full denture patient.

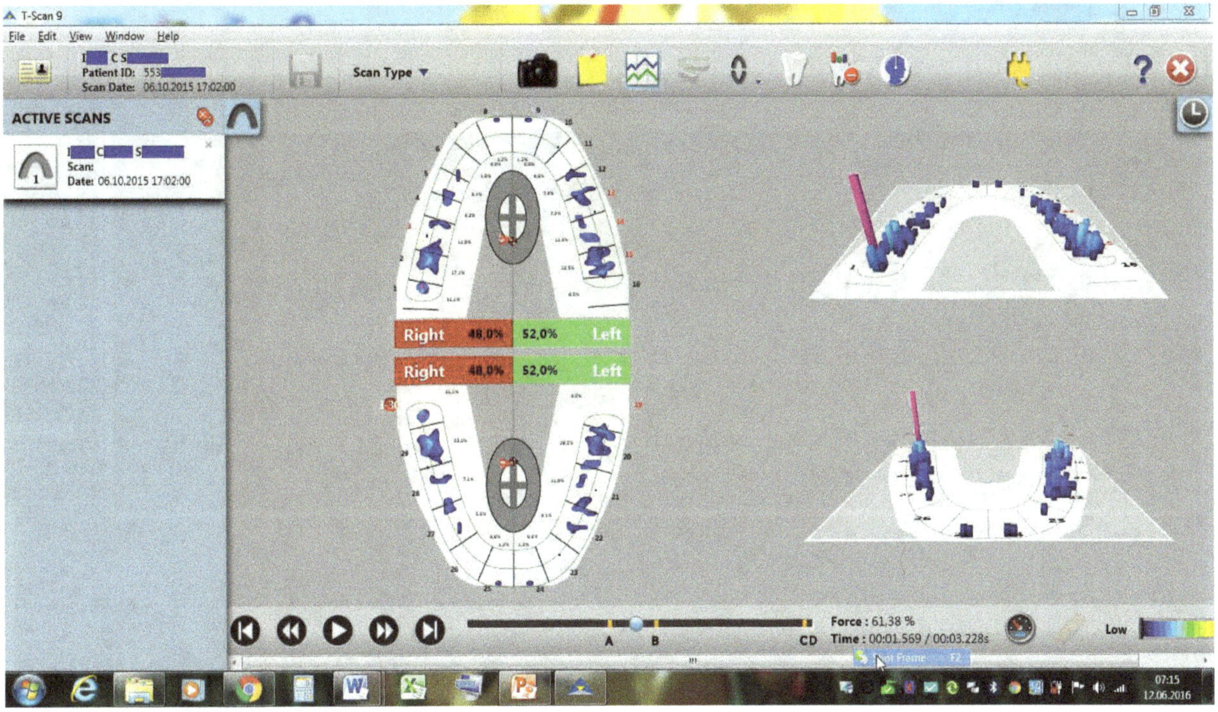

Figure 17. Discrepancy in masticatory occlusion is a trigger mechanism for the muscle pain dysfunction syndrome. Premature contacts may stimulate neural mechanism in masticatory MPD syndrome will be developed if premature contacts are not removed from the occlusion. We use also T-scan occlusal analysis system to find and remove the premature contacts from masticatory occlusion [68].

Total quantity in mastication analysis is the chewing cycle, representing the motion of the mandible from occlusion to open and from open, back to maximum masticatory occlusion. The turning point (TP) is defined to be the masticatory open position of the mandible in the middle of a chewing cycle. It averages about 2 mm laterally toward the working (chewing) side and nominally 16 mm open from centric occlusion. The terminal chewing position (TCP) is defined as the most closed position of the mandible as it approaches occlusion during mastication (masticatory occlusion).

Chewing rhythm is closely related to the patients' average chewing pattern (ACP). Average values of parts of chewing pattern are as follows:

1. Opening time is around 250 ms (± 50 ms), (one-third of total chewing cycle approx.)
2. Closing time is around 220 ms (± 50 ms), (one-third of total chewing cycle approx.)
3. Occlusion time is around 200 ms (± 50 ms), (one-third of total chewing cycle approx.)

We must consider a problem regarding to the joints if cycle time, opening, closing and occlusal time have an unusually longer or shorter value than normal.

Masticatory movements end in an occlusal phase. In an occlusal movement, lower teeth glide on upper teeth's occlusal surface and stop at top maximum contact position of masticatory movement. This is not a maximum force position because maximum force position is not a functional situation but a conscious action. Maximum top position of masticatory movement can also be named as "reverse turning point" (RTP) of masticatory movement. Upper and

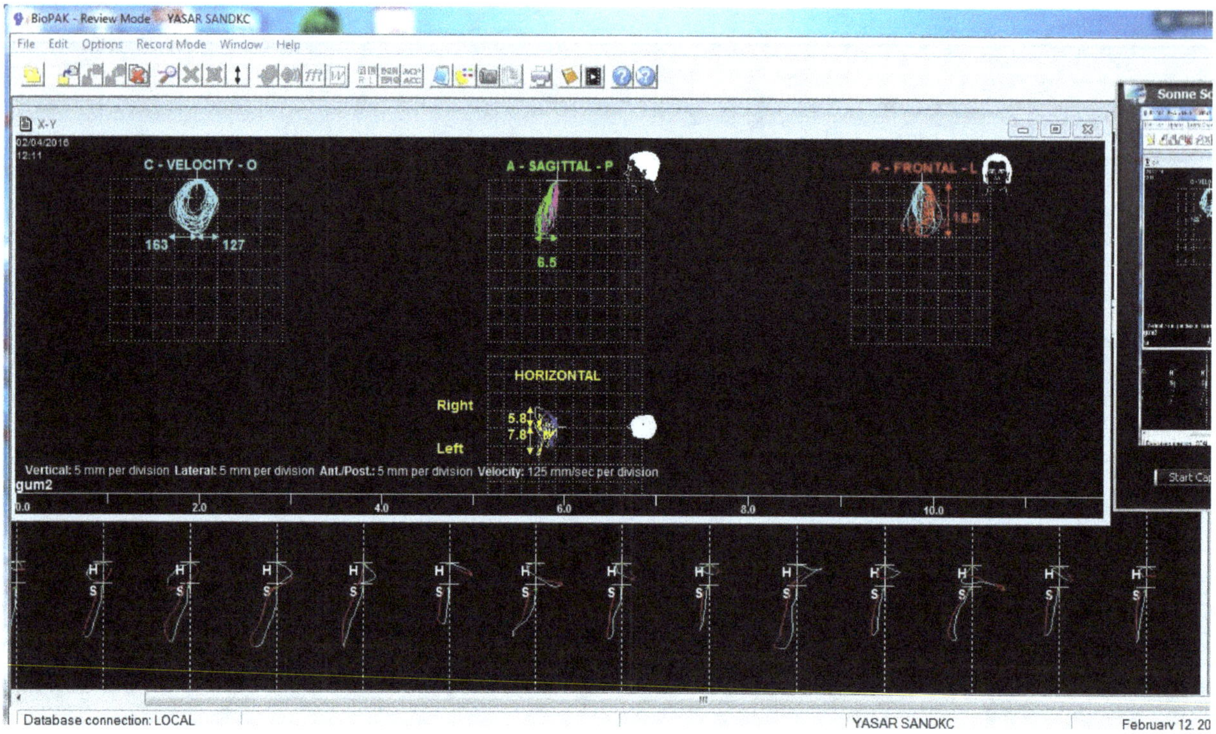

Figure 18. Opening phase of mastication starts from reverse turning point.

lower teeth are contacted slightly, or not any contact, and opening phase of mastication starts from this point. RTP point is illustrated in **Figure 18**:

Reverse turning position is not a harmful situation. Furthermore, the CNS reflex (Jaw Jerk Reflex) will form an early RTP point and will escape from excessive contact. This point is variable according to the harmonic masticatory movements of mandible. Normally, this

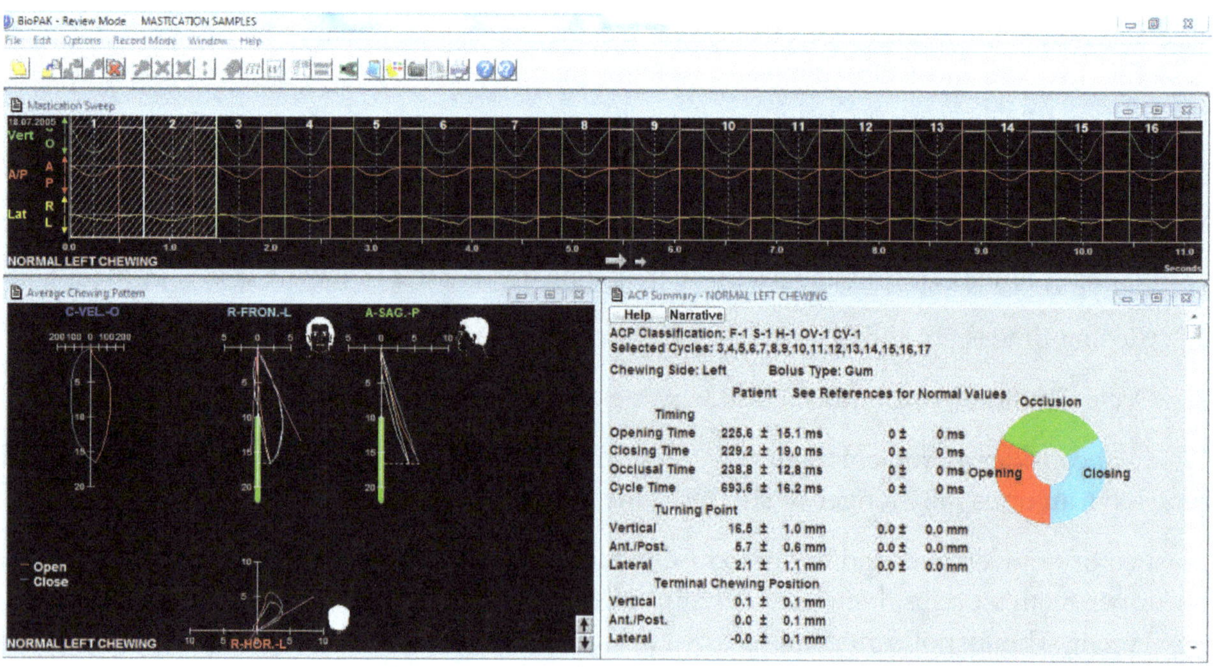

Figure 19. The chewing record formed by RTP, and the pattern of the chewing movement was also affected.

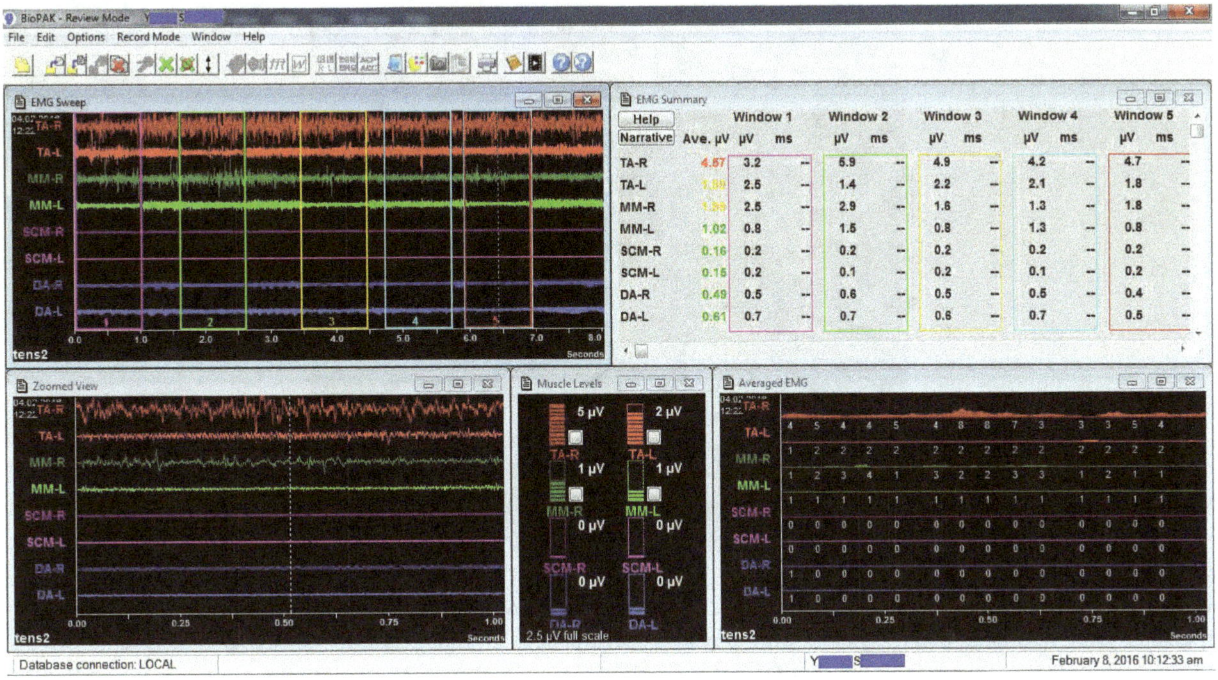

Figure 20. EMG record of a patient with RTP; right temporal and masseter muscles have hyper-activities. Right side of the joint will be under overload. At the beginning, this situation may not be harmful, though in time the condition may lead to impairment of the right-side condyle.

neuromuscular behavior will protect the teeth and will not cause a problem in the joints. But if it lasts for a long time, the working side condenses will be under constant overpressure, which will cause the working joint to eventually break down. The early occurrence of the RTP point should be seen as an adverse symptom that should be corrected clinically for joints. EMG records (**Figures 20**) of unbalanced muscle force application with the chewing record (**Figure 19**) of a person in this situation can be seen below:

6. Computerized occlusal analysis

"To look at the occlusion and to see the occlusion."

Occlusion analysis is one of the most complicated and sophisticated areas of dentistry. According to Prof. Dr. Senih Calikkocaoglu[*] "Occlusion is a phenomenon related with bones, teeth, muscles and neurons." It has four main key points:

1. Mandibular movements: controlled by joints, muscles and neural receptors,
2. Upper and lower teeth: end point of the movement - like a stopper, System likes a nut-crucker (**Figure 21**).
3. Masticatory muscles: apply force in a harmonized manner,
4. Neural system: controls the magnitude, duration and direction of forces.

[*]Prof. Dr. Senih Calıkkocaoglu, Retired from Dentistry Faculty of Istanbul University, died in the year of 2016.

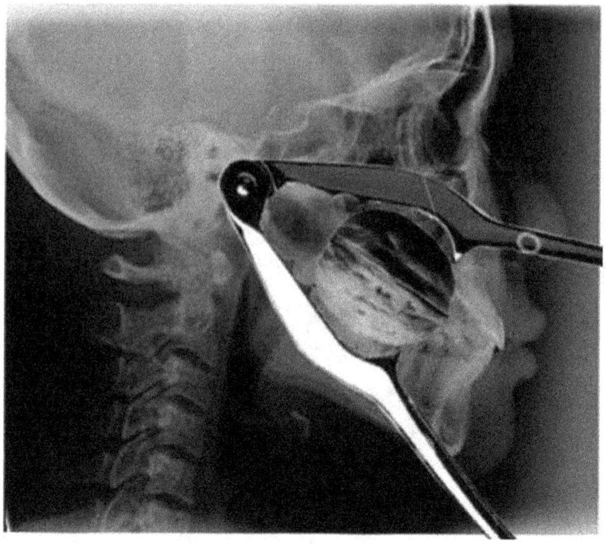

Figure 21. The system is like a second class leverage system and is similar to a nuts breaker. Masticatory muscles apply the force in a harmonic manner, joints bear forces which applied by muscles and the neural system controls the magnitude, duration, direction and peak time of that forces.

There are many dental disturbances to be linked to the occlusion: bruxism, attrition, erosion, abfraction, muscle pain dysfunction syndrome, TMJ problems, and so on, are typical examples [5, 13, 24, 61, 71–76]. Whether these disorders are related to occlusal discrepancies is the subject of occlusal analysis.

Occlusion analysis is simply the analysis of all contact positions based on the time vector during closing and departing of upper and lower teeth. Occlusal analysis gives to the clinician teeth position, relative force and time data. Additionally, occlusion analysis gives the sequential time and relative force data of occlusion. Occlusal analysis data present potential to make chance of commentary on pathological reasons of stomatognathic system. Occlusal papers and/or another occlusal indicators do not have that kind of ability.

The most disturbing situation about occlusion in dentistry is premature contact. As a dentist, we make restorations, bridges, crowns, orthodontic treatment, tooth extraction, and so on, and we may change the occlusion. In proprioceptive mechanism, premature contacts detected by mechanoreceptors in the periodontal ligaments may be harmful for teeth and other structures of stomatognathic system. Normally, temporomandibular joints are not affected immediately by this irregularity. During movements of the mandible, the inputs to muscle spindles and Golgi tendon organs change. But their outputs are differently related to their respective inputs [77]. The reflex control of the mandible is of vital importance for the normal masticatory functioning of humans. Excitatory jaw reflexes are responsible for the rapid reaction to external stimuli to the masticatory muscles [67], while inhibitory jaw reflexes protect the system when sudden loads are applied to the muscles. The fine coordination of the mandibular function is the result of the balanced activation of these reflexes together with the activity of the masticatory muscles, the temporomandibular joints and the associated tissues [78]. *Premature contacts are one of the most prominent jaw jerk reflex triggers [68].* The jaw jerk reflex is another protection control mechanism of the stomathognathic system, but it has slightly more rapid and more reflex characteristics than the RTP mechanism of the masticatory movements. After the first reaction, the Jaw Jerk Reflex turns to a RTP mechanism [79]. As we mentioned in the Mastication Analysis section of this chapter, if the reasons for the jaw jerk reflex persists for a long time, the working side condenses will be under constant overload and will cause the working joint to break down.

"Best Occlusion Analysis starts from Temporomandibular Joints" Peter Dawson [75, 80].

For many years, scientists created many theories on dental occlusion and its links to the occlusal problems and temporomandibular pathology. Occlusal theories have been focused on two principal matters:

1. Analysis of occlusion using simulation tools and articulators.
2. Working on the chairside, the computerized occlusal analysis technique.

There are many advantages in the second method. In-vitro occlusion analysis techniques are extremely difficult and long procedures. The main advantage of the first method is that it does not contain any risks, and dentist can work under very controlled conditions. But there are a lot of question on the details of the procedures; traditionally, more than one visit is required to complete analyzing and treatment. Working on stomatognathic system needs to be considered together with the neuromuscular mechanism. Articulators may be most useful tools for the production of dental restorations, but they cannot simulate the neuromuscular mechanism [81].

Computerized occlusal analysis systems are the fastest and safest way to check the dental occlusion. If not intervened, all occlusal contacts can be controlled in detail and sequentially together with relative force info. Analysis of the occlusion can be performed under maximum physiological conditions. Each intervention will be perceived by the neuromuscular mechanism, and the movement will not be a physiological function. Computerized occlusal analysis systems give us control of extreme physiologic occlusion [35, 82–86]. Actually, occlusal papers and similar indicators (wax, powder, shimstock, foil, etc.), which using intraoral indicators, are also not proper materials for occlusal diagnostics [87].

Because contact "hold" resistance levels are subjective. Therefore, it is a difficult guiding factor to utilize when selecting contacts to adjust the demonstrated variable forces are within occlusal contacts. Because shim stock foil does not mark the selected teeth, the articulating paper markings are the primary guide for the operator when selecting which contact(s) require adjustment.

It has been advocated in textbooks on occlusion [2, 3, 5–7] that mark area is a representative of the load contained within the mark. Legends to photographs depicting occlusal adjustment technique end results and paper mark appearance describe that large and dark marks indicate heavy load, and that smaller and light marks indicate lesser loads [5–7]. Additionally, the presence of many similar sized marks spread around the contacting arches is purported to indicate equal occlusal contact intensity, evenness, and simultaneity [1, 3].

Though occlusal indicators show prints of the end of the occlusion, they cannot provide important information such as which tooth tubercle is first in occlusion, which one is second or which one is last and the force differences between these points (**Figures 22**).

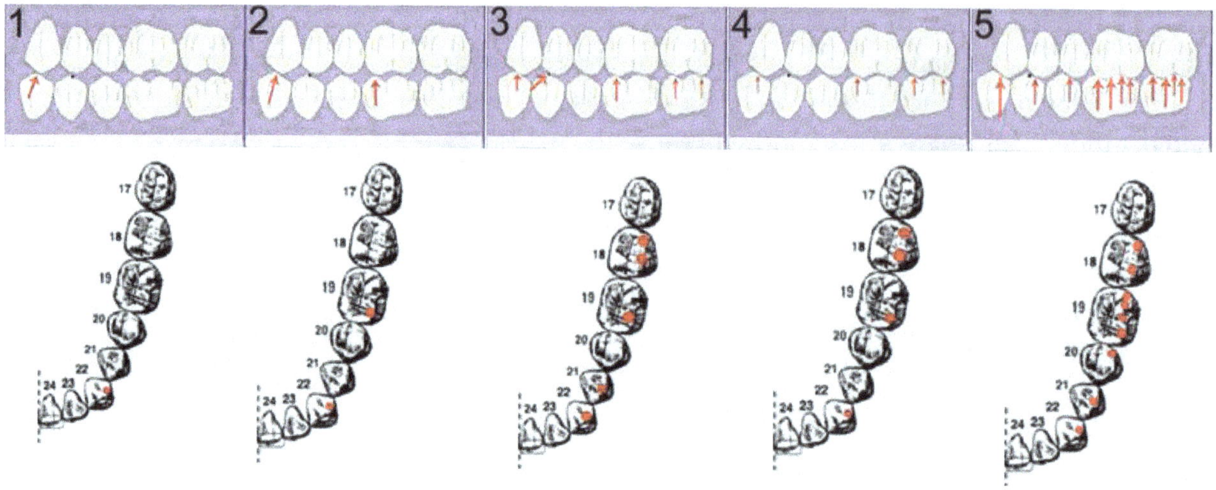

Figure 22. Occlusal indicators such as occlusion paper may first show contacts first followed by consecutive contacts, but we can only see the last picture and not the events that occurred before [88]. Which is first, second and last? Occlusal paper is like a stamp that shows the static photo of a last step.

Owing to the computer technologies developed in recent years, we now have the chance to examine the intraoral occlusion as detailed as possible.

Computerized occlusion is the system that can be best examined today without disrupting the neuromuscular mechanism of the occlusion [20, 23, 38, 39, 83]. In this method, dynamic information of all occlusal contacts that occur when the patient closes and opens mouth is recorded digitally. T-Scan computerized occlusal analysis system (COAS) is one of the most advanced devices in the market today (Tekscan Inc., Boston, USA.) It is a unique system that allows the occlusion to be recorded from the beginning to the end.

COAS basically consists of three main parts as follows:

1. Sensor,
2. Hardware: handle and computer,
3. Software.

The sensor used in the system is ultra-fine plastic with a thickness of 0.1 mm (0.004 inch). This thin **Figure 23** sensor does not change the neuromuscular pattern that defines the occlusion of the patient. When the patient bites the sensor, the mandibular functional movement is not changed. The occlusion phenomenon occurs physiologically and with the neuromuscular orientation of the patient at that time. Thus, the clinician can accurately see the functional occlusion at that time. **Figure 24** shows the sensor used in the T-Scan computerized occlusal analysis system.

Case No.2.

Patient S.S. Age: 68, Male.

The patient with headache around anterior temporal area for approximately 7 years, occurring usually on mornings due to clenching of his teeth. There was a click sound on left TMJ.

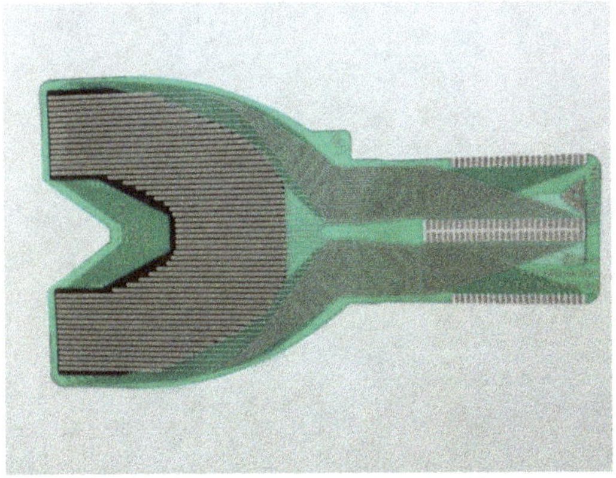

Figure 23. The T-scan sensor is an ultra-thin (0.004 inch, 0.1 mm), flexible printed circuit that detects your patient's occlusal forces. These sensors are made up of 1370 active pressure sensing locations for the large sensor (#2002 for the Novus Handpiece, and #2001 for the Evolution Handle), and 1122 pressure sensing locations for the small sensor (#2502 for the Novus Handpiece, and #2501 for the Evolution Handle). These sensing locations are referred to as "sensing elements" or "sensels." the "sensels" are arranged in rows and columns on the sensor. Each sensel can be seen as an individual square on the computer screen by selecting the 2D display mode (text is from company user manual, Teksan Inc. USA) [95] (**Figures 24** and **25**).

Radiographic (**Figure 25**) and intraoral examination: A remarkable abfraction detected and restored by fillings 3–4 times but the fillings dropped every time.

When the occlusal analysis was performed, disclussion time was found to be 0.48 s (**Figure 26**). Premature contacts identified after the evaluation of the occlusion. The premature contacts are eliminated using a fine diamond bur, and the disclussion time was reduced to 0.23 s. (**Figure 27**).

After equilibration of occlusion, composite restorations were performed on teeth with abfraction. For the next month, the patient was given another follow-up appointment. When he arrives a month later for his follow-up appointment; filling restorations are still standing. There was no headache, and the click sound was gone.

T-Scan records of before and after the occlusal stabilization of the patient are given as follows:

In the computerized occlusal analysis software, the graphic arc dimensions are automatically adjusted according to the size of the anterior teeth in routine clinical trials. (**Figure 28**).

However, if you need an in detail work and you need to see the occlusion in maximum precision you can choose to work with STL (**ST**ereo**L**ithography) data. The great advantage of this method is that the tooth copies can be loaded automatically and individually. All teeth sizes are the same with the real dimensions. In this technique, upper and lower stone models are digitally scanned with an STL data ability scanner, and output data in the STL format are uploaded on the computer. Now, the clinician is able to analyze the occlusion in the real dimensions and locate the possible premature contacts precisely. (**Figure 29**).

Computerized occlusal analysis is currently the most powerful method of TMD clinics for the treatment of patients with muscle pain dysfunction syndrome [23, 68, 89, 90]. Especially with JAVA, it is now frequently used in clinical routine. Computerized occlusal analysis allows us to perform the following treatments [91]:

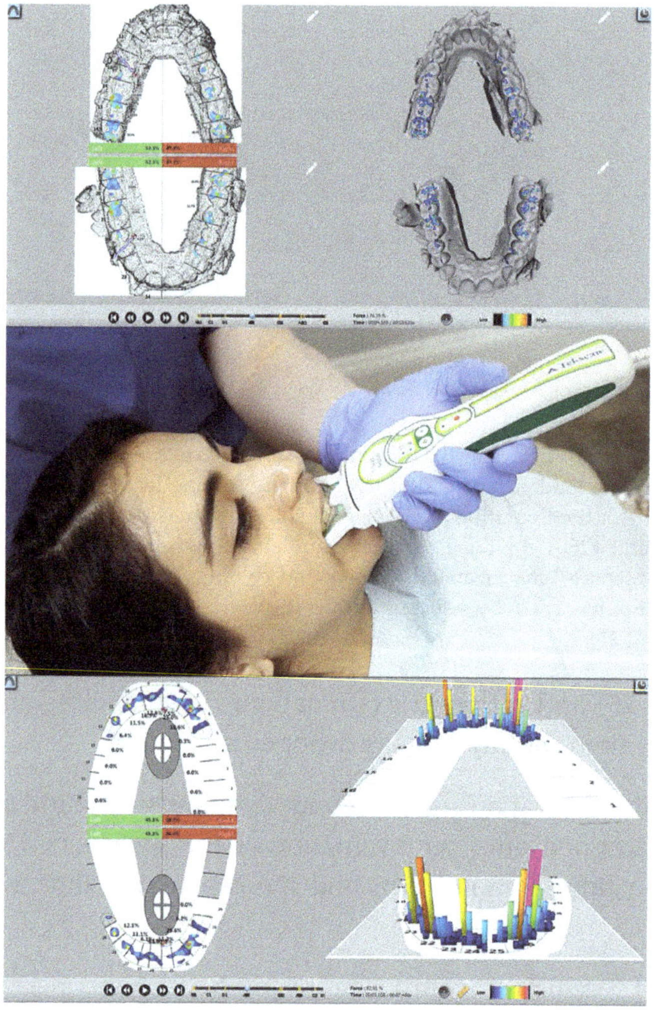

Figure 24. Application of computerized occlusal analysis system. In this case, patient's stone model was scanned and model's stl (STereoLithography) data were imported to the T-scan software. The occlusion analysis was performed on the real model's 3D image.

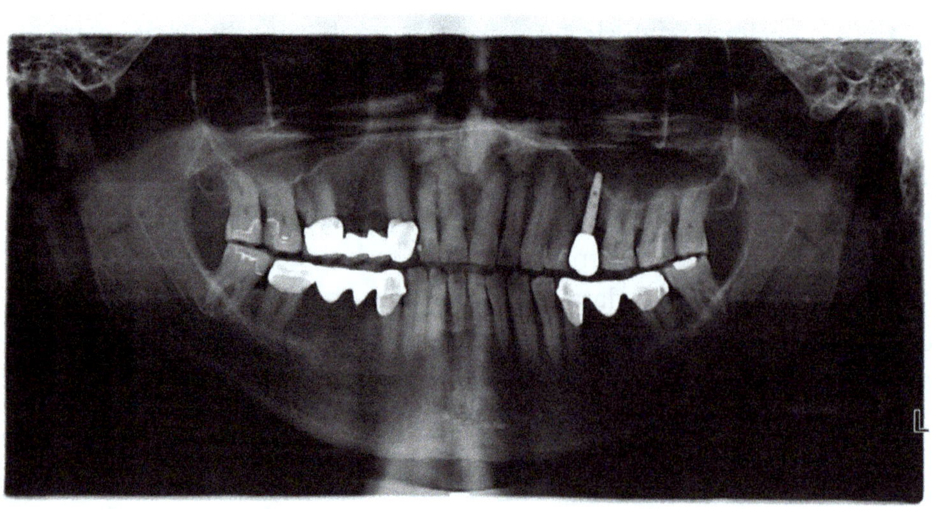

Figure 25. Panoramic X-ray of the patient. He has various restorations both the upper and lowers of the posterior area.

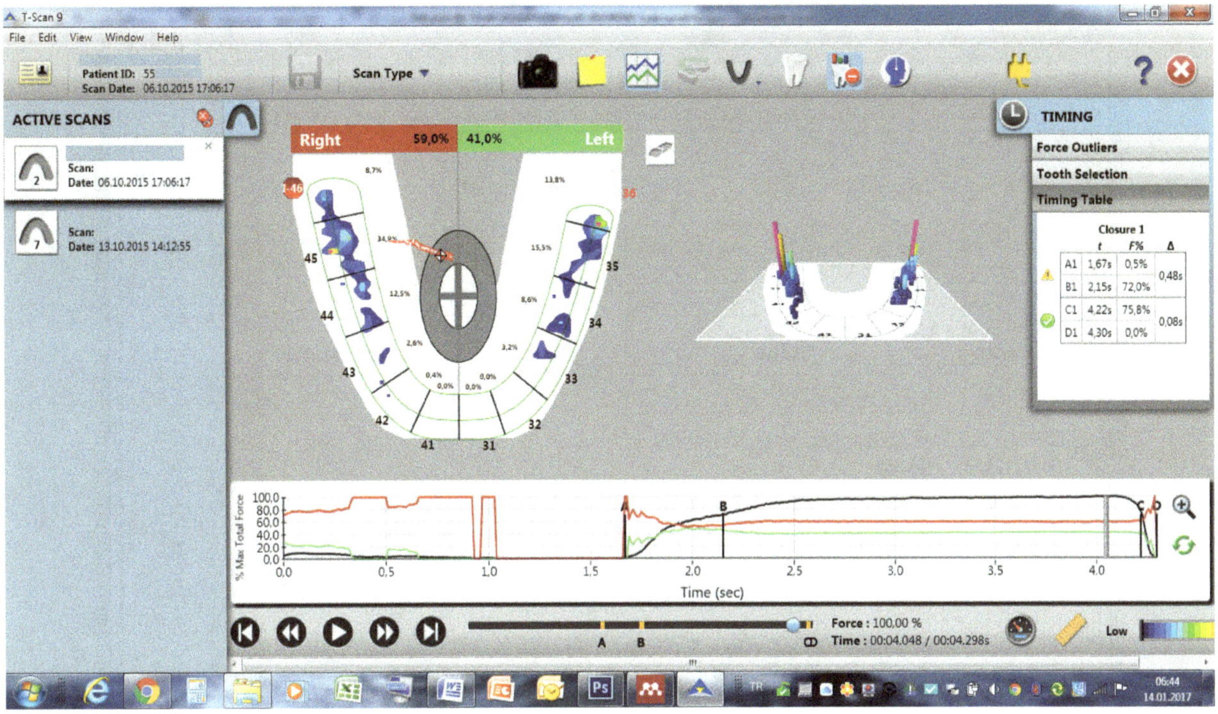

Figure 26. Before occlusal equilibration.

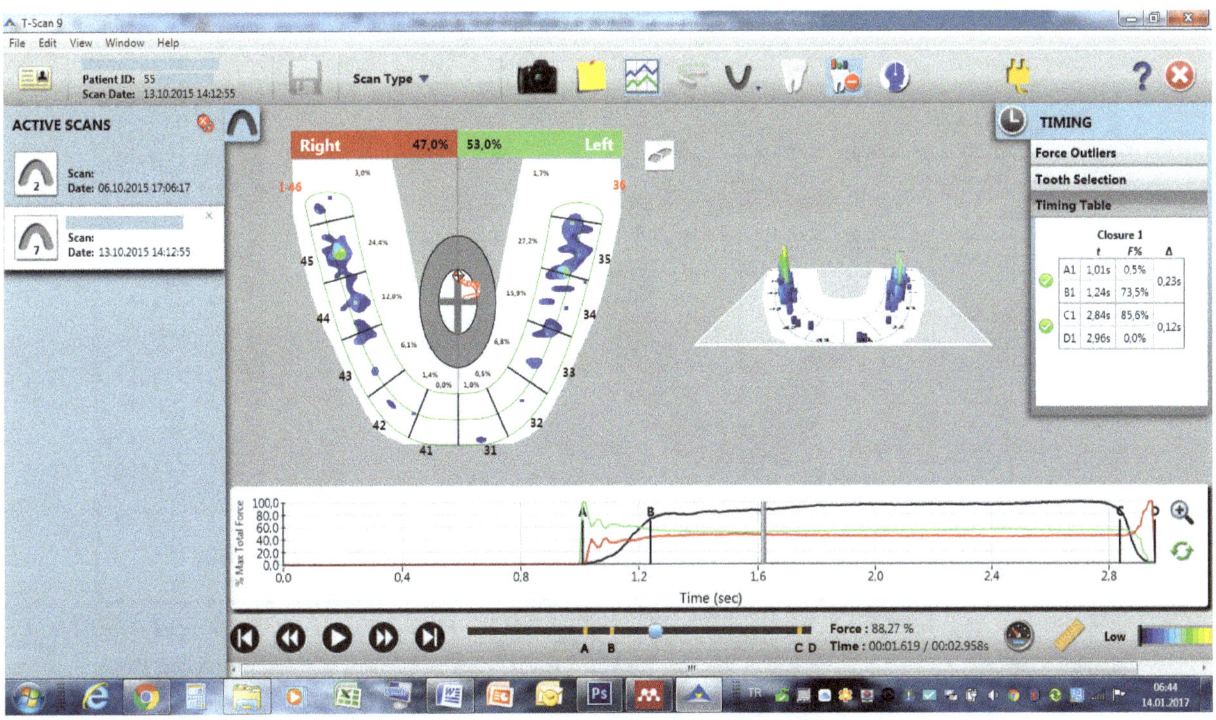

Figure 27. After occlusal equilibration.

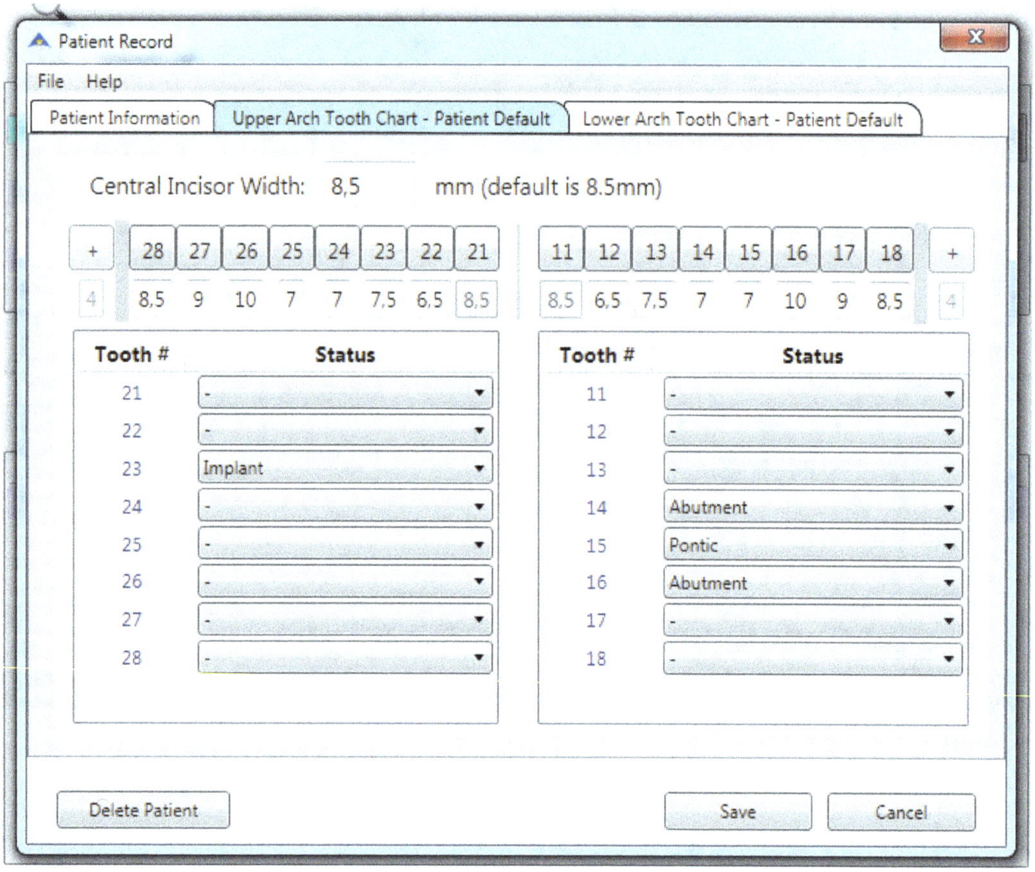

Figure 28. Central teeth dimensions are determinative; after the mesiodistal distance of the central teeth is entered, the dimensions of the other teeth are automatically calculated and the dental arch is formed.

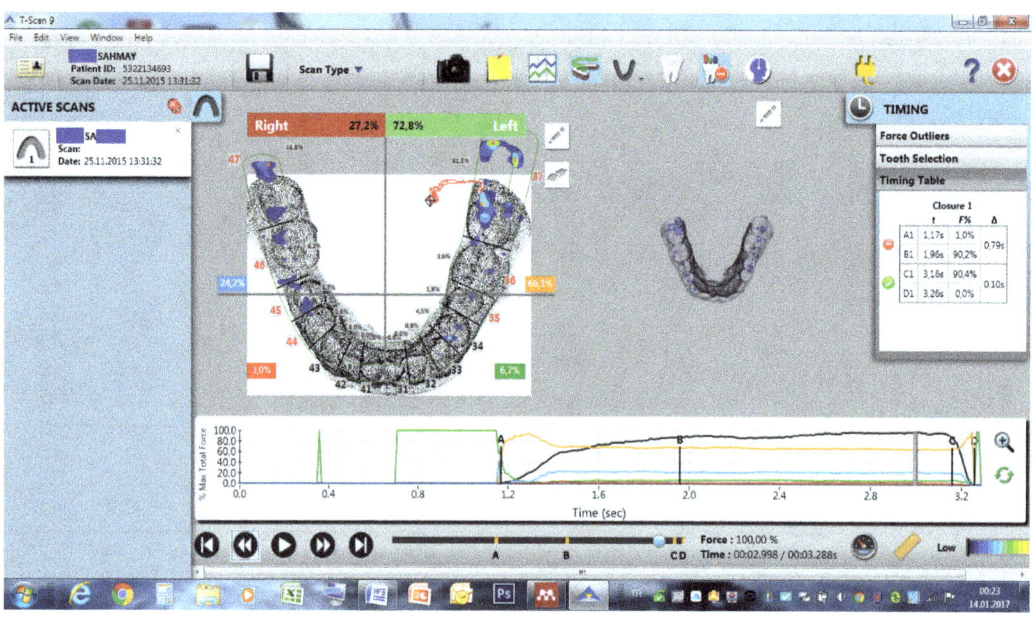

Figure 29. Computerized Occlusion Analysis is currently the most powerful method of TMD clinics for treatment of patients with muscle pain dysfunction syndrome.

1. Muscle pain dysfunction syndrome can be removed very quickly,
2. Splint dependence at unbalanced anterior dislocations can be minimized,
3. Allows for occlusion stabilization in full mouth restorations [84],
4. Allows to keep occlusal stress within physiological limits in implant prosthetic studies [7].

The impact of occlusal forces on teeth is variable. Occlusal derangements in physiological limits are absorbed with the buffer ability of periodontal ligaments [92]. However, impact of premature contacts on periodontium is like jigging, and this effect causes the enlargement of the alveolar space of teeth causing the teeth to loosen in alveolar space [93]. Therefore, it seems important to remove the occlusal traumas without causing any disruption on temporomandibular joints.

Author details

Serdar Gözler

Address all correspondence to: serdargozler@aydin.edu.tr

Dentistry Faculty of Istanbul Aydin University, Istanbul, Turkey

References

[1] Buescher J. Temporomandibular joint disorders. In: Am Fam Physician [Internet]. Elsevier; 2007 [cited 2016 Dec 15]. pp. 1477-1482. Available from: http://linkinghub.elsevier.com/retrieve/pii/B9780323045742500144

[2] Scrivani SJ, DAS K, Kaban LB. Temporomandibular disorders. New England Journal of Medicine. 2008:2693-2705

[3] Yuasa H, Kino K, Kubota E, Kakudo K, Sugisaki M, Nishiyama A, et al. Primary Treatment of Temporomandibular Disorders : The Japanese Society for the Temporomandibular Joint Evidence-Based Clinical Practice Guidelines. 2013

[4] Fletcher, Piecuch, Lieblich. Anatomy and pathophysiology of the Temporomandibular joint. In: Peterson's Principles of Oral and Maxillofacial Surgery [Internet]. 2004 [cited 2016 Dec 15]. pp. 933-948. Available from: http://dx.doi.org/10.1016/B978-0-7234-3809-0.00006-1

[5] McNeill C. Management of temporomandibular disorders: Concepts and controversies. The Journal of Prosthetic Dentistry. 1997;**77**(5):510-522

[6] Issa TS, Huijbregts PA. Physical therapy diagnosis and Management of a Patient with chronic daily headache: A case report. The Journal of Manual & Manipulative Therapy. 2006;**14**(4):E88-123

[7] Advisors E. Principles of Occlusion. Vol. 172006

[8] Gonzalez YM, Greene CS, Mohl ND. Technological devices in the diagnosis of Temporomandibular disorders. Oral and Maxillofacial Surgery Clinics of North America. 2008; **20**(2):211-220

[9] Lund JP, Widmer CG, Feine JS. Validity of diagnostic and monitoring tests used for temporomandibular disorders. Journal of Dental Research. 1995;**74**(4):1133-1143

[10] Baba K, Tsukiyama Y, Yamazaki M, Clark GT. A review of temporomandibular disorder diagnostic techniques. The Journal of Prosthetic Dentistry. 2001;**86**(2):184-194

[11] Dergin DO. SÜT, KARIŞIK VE DAİMİ DİŞLENME DÖNEMİNDE TEMPOROMANDİBULAR RAHATSIZLIKLARIN GÖRÜLME SIKLIĞI, ETİYOLOJİSİ VE DAĞILIMININ İNCELENMESİ. University of Marmara; 2014

[12] Köse G. BRUKSIZMLI HASTALARD a OKLUZAL TEMAS VE TME SESLERI ARASINDAKI ILISKININ DEĞERLENDIRILMESI. Ankara Üniversitesi Sağlık Bilimleri Enstitüsü Protetik Diş Tedavisi; 2015

[13] Clark GT, Tsukiyama Y, Baba K, Simmons M. The validity and utility of disease detection methods and of occlusal therapy for temporomandibular disorders. Oral Surgery, Oral Medicine, Oral Pathology, Oral Radiology Endodontology [Internet]. 1997;**83**(1):101-106. Available from: http://www.sciencedirect.com/science/article/pii/S1079210497900998

[14] Ishigaki S, Basette R, Maruyama T. Vibration of the temporomandibular joints with normal radiographic imagings: Comparison between asymptomatic volunteers and symptomatic patients. Cranio Journal of Craniomandibular Practice. 1993;**11**(2):88-94

[15] Nascimento MM, Dilbone DA, Pereira PN, Duarte WR, Geraldeli S, Delgado AJ. Abfraction lesions: Etiology, diagnosis, and treatment options. Clinical, Cosmetic and Investigational Dentistry [Internet]. 2016 [cited 2016 Dec 22];**8**:79-87. Available from: http://www.ncbi.nlm.nih.gov/pubmed/27217799%0Ahttp://www.pubmedcentral.nih.gov/articlerender.fcgi?artid=PMC4861607

[16] Mamoun JS, Napoletano D. Cracked tooth diagnosis and treatment: An alternative paradigm. European Journal of Dentistry. 2015;**9**(2):293-303

[17] Dym H, Israel H. Diagnosis and treatment of Temporomandibular disorders. Dental Clinics of North America. 2012;**56**:149-161

[18] Olesen J. The international classification of headache disorders, 3rd edition. Cephalagia [Internet]. 2013;**33**(9):629-808. Available from: http://www.ncbi.nlm.nih.gov/pubmed/18808500%5Cnhttp://www.ncbi.nlm.nih.gov/pubmed/24409431%5Cnhttp://www.ncbi.nlm.nih.gov/pubmed/22325197%5Cnhttp://www.ncbi.nlm.nih.gov/pubmed/16805756%5Cnhttp://www.ncbi.nlm.nih.gov/pubmed/24238370%5Cnhttp://www.ncbi.nlm

[19] López-Frías FJ, Castellanos-Cosano L, Martán-González J, Llamas-Carreras JM, Segura-Egea JJ. Clinical measurement of tooth wear: Tooth wear indices. Journal of Clinical and Experimental Dentistry. 2012;**4**(1):48-53

[20] Di Berardino F, Filipponi E, Schiappadori M, Forti S, Zanetti D, Cesarani A. The occlusal imaging and analysis system by T-scan III in tinnitus patients. Biomed Journal [Internet]. 2016;**39**(2):139-144. Available from: http://dx.doi.org/10.1016/j.bj.2016.04.001

[21] Pokorny PH, Wiens JP, Litvak H, Pokorney P, Weins J, Litvak H. Occlusion for fixed prosthodontics: A historical perspective of the gnahological influence. The Journal of Prosthetic Dentistry. 2008;**99**(4):299-313

[22] Okeson JP. Evolution of occlusion and temporomandibular disorder in orthodontics: Past, present, and future. American Journal of Orthodontics and Dentofacial Orthopaedic [Internet]. 2015;**147**(5):S216-S223. Available from: http://dx.doi.org/10.1016/j.ajodo.2015.02.007

[23] Wang C, Yin X. Occlusal risk factors associated with temporomandibular disorders in young adults with normal occlusions. Oral Surgery, Oral Medicine, Oral Pathology, Oral Radiology [Internet]. 2012;**114**(4):419-423. Available from: http://dx.doi.org/10.1016/j.oooo.2011.10.039

[24] McNamara JA. Orthodontic treatment and temporomandibular disorders. Oral Surgery, Oral Medicine, Oral Pathology, Oral Radiology Endodontology [Internet]. 1997;**83**(1):107-117. Available from: http://www.sciencedirect.com/science/article/pii/S1079210497901001

[25] Travess H, Roberts-Harry D, Sandy J. Orthodontics. Part 6: Risks in orthodontic treatment. British Dental Journal [Internet]. 2004;**196**(2):71-77. Available from:http://www.ncbi.nlm.nih.gov/pubmed/14739957

[26] Clark JR, Hutchinson I, Sandy JR. Functional occlusion: II. The role of articulators in orthodontics. Journal of Orthodontics. 2001;**28**:173-177

[27] Luther F. Orthodontics and the temporomandibular joint: Where are we now? Part 2. Functional occlusion, malocclusion, and TMD. Angle Orthodontist. 1998;**68**:305-318

[28] Alarabawy RA, El Ahwal HM, El Sergany MAES, Mehrez WW. Magnetic resonance imaging evaluation of temporo-mandibular joint disorders, criterial analysis and significance in comparison with arthroscopy. Egypt Journal of Radiology and Nuclear Medicine [Internet]. 2016;**47**(2):467-475. Available from: http://dx.doi.org/10.1016/j.ejrnm.2016.01.002

[29] Bas B, Ylmaz N, Gkce E, Akan H. Diagnostic value of ultrasonography in temporomandibular disorders. Journal of Oral and Maxillofacial Surgery. 2011;**69**(5):1304-1310

[30] Chen H, Slade G, Feng Lim P, Miller V, Maixner W, Diatchenko L. Relationship between Temporomandibular disorders, widespread palpation tenderness, and multiple pain conditions: A case-control study perspective: TMD subjects with WPT experience a greater level of multiple comorbid pain condition. The Journal of Pain. 2012;**13**(10):1016-1027

[31] Dolwick FM, Ambramowicz S, Bagheri SC. Diagnosis and Management of Temporomandibular Joint Pain and Masticatory Dysfunction. Current Therapy in Oral and Maxillofacial Surgery. 2012:859-868

[32] Drum R. FUNCTION spectral analysis of temporomandibular. 1985;7083

[33] Elfving L, Helkimo M, Magnusson T. Prevalence of different temporomandibular joint sounds, with emphasis on disc-displacement, in patients with temporomandibular disorders and controls. Swedish Dental Journal [Internet]. 2002 [cited 2016 Dec 22];**26**(1):9-19. Available from http://www.ncbi.nlm.nih.gov/pubmed/12090160

[34] Fushima K, Gallo LM, Krebs M, Palla S. Analysis of the TMJ intraarticular space variation: A non-invasive insight during mastication. Medical Engineering & Physics. 2003; **25**(3):181-190

[35] Iwase M, Ohashi M, Tachibana H, Toyoshima T, Nagumo M. Bite force, occlusal contact area and masticatory efficiency before and after orthognathic surgical correction of mandibular prognathism. International Journal of Oral and Maxillofacial Surgery. 2006;**35**(12):1102-1107

[36] Aras K, Hasanreisoğlu U, Shinogaya T. Masticatory performance, maximum occlusal force, and occlusal contact area in patients with bilaterally missing molars and distal extension removable partial dentures. International Journal of Prosthodontics [Internet]. 2011;**22**(2):204-209. Available from: http://www.ncbi.nlm.nih.gov/pubmed/19418870

[37] Lepley CR, Throckmorton GS, Ceen RF, Buschang PH. Relative contributions of occlusion, maximum bite force, and chewing cycle kinematics to masticatory performance. American Journal of Orthodontics and Dentofacial Orthopedics [Internet]. 2011;**139**(5): 606-613. Available from: http://dx.doi.org/10.1016/j.ajodo.2009.07.025

[38] Svetlana K. EC DENTAL SCIENCE case report T-scan III computed guided Occlusal adjustment in orthodontic relapse patient. The procedure description. EC Dental Science. 2016;**2**(Figure 2):1297-1308

[39] Gozler S, Vanlioglu B, Evren B, Gozneli R, Yildiz C, Ozkan YK. The effect of temporary hydrostatic splint on occlusion with computerized occlusal analysis system. Indian Journal of Dental Research. 2012;**23**(5):617-622

[40] Sutton DI, Sadowsky PL, Bernreuter WK, McCutcheon MJ, Lakshminarayanan AV. Temporomandibular joint sounds and condyle/disk relations on magnetic resonance images. American Journal of Orthodontics and Dentofacial Orthopedics. 1992;**101**(1):70-78

[41] Krohn S, Gersdorff N, Wassmann T, Merboldt KD, Joseph AA, Buergers R, et al. Real-time MRI of the temporomandibular joint at 15 frames per second???A feasibility study. European Journal of Radiology [Internet]. 2016;**85**(12):2225-2230. Available from: http://dx.doi.org/10.1016/j.ejrad.2016.10.020

[42] von Piekartz H. Craniomandibular region: Clinical patterns and management. Craniofacial Pain. 2007;215-284

[43] Shu L, Building F, Shu L, Building F, Kong H. Characterization of sounds emanatIng from the human temporom and Ibular joints. Archives of Oral Biology. 1996;**41**(7):631-639

[44] Wänman A, Agerberg G. Temporomandibular joint sounds in adolescents: A longitudinal study. Oral Surgery, Oral Medicine, Oral Pathology. 1990;**69**(1):2-9

[45] Widmalm SE, Westesson PL, Brooks SL, Hatala MP, Paesani D. Temporomandibular joint sounds: Correlation to joint structure in fresh autopsy specimens. American Journal of Orthodontics and Dentofacial Orthopedics. 1992;**101**(1):60-69

[46] Rohlin M, Westesson PL, Eriksson L. The correlation of temporomandibular joint sounds with joint morphology in fifty-five autopsy specimens. Journal of Oral and Maxillofacial Surgery. 1985;**43**(3):194-200

[47] Tallents RH, Hatala M, Katzberg RW, Westesson PL. Temporomandibular joint sounds in asymptomatic volunteers. The Journal of Prosthetic Dentistry. 1993;**69**(3):298-304

[48] Leader JK, Boston JR, Rudy TE, Greco CM, Zaki HS. Relation of jaw sounds and kinematics visualized and quantified using 3-D computer animation. Medical Engineering & Physics. 2003;**25**(3):191-200

[49] Oster C, Katzberg RW, Tallents RH, Morris TW, Bartholomew J, Miller TL, et al. Characterization of temporomandibular joint sounds. A preliminary investigation with arthrographic correlation. Oral Surgery, Oral Med Oral Pathol. 1984;**58**(1):10-16

[50] Time AA. Frequency analysis and classification of temporomandibular joint sounds ☋ Aydin Akan *, R. Bas7 ar U. Journal of the Franklin Institute. 2000;**337**

[51] Akan A, Ergin A, Yildirim M, Öztaş E. Analysis of temporomandibular joint sounds in orthodontic patients. Computers and Electrical Engineering. 2006;**32**(4):312-321

[52] Gay T, Bertolami CN, Donoff RB, Keith DA, Kelly JP. The acoustical characteristics of the normal and abnormal temporomandibular joint. Journal of Oral Maxillofacial Surgery [Internet]. 1987 [cited 2016 Dec 16];**45**(5):397-407. Available from: http://www.ncbi.nlm.nih.gov/pubmed/3471925

[53] Paesani D, Westesson P-L, Hatala MP, Tallents RH, Brooks SL. Accuracy of clinical diagnosis for TMJ internal derangement and arthrosis. Oral Surgery, Oral Medicine, Oral Pathology [Internet]. 1992 Mar;**73**(3):360-363. Available from: http://www.sciencedirect.com/science/article/pii/003042209290135D

[54] Dimitroulis G. The prevalence of osteoarthrosis in cases of advanced internal derangement of the Temporomandibular joint: A clinical, surgical and histological study. International Journal of Oral and Maxillofacial Surgery. 2005;**34**(4):345-349

[55] Mapelli A, Zanandréa Machado BC, Giglio LD, Sforza C, De Felício CM. Reorganization of muscle activity in patients with chronic temporomandibular disorders. Archives of Oral Biology [Internet]. 2016;**72**:164-171. Available from: http://dx.doi.org/10.1016/j.archoralbio.2016.08.022

[56] Shimshak DG, DeFuria MC. Health care utilization by patients with temporomandibular joint disorders. Cranio. 1998;**16**(3):185-193

[57] De Rossi SS, Stern I, Sollecito TP. Disorders of the masticatory muscles. Dental Clinics of North America [Internet]. 2013;**57**(3):449-464. Available from: http://dx.doi.org/10.1016/j.cden.2013.04.007

[58] Kuninori T, Tomonari H, Uehara S, Kitashima F, Yagi T, Miyawaki S. Influence of maximum bite force on jaw movement during gummy jelly mastication. Journal of Oral Rehabilitation. 2014;**41**(5):338-345

[59] Abduo J, Tennant M. Impact of lateral occlusion schemes: A systematic review. Journal of Prosthetic Dentistry [Internet]. 2015;**114**(2):193-204. Available from: http://dx.doi.org/10.1016/j.prosdent.2014.04.032

[60] Rossi SS De, Greenberg MS, Rcsd FDS, Liu F, Steinkeler A. Temporomandibular Disorders evaluation and management. The Medical Clinics of North America. 2014;**98**(2014): 1353-1384

[61] Rinchuse DJ, Kandasamy S, Sciote J. A contemporary and evidence-based view of canine protected occlusion. American Journal of Orthodontics and Dentofacial Orthopedics. 2007;**132**(1):90-102

[62] Slavicek G. Human mastication. International Journal of Stomatology and Occlusion Medicine [Internet]. 2010;**3**(1):29-41. Available from: http://dx.doi.org/10.1007/s12548-010-0044-6

[63] van der Bilt A, Engelen L, Pereira LJ, van der Glas HW, Abbink JH. Oral physiology and mastication. Physiology & Behavior. 2006;**89**(1):22-27

[64] Kubein-Meesenburg D, Fanghänel J, Ihlow D, Lotzmann U, Hahn W, Thieme KM, et al. Functional state of the mandible and rolling-gliding characteristics in the TMJ. Annals of Anatomy. 2007;**189**(4):393-396

[65] Hill L. An Introduction to Mastication Analysis in General Practice 2015. pp. 1-5. Available from: http://www.oralhealthgroup.com/news/anintroductiontomasticationanalysisingeneralpractice/1002121139/?&er=NA

[66] Kumbuloglu O, Saracoglu A, Bingol P, Hatiopglu A, Ozcan M. Clinical study on the comparison of masticatory efficiency and jaw movement before and after temporomandibular disorder treatment. Cranio – Journal of Craniomandibular Practice. 2013;**31**(3):190-201

[67] Gözler S. Stomatognatik Sistemin Nöromüsküler Fizyolojisi. In: Çalıkkocaoğlu PDS, editor. Tam Protezler. 5th ed. Istanbul: Gnatoloji Derneği; 1989. pp. 89-105

[68] Gözler S. Aggregating stimulus increases the activity in motoneurons causing spasms. Pdf. In: Turker K, editor. 10th biennial international motoneuron meeting, Istanbul [Internet]. Istabul: Koc University; 2016. p. 76. Available from: https://neurist.ku.edu.tr/

[69] Türker KS, Sowman PF, Tuncer M, Tucker KJ, Brinkworth RSA. The role of periodontal mechanoreceptors in mastication. Archives of Oral Biology. 2007;**52**(4):361-364

[70] Herring SW, Rafferty KL, Liu ZJ, Marshall CD. Jaw muscles and the skull in mammals: The biomechanics of mastication. Comparative Biochemistry and Physiology - A Molecular and Integrative Physiology. 2001:207-219

[71] Ferreira LA, Grossmann E, Januzzi E, de Paula MVQ, Carvalho ACP. Diagnosis of temporomandibular joint disorders: Indication of imaging exams. Brazilian Journal of Otorhinolaryngology. 2016;**82**(3):341-352

[72] Cooper BC, Kleinberg I. Relationship of temporomandibular disorders to muscle tension-type headaches and a neuromuscular orthosis approach to treatment. Cranio – Journal of Craniomandibular Practice. 2009;**27**(2):101-108

[73] Yamada K, Hanada K, Fukui T, Satou Y, Ochi K, Hayashi T, et al. Condylar bony change and self-reported parafunctional habits in prospective orthognathic surgery patients with temporomandibular disorders. Oral Surgery, Oral Medicine, Oral Pathology, Oral Radiology, and Endodontics. 2001;**92**(3):265-271

[74] Baldini A, Nota A, Cozza P. The association between occlusion time and Temporomandibular disorders. Journal of Electromyography and Kinesiology. 2015;**25**(1):151-154

[75] Dawson PE. A classification system for occlusions that relates maximal intercuspation to the position and condition of the temporomandibular joints. The Journal of Prosthetic Dentistry. 1996;**75**(1):60-66

[76] Wieckiewicz M, Boening K, Wiland P, Shiau Y-Y, Paradowska-Stolarz A. Reported concepts for the treatment modalities and pain management of temporomandibular disorders. Journal of Headache Pain [Internet]. 2015;**16**(1):106. Available from: http://www.thejournalofheadacheandpain.com/content/16/1/106

[77] Windhorst U. Muscle proprioceptive feedback and spinal networks. Brain Research Bulletin. 2007;**73**(4-6):155-202

[78] Palla S. Trigger points as a cause of Orofacial pain. Journal of Musculoskeletal Pain. 2004; **12**(3-4):29-36

[79] Kurose M, Yamamura K, Noguchi M, Inoue M, Ootaki S, Yamada Y. Modulation of jaw reflexes induced by noxious stimulation to the muscle in anesthetized rats. Brain Research. 2005;**1041**(1):72-86

[80] Dawson PE, Rinchuse DJ, Rinchuse DJ, Kandasamy S. Evidence-based versus experience-based views on occlusion and TMD [4] (multiple letters). American Journal of Orthodontics and Dentofacial Orthopedics. 2005;**128**(2):150-152

[81] Panigrahi D, Satpathy A, Patil A, Patel G. Occlusion and occlusal indicating materials. 2015;**1**(4):23-26

[82] Ruge S, Quooss A, Kordass B. Variability of closing movements, dynamic occlusion, and occlusal contact patterns during mastication. International Journal of Computerized Dentistry. 2011;**14**(2):119-127

[83] Qadeer S, Yang L, Sarinnaphakorn L, Kerstein RB. Comparison of closure occlusal force parameters in post-orthodontic and non-orthodontic subjects using T-scan(R) III DMD occlusal analysis. Cranio [Internet]. 2016;**9634**(April):1-7. Available from: http://dx.doi.org/10.1080/08869634.2015.1122277

[84] Gözler S. Courtesy of Dr Serdar Gözler. In: Erdemir U, Yildiz E, editors. Esthetic and Functional Management of Diastema: A Multidisciplinary Approach [Internet]. 1st ed. Istanbul: Springer; 2015. p. 35. Available from: https://books.google.com/books?id=FawvCwAAQBAJ&pgis=1

[85] Kürklü D, Yanikoglu N, Gözler S. Oklüzal Analiz Metodları ve T-scan. Atatürk Üniv Diş Hek Fak Derg. 2009;**19**(1):55-60

[86] Suit SR, Gibbs CH, Benz ST. Study of gliding tooth contacts during mastication. Journal of Periodontology [Internet]. 1976;**47**(6):331-334. Available from: http://www.ncbi.nlm.nih.gov/pubmed/1064720

[87] Carey J, Craig M, Kerstein R, Radke J. 2_EPA articulating paper study presentation. The Open Dentistry Journal. 2007;**1**(1):1-7

[88] Carey JP, Craig M, Kerstein RB, Radke J. Determining a relationship between applied occlusal load and articulating paper mark area. Open Dentistry Journal [Internet]. 2007;**1**: 1-7. Available from: http://www.pubmedcentral.nih.gov/articlerender.fcgi?artid=2581523&tool=pmcentrez&rendertype=abstract

[89] Solow RA. Customized anterior guidance for occlusal devices: Classification and rationale. The Journal of Prosthetic Dentistry. 2013;**110**(4):259-263

[90] Thumati P, Thumati R. The effect of disocclusion time-reduction therapy to treat chronic myofascial pain: A single group interventional study with 3 year follow-up of 100 cases. Journal of Indian Prosthodontic Society [Internet]. 2016;**0**(0):0. Available from: http://www.j-ips.org/preprintarticle.asp?id=176529

[91] Clark JR, Evans RD. Functional occlusion: I. A review. Journal of Orthodontics. 2001;**28**: 76-81

[92] Karibe H, Ogata K, Hasegawa Y, Ogihara K. Relation between clenching strength and occlusal force distribution in primary dentition. Journal of Oral Rehabilitation. 2003;**30**(3): 307-311

[93] Daegling DJ, Hylander WL. Occlusal forces and mandibular bone strain: Is the primate jaw "overdesigned"? Journal of Human Evolution [Internet]. 1997;**33**(6):705-717. Available from: http://www.ncbi.nlm.nih.gov/pubmed/9467777

[94] Biopak User Guide, Ver.7. 9275 N. 49th Street, Suite 150 Milwaukee, WI 53223 USA: BioResearch Associates, Inc.; 2011

[95] T-Scan User Manual (Help File in T-Scan Software 9.1). 307 West First Street. South Boston, MA 02127–1309: Tekscan, Inc; 2015

Permissions

All chapters in this book were first published in TJPCAU, by InTech Open; hereby published with permission under the Creative Commons Attribution License or equivalent. Every chapter published in this book has been scrutinized by our experts. Their significance has been extensively debated. The topics covered herein carry significant findings which will fuel the growth of the discipline. They may even be implemented as practical applications or may be referred to as a beginning point for another development.

The contributors of this book come from diverse backgrounds, making this book a truly international effort. This book will bring forth new frontiers with its revolutionizing research information and detailed analysis of the nascent developments around the world.

We would like to thank all the contributing authors for lending their expertise to make the book truly unique. They have played a crucial role in the development of this book. Without their invaluable contributions this book wouldn't have been possible. They have made vital efforts to compile up to date information on the varied aspects of this subject to make this book a valuable addition to the collection of many professionals and students.

This book was conceptualized with the vision of imparting up-to-date information and advanced data in this field. To ensure the same, a matchless editorial board was set up. Every individual on the board went through rigorous rounds of assessment to prove their worth. After which they invested a large part of their time researching and compiling the most relevant data for our readers.

The editorial board has been involved in producing this book since its inception. They have spent rigorous hours researching and exploring the diverse topics which have resulted in the successful publishing of this book. They have passed on their knowledge of decades through this book. To expedite this challenging task, the publisher supported the team at every step. A small team of assistant editors was also appointed to further simplify the editing procedure and attain best results for the readers.

Apart from the editorial board, the designing team has also invested a significant amount of their time in understanding the subject and creating the most relevant covers. They scrutinized every image to scout for the most suitable representation of the subject and create an appropriate cover for the book.

The publishing team has been an ardent support to the editorial, designing and production team. Their endless efforts to recruit the best for this project, has resulted in the accomplishment of this book. They are a veteran in the field of academics and their pool of knowledge is as vast as their experience in printing. Their expertise and guidance has proved useful at every step. Their uncompromising quality standards have made this book an exceptional effort. Their encouragement from time to time has been an inspiration for everyone.

The publisher and the editorial board hope that this book will prove to be a valuable piece of knowledge for researchers, students, practitioners and scholars across the globe.

List of Contributors

Oksana Ivask and Ülle Voog-Oras
Department of Stomatology, University of Tartu, Estonia

Edvitar Leibur
Departments of Stomatology and Internal Medicine, University of Tartu, Estonia

Mohammad Esmaeelinejad
Department of Oral and Maxillofacial Surgery, School of Dentistry, Semnan University of Medical Sciences, Semnan, Iran

Maryam Sohrabi
Department of Oral and Maxillofacial Surgery, School of Dentistry, Azad University of Medical Sciences, Tehran, Iran

José Thiers Carneiro Junior and Francisco de Sousa Neves Filho
Federal University of Pará (UFPA), Belém, Brazil

Dênis Pimenta e Souza
University of São Paulo (USP), São Paulo, Brazil

Diogo Souza Ferreira Rubim de Assis
Federal University of Maranhão (UFMA), Brazil

Paulo Hemerson de Moraes
University of Campinas (UNICAM), Brazil

Mehmet Emre Yurttutan, Ayşegül Tüzüner Öncül and Hakan Alpay Karasu
Faculty of Dentistry, Department of Oral and Maxillofacial Surgery, Ankara University, Ankara, Turkey

Serdar Gözler
TMD Clinic, Dentistry Faculty of Istanbul Aydin University, Istanbul, Turkey

Ufuk Tatli
Department of Oral and Maxillofacial Surgery, Çukurova University Faculty of Dentistry, Adana, Turkey

Vladimir Machon
Department of Oral and Maxillofacial Surgery, Charles University and General University Hospital, Prague, Czech Republic

Buket Aybar and Yusuf Emes
Faculty of Dentistry, Department of Oral and Maxillofacial Surgery, Istanbul University, Turkey

Guhan Dergin
Faculty of Dentistry, Department of Oral and Maxillofacial Surgery, Marmara University, Turkey

Bakr M.Rabie
Faculty of Dentistry, The University of Hong Kong, Hong Kong

Jeremy Ho and Qianfeng Li
The University of Hong Kong, Hong Kong

Gustavo Monasterio and Francisca Castillo
Periodontal Biology Laboratory, Faculty of Dentistry, Universidad de Chile, Chile

Daniel Betancur
Molecular Immunology Laboratory, Faculty of Biological Sciences, Universidad de Concepción, Chile

Arnoldo Hernández
Anatomy and Biology Program, Faculty of Medicine, Universidad de Chile, Chile

Guillermo Flores and Walter Díaz
Department of Prosthesis, Faculty of Dentistry, Universidad de Chile, Chile

Marcela Hernández
Periodontal Biology Laboratory, Faculty of Dentistry, Universidad de Chile, Chile
Department of Pathology and Oral Medicine, Faculty of Dentistry, Universidad de Chile, Chile

Rolando Vernal
Periodontal Biology Laboratory, Faculty of Dentistry, Universidad de Chile, Chile
Department of Conservative Dentistry, Faculty of Dentistry, Universidad de Chile, Chile

Serdar Gözler
Dentistry Faculty of Istanbul Aydin University, Istanbul, Turkey

Index

A

Alloplastic Materials, 38, 51, 121

Ankylosis Relapse, 38

Apoptosis, 4, 149, 158, 178

Arthralgia, 3, 142, 171, 173, 177

Arthroscopic Biopsy, 112-113

Articular Fossa, 38, 123, 130

B

Biochemical Markers, 1-2, 10, 12, 18-19, 186

Biocompatibility, 38, 41, 48

Bone Markers, 1-2, 7, 9

C

Cartilage Tumors, 54-55

Chondroma, 54-57, 59, 69, 71-72

Chronic Inflammation, 37, 69

Computed Tomography, 5-6, 12, 18, 21, 65, 70, 113-114, 173, 175, 184, 187-189

Condylar Growth, 146, 148-149, 151

Condylectomy, 25, 27, 33, 35, 56, 59, 62-63, 68, 122-123, 140

Conservative Treatment, 108, 112, 115, 118, 133, 165

E

Endocrinological Disturbances, 4

Esterolitografia, 40, 45

Etiological Risk, 2

F

Facial Asymmetry, 50, 56, 58, 62

Fibrohistiocytic Tumors, 55, 68

G

Giant Cell Tumor, 55, 66-69, 72, 74-75, 77

Glenoid Fossa, 23, 40-41, 69, 81, 113-114, 119-120, 123, 144, 198, 201

H

Hemangioma, 55, 67, 69, 76

I

Internal Derangement, 15, 81, 108-109, 111, 113, 125-126, 128, 134-136, 140, 170, 177, 188-190, 195, 223

Intraosseous Lipoma, 68, 76

Ischemic, 2, 174

J

Juxta-articular Myxoma, 54-55, 70, 78

L

Lipogenic Tumors, 55, 68

M

Magnetic Resonance Imaging, 17, 59-60, 109, 113, 126, 130, 135, 187-188, 195, 221

Malocclusion, 3-4, 15-16, 54, 56, 62, 103, 117, 155, 162, 168, 204, 221

Mandible, 5, 10, 17, 21-22, 25, 29-32, 36, 47-49, 62, 66-68, 73-74, 76, 80, 83, 86, 98, 113, 142, 144-145, 152-154, 156, 162-163, 201, 204-206, 208-210, 212, 224

Mandibular Branch, 25, 35, 41

Mandibular Condyle, 7, 22-23, 25, 28, 33, 37, 55-56, 59, 70-74, 76-77, 110, 124, 129, 166, 173, 186, 188

Mastication, 3, 82, 85, 88, 103-105, 107, 145, 170, 194-195, 203-210, 213, 222, 224-226

Masticatory Muscle Problems, 79

Maxillary Sinusitis, 3, 113

Maxillofacial Surgery, 22, 34-35, 51, 70-74, 76, 78, 103, 125-128, 135-140, 186-187, 189-191, 219-223

Menisci, 4

N

Neuronal Mechanism, 82-83

Neuropathic, 2

Nociceptive, 2, 86, 88-91

O

Occlusal Splint, 102, 117-118, 137

Odontogenic Infections, 4

Orthodontics, 97, 141, 156-157, 159-164, 187-189, 221-226

Orthopantomograph, 1

Ossifying Fibroma, 55, 59, 67-68, 77

Osteochondroma, 54-59, 70-71, 113

Osteoclastic Enzyme, 7

Osteogenic Tumors, 54-55, 62

Osteoma, 54-56, 59, 62-66, 73-74, 77

Osteoporosis, 1, 6-7, 9-11, 18-19, 21, 132

Otitis, 3, 29, 113

P

Pain Measurement, 1

Primary Neoplasms, 54

Prosthetic Reconstruction, 36, 52

Psoriatic Arthritis, 3, 37, 39, 112

R

Radiographic Changes, 1, 5-6, 10-11, 14, 18, 174

Radiographic Imaging, 5

Rheumatoid Arthritis, 3, 13, 16, 18-19, 37, 39, 112, 114, 120, 124, 174, 178, 182, 191-192

Rheumatology, 5, 77, 102, 104, 131, 136, 190-192

S

Stock Prosthesis, 36, 42, 123

Stomatognathic System Problems, 79

Subchondral Bone, 4, 145

Subchondral Cysts, 6

Subperiosteal Dissection, 33

Superficial Musculoaponeurotic System, 22

Synovial Chondromatosis, 54-55, 59, 69, 72-73, 113, 171, 187

Synovial Joint, 23, 119, 166

Synovium, 4, 70, 117, 119, 177, 191, 196

T

Temporomandibular Disorders, 12-17, 36-37, 51, 59, 66, 70, 75, 79-80, 82, 102-104, 106, 108, 125-127, 129-130, 135-139, 141, 156, 168-169, 171, 174, 176, 185-187, 189, 191, 194-195, 205, 219-225

Temporomandibular Joint Disorders, 1-4, 16, 137, 139-140, 170-171, 186-187, 189-191, 195, 197, 219, 223-224

Trabecular Pattern, 10, 17

Treg Cells, 165

Trigeminal Nerve, 25, 88

Trismus, 54, 59, 66, 69, 114

V

Vertical Osteotomy, 41

Visual Analogue Scale, 4-5

Z

Zygomatic Arch, 24, 26, 28, 40, 42-43, 45, 47, 123

www.ingramcontent.com/pod-product-compliance
Lightning Source LLC
LaVergne TN
LVHW060550210926
848485LV00005B/1291